ISLAM AND ASSISTED REPRODUCTIVE TECHNOLOGIES:
SUNNI AND SHIA PERSPECTIVES

Fertility, Reproduction and Sexuality

GENERAL EDITORS:

Soraya Tremayne, Founding Director, Fertility and Reproduction Studies Group, and Research Associate, Institute of Social and Cultural Anthropology, University of Oxford
Marcia C. Inhorn, William K. Lanman, Jr. Professor of Anthropology and International Affairs, Yale University
Philip Kreager, Director, Fertility and Reproduction Studies Group, and Research Associate, Institute of Social and Cultural Anthropology and Institute of Human Sciences, University of Oxford

ISLAM AND ASSISTED REPRODUCTIVE TECHNOLOGIES
SUNNI AND SHIA PERSPECTIVES

Edited by

Marcia C. Inhorn and Soraya Tremayne

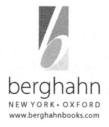

berghahn
NEW YORK • OXFORD
www.berghahnbooks.com

First published in 2012 by
Berghahn Books
www.BerghahnBooks.com

© 2012, 2015 Marcia C. Inhorn and Soraya Tremayne
First paperback edition published in 2015

Library of Congress Cataloging-in-Publication Data

Islam and assisted reproductive technologies : Sunni and Shia
perspectives / edited by Marcia C. Inhorn and Soraya Tremayne.
    p. cm. — (Fertility, reproduction, and sexuality ; v. 23)
ISBN 978-0-85745-490-4 (hardback : alk. paper)-- ISBN 978-1-78533-
045-2 (paperback : alk. paper) -- ISBN 978-0-85745-491-1 (ebook)
    1. Human reproductive technology—Islamic countries—Congresses.
2. Fertility, Human—Islamic countries—Congresses. 3. Human
reproduction—Religious aspects—Islam—Congresses. I. Inhorn,
Marcia Claire, 1957– II. Tremayne, Soraya.
    RG133.5.I74 2012
    618.1'7806—dc23

                                                    2011052129

British Library Cataloguing in Publication Data

A catalogue record for this book is available from the British Library.

Printed in the United States on acid-free paper

ISBN 978-0-85745-490-4 (hardback)
ISBN 978-1-78533-045-2 (paperback)
ISBN 978-0-85745-491-1 (ebook)

CONTENTS

PART III
Islamic Biopolitics and the "Modern" Nation-state:
Comparative Case Studies of ART

LIST OF FIGURES

Tables

Illustration

ACKNOWLEDGMENTS

This edited volume is the result of a wonderful conference workshop, held at Yale University in New Haven, Connecticut, on the theme of "Islam and the Biotechnologies of Human Life." Following a day of public presentations, the contributors to this volume remained at Yale for an intensive, two-day workshop discussion of their conference papers, which have ultimately become the polished chapters of this edited volume.

To our knowledge, this volume is unique, for it represents the work of nearly all of those scholars whose research focuses on Islam and assisted reproductive technologies (ARTs). Only two scholars—Ebrahim Moosa of Duke University, who has worked on Islam and human cloning, and Vardit Rispler-Chaim of the University of Haifa, who has worked on ARTs and Islamic bioethics—were unable to participate in the project, due to previous commitments. For the rest of us, meeting (often for the first time), discussing our work, and producing this volume together has been an immensely rewarding experience. For me and for my co-convener, Soraya Tremayne, the project and the process have been especially gratifying, for we have been able to bring together our junior colleagues, many of whom are producing nuanced, field-based research on ARTs in a variety of Islamic settings. As a result, all of the chapters in this volume can be said to be original, timely, and "cutting edge," reflecting the rapidly evolving ART landscape in the Muslim world in the new millennial second decade.

This volume would not have been possible without the support of a number of institutions and individuals. First, I would like to acknowledge the tremendous support of Yale University, particularly The Whitney and Betty MacMillan Center for International and Area Studies, and the MacMillan Center's Council on Middle East Studies, which I directed at the time of the original conference.

Ian Shapiro, Sterling Professor of Political Science and the Henry R. Luce Director of the MacMillan Center, generously funded the conference and also committed resources for hiring a copyeditor.

I am also grateful to the staff of our council, Lora LeMosy and Amaar Al-Hayder, for helping with the conference logistics. Special thanks go to Mikaela Rogozen-Soltar, my visiting assistant in research at Yale, for being an excellent workshop rapporteur, and to Molly K. Moran for her exceptional editorial assistance with the volume. I also extend my thanks to Yale's Department of Anthropology for providing a beautiful setting for our workshop.

At Yale, I am fortunate to be surrounded by an extraordinary group of colleagues and students in Middle East Studies, Islamic Studies, and medical anthropology. In the midst of their busy schedules, several of them accepted our invitations to serve as conference moderators and discussants. They include: Abbas Amanat, P. Sean Brotherton, Narges Erami, Zareena Grewal, Frank Griffel, Kaveh Khoshnood, and Noah Salomon. In this volume, we have chosen to publish the excellent section introductions provided by several of these fine Yale scholars.

Finally, I am most grateful to my dear colleague and friend, Soraya Tremayne, founding director of the Fertility and Reproduction Studies Group in the Institute for Social and Cultural Anthropology at the University of Oxford. Soraya has been working for many years on reproductive health issues in Iran, and it was she who first opened my eyes to the incredible developments in third-party reproductive assistance going on in that country. In February 2006, we both traveled to Iran to serve as keynote speakers in a conference on "Embryo and Gamete Donation," which was simply fascinating. Since then, we have been close colleagues in our ART scholarship and in this book series on "Fertility, Reproduction, and Sexuality," which Soraya founded at Berghahn. Sometimes in the academy, we are simply lucky to find true "intellectual soul mates." Soraya has been that, and much more for me, over the past decade. Thus, I am delighted that we have published our first book together.

Marcia C. Inhorn
Yale University

GLOSSARY OF ARABIC, PERSIAN, AND TURKISH TERMS

Arabic

ajnabi—stranger; man other than the husband in the context of arguments over donor sperm

'alaqa—clot of blood; a stage in the Qur'anic account of embryogenesis

'aql—intellectual reasoning

'awra—private parts that should not be revealed to others (i.e., could be male or female, and includes but is not confined to the genitalia)

Ash'ari—Traditionalists, constitute the majority of Sunni Muslims; believe that human actions were predetermined, that the Qur'an was eternal, and that humanity was not capable of deciding what was right and what was wrong

Ayatollah—high-ranking Shia religious authority

baraka—God's grace

bint (pl. *banat*)—daughter(s)

bint al-zina—daughter born out of wedlock

bint min al-rida'—"milk daughter"; the term for the relationship between a man, whose wife had breastfed a female child, and that female child

bunuwa—childship

dakhala—to penetrate

darura (pl. *darurat*)—necessity

daruriyyat al-khamsa, al- —"the five essential principles," posited as fundamental to Islamic law: religion, life, intellect, offspring, and property

di'wa—in which the nasab link is changed from one father to
   another by claim and mutual consent

dukhul—sexual penetration; intercourse

dunya—mundane world

fahisha—adultery, fornication

faqih (pl. *fuqaha*)—legal scholar, experts in fiqh

fard kifaya—absolute moral obligation; collective moral duty

fatwa—religious proclamation outlining which attitudes and practices are halal (permitted) or haram (prohibited); a non–legally
   binding but authoritative Islamic religious opinion, offered by an
   Islamic cleric who is considered to be an expert concerning the
   Islamic scriptures and jurisprudence

fiqh—Islamic jurisprudence

fiqh al-tibb—the jurisprudence of medicine

firash—literally "bed"; matrimonial bed; a broad concept that is not
   restricted to marriage and also includes intercourse with a slave

hadith–sayings of the Prophet Muhammad

haja—need

halal—permitted

Hanafi—one of the four schools of Islamic jurisprudence within the
   Sunni branch of Islam

Hanbali—one of the four schools of Islamic jurisprudence within
   the Sunni branch of Islam

haqiqa—the truth; reality

haqq (pl. *huquq*)—right

haqq al-abawayn—right of the parents

haqq al-janin—right of the fetus

haqq al-mujtama'—right of society

haqq shakhsi—personal right

haram—prohibited

hartaqa—heresy

hijra—the migration of the Prophet Muhammad and his followers
   to the city of Medina in 622 CE

hiyal—legal stratagems to get around sharia rules

hurma—sacredness

'ibadat—worship; religious observances that occur between the
   believer and God (such as prayer and fasting)

ibaha—permissibility

ibn—son

'idda—waiting period enjoined after divorce or widowhood before
   remarriage, in order to establish presence or absence of pregnancy

ijtihad—religious reasoning

ijma'—consensus or agreement of Islamic jurists

'illa—legal cause

imam—Muslim community leader

istihsan—juristic preference; seeking an equitable and just solution

istilhaq—the point at which a child has the rights to receive a share of inheritance

Jafari—the Shia school of Islamic jurisprudence

jahiliyya—state of ignorance; a term used to refer to pre-Islamic times

li'an–repudiation of one's wife, which may include repudiation of a child born to her

lughawi—linguistic

madhhab—Islamic legal school

mahram—someone forbidden to you in marriage (e.g., a woman's brother), affecting gender comportment in family life (e.g., no requirement to veil before him)

majaz—metaphorical

makruh—a practice that is reprehensible and should be avoided, but is not absolutely prohibited (*haram*)

Maliki—one of the four schools of Islamic jurisprudence within the Sunni branch of Islam

maqsud—purpose

marja' al-taqlid—source of emulation; usually contracted to *marja'*; Shia religious authority of the highest rank; source of guidance for Shia Muslims

mashhur—commonly accepted, established (legal opinion)

maslaha—public interest; a concept in Islamic law invoked to permit something based on whether it serves the common good

mu'amalat—realm of social transactions and the location of social ethics in Islam

mu'asir—contemporary

mudgha—lump of flesh; stage in the Qur'anic account of embryogenesis

mujtahid—Muslim religious scholars who undertake *ijtihad*

munfatih—open-minded

mut'a—a fixed term contract of temporary marriage in Shia Islam

muta'akhkhirun—the term in Islamic legal theory that signifies the scholars who came after the first three centuries

mutaqaddimun—the term in Islamic legal theory that signifies the scholars who lived during the first three centuries

Mu'tazalites—Rationalists; claim that humanity was endowed with reason and can therefore differentiate right from wrong

Muwatta—early collection of hadith edited by the Imam Malik ibn
    Anas
nasab (pl. *ansab*)—filiation; lineage; relations by blood; genealogy
nikah—"marriage," contested word in Islamic jurisprudence, taken
    to mean either marriage contract, marriage consummation, or
    "uniting between two things"
nikah fasid—defective marriage
nutfa—sperm
qawa'id al-fiqh—legal maxims
qiyas—drawing an analogy from the Qur'an or hadith
Qur'an—the sacred writings of Islam revealed by God to the
    Prophet Muhammad
raghba—desire
rida'—milk kinship
ruh—spirit
sadd al-dhara'i'—blocking the means to do a later harm
sabab—cause
Shafi'i—one of the four schools of Islamic jurisprudence within the
    Sunni branch of Islam
shar'i—legal
Shaykh—honorific term for an elder, an Islamic scholar, or a person
    of royal lineage
sharia—body of religious law in Islam
Shia—the minority branch of Islam, constituting slightly more than
    10 percent of the world's Muslim population
siyasa shar'iyya—government in accordance with the goals and
    objectives of sharia
Sunna—the way of the Prophet Muhammad
Sunni—the majority branch of Islam
tabanni—adoption
tafsir—interpretation of the Qur'an
takhayyur—borrowing a doctrine from another school of Islamic
    law (*madhhab*)
takhalluf—backwardness
ta'wil—explanation of the inner meaning of the Qur'an
ulama—Muslim legal scholars
umm al-hadina, al- —"the nursing mother," i.e., the woman who
    carries the child; the gestational carrier
umm walad—the mother of a child; used to refer to a slave wife
    who had born a child to her master and thereby acquires a new,
    more elevated status
'urf—custom

usul al-fiqh—sources of Islamic jurisprudence

wa'da—infanticide; literally "of being buried alive," a practice deemed characteristic of pre-Islamic Arabia

walad al-zina—child of adultery; an out-of-wedlock bastard

walad li-l-firash, al- —"the child to the (marital) bed," a hadith used to assign paternity to the husband

wali—legal guardian

waqi', al- —reality

wat' bi-shabh—intercourse in doubtful circumstances; when two people erroneously assumed to act within a legitimizing framework

zihar—lit. means "back" in Arabic; a pre-Islamic custom of repudiation or divorce, in which a husband could divorce his wife by verbally declaring to his wife, "You are to me as the back of my mother."

zina—illicit sexuality in Islam, including adultery

Persian

adab—ethical codes

ahkam—rules

ahkam-e erth—rules of inheritance

ahkam-e ezdewaj—rules of marriage

ahkam-e nasabi—progeny laws

amanat—deposit

biganeh—stranger

ehday-e janin—embryo donation

en'eqad-e nutfah—conception; coagulation of male and female semen

ertebat-e takwini—a relation through the act of bringing into being and formation

fe'el-e haram—forbidden act

farhang sazi—creating a culture

hamli—gestational; through gestation

ja andakhtan—literally means making two parts fit into each other; in the context of this volume, it means making the ARTs fit into the Iranian culture

ja'ez nist—not allowed

janin—fertilized egg

khoda—God

leqah-e masnu'i—artificial insemination

ma' al-mar'at—female fluids (derived from Arabic)
ma' al-rajol—male fluids (derived from Arabic)
madar-e rida'i—milk mother
mahramiyat—marriage prohibition
majlis—council; the term used for the Iranian parliament
maniyy—seminal fluid of a man or a woman produced by orgasm;
    also man's sperm
mavazin-e islami—Islamic principles
me'yar-e madari—determination of maternity
nasab-e madari—maternal filiation
nasab-e pedari—paternal filiation
na-zai—inability to give birth. also: infertility
nutfah emshaj—zygote
qerabat-e nasabi—kinship relations created by *nasab*
qerabat-e rida'i—kinship relations created by the act of suckling
rahem—uterus
shabih-sazi—cloning
saheb-e tokhmak—contributor of the egg
sahib-e rahim—gestational carrier
Shora-ye negahban—Guardian Council in Iran
takwin—to cause to exist; bring into being and formation; creation
talqih—insemination
tokhmak—woman's egg
ulum-e qor'ani—Qur'anic sciences
wajib—necessary
weladati—through birth
zan-e hamel—gestational carrier
zayeman—the act of giving birth to a child
zina-ye ba maharem—incestuous adultery

Turkish

çağdaş—modern, contemporary
Diyanet—short for Diyanet İşleri Başkanlığı, Turkey's Department
    of Religious Affairs
laiklik—state secularism
muhafazakâr—conservative
tüp bebek—IVF, literally "tube baby"
tutucu—conservative
yasaklar—prohibitions

Introduction

ISLAM AND ASSISTED REPRODUCTIVE TECHNOLOGIES

Soraya Tremayne and Marcia C. Inhorn

Introduction: Islam and ARTs

Since the birth in 1978 of England's Louise Brown, the world's first "test-tube baby," assisted reproductive technologies (ARTs) designed to create human life have proliferated and spread around the globe. Over the past thirty-five years, the world has seen the rapid expansion of a whole host of reproductive technologies, including:

- *in vitro fertilization* (IVF) to overcome female infertility, especially blocked fallopian tubes;
- *intracytoplasmic sperm injection* (ICSI) to overcome male infertility;
- *third-party donation* (of eggs, sperm, embryos and uteruses, as in *surrogacy*) to overcome absolute sterility;
- *multifetal pregnancy reduction* to selectively abort multiple-gestation IVF pregnancies;
- *ooplasm transfer* (OT), of cytoplasm from a younger to an older woman's oocytes, to improve egg quality in perimenopausal women;
- *cryopreservation* (freezing) and storage of unused sperm, embryos, oocytes, and now ovarian tissue;

- *preimplantation genetic diagnosis* (PGD) to identify genetic defects in embryos created through IVF or ICSI before their transfer into the uterus; controversial uses of PGD include sex selection and the creation of "savior siblings" for children with life-threatening illnesses;

- *human embryonic stem cell* (hESC) research on unused embryos for the purposes of therapeutic intervention; and

- *human cloning*, or the possibility for asexual, autonomous reproduction, which has already occurred in other mammals (e.g., Dolly the sheep).

With virtually all of these technologies, sperm and eggs are retrieved from bodies, embryos are returned to bodies, and sometimes these reproductive materials are donated to other bodies or are used and discarded for the purposes of medical research (Franklin 1996; Kahn 2000; Kirkman 2003; Konrad 1998). Numerous infertility scholars have noted in recent years that ARTs exact a significant toll on the body, especially for women as both recipients of ARTs and as oocyte donors, but also for men in the era of ICSI (Inhorn 2003, 2012; Kahn 2000; Lorber 1989; Storrow 2005; van der Ploeg 1995). Moreover, despite the existence of national and international statements opposing the commercialization of ART services, significant commodification has occurred, as gametes and embryos are increasingly sold on the open market through Internet websites and college newspapers (Blank 1998; Braverman 2001; Carmeli and Birenbaum-Carmeli 2000; Pollock 2003; Shanley 2002; Thompson 2005). Indeed, Ruth Deech, former chairperson of the UK Human Fertilization and Embryology Authority, questions the human rights implications of the documented massive global transfer within the European Union (EU) of gametes and embryos "passed from country to country in search of one that permits the desired treatment or allows the chosen gametes to be used" (Deech 2003: 425).

The Muslim countries are different from both the EU nations and the United States in terms of their enthusiastic embrace of ARTs *without* this commodification and transfer of human gametes. Since 1986, a Middle Eastern ART industry has been flourishing, with hundreds of mostly private IVF clinics in countries ranging from the small, wealthy Arab Gulf states to the larger but less prosperous nations of North Africa (Inhorn 2003; Serour 1996, 2008; Serour and Dickens 2001). This fluorescence of a Middle Eastern ART industry is not surprising: Islam encourages the use of science and medicine as solutions to human suffering and is a religion that can be described as "pronatalist," encouraging the growth of an Islamic "multitude" (Brockopp 2003; Brockopp and Eich 2008; Inhorn 1994; Musallam 1986). Hence, biotechnologies to assist in the conception of human life have implicit appeal in the Muslim world.

However, as noted by Islamic studies scholar Ebrahim Moosa (2003: 23),

> In terms of ethics, Muslim authorities consider the transmission of reproductive material between persons who are not legally married to be a major violation of Islamic law. This sensitivity stems from the fact that Islamic law has a strict taboo on sexual relations outside wedlock (*zina*). The taboo is designed to protect paternity (i.e., family), which is designated as one of the five goals of Islamic law, the others being the protection of religion, life, property, and reason.

Accordingly, at the ninth Islamic law and medicine conference, held under the auspices of the Kuwait-based Islamic Organization for Medical Sciences (IOMS) in Casablanca, Morocco, in 1997, a landmark five-point declaration included recommendations to prevent human cloning and to prohibit all situations in which a third party invades a marital relationship through donation of reproductive material (Moosa 2003). Such a ban on third-party gamete donation is effectively in place among the Sunni branch of Islam, which represents approximately 80–90 percent of the world's more than 1.5 billion Muslims (see Inhorn et al., this volume).

The situation has changed quite dramatically, however, within the minority Shia branch of Islam. In 1999, the Supreme Leader of the Islamic Republic of Iran, Ayatollah Ali Hussein Khamene'i—the hand-picked successor to Iran's Ayatollah Khomeini—issued a fatwa, or nonbinding but authoritative religious proclamation, allowing donor technologies to be used (Inhorn 2005). As a result, since the new millennium, donor gametes are now being purchased by infertile couples in IVF clinics in Shia-majority Iran and Lebanon, currently the only two countries in the Muslim world to allow this practice.

Understanding this rapidly evolving moral-religious climate surrounding ARTs in the Muslim world is imperative for scholars, policymakers, and the public. To do so requires examining the Islamic scriptures themselves, the contemporary fatwas that have been issued on these ARTs, as well as the subsequent bioethical and legal rulings that are being used to enforce or, in some cases, to override these fatwas. For example, in a rather surprising turn of events, Iran's parliament decided against sperm donation in 2003, equating it with polyandry (i.e., marriage of one woman to more than one man, which is illegal in Islam). Thus, the Iranian parliament effectively overturned the Khamene'i fatwa. However, in an even more unprecedented turn of events, gestational surrogacy arrangements have been permitted in Iran, with several cases highlighted in the Iranian media (see Garmaroudi Naef, this volume; Tremayne 2005, 2008, 2009). Furthermore, Iran is at the forefront of a nascent Middle Eastern stem cell industry, highlighting a moral attitude toward abortion that is very different from that found currently in the United States (Saniei, this volume).

In the future, human reproductive cloning may also have great potential in the Muslim world, as it bypasses sexual reproduction and, hence, concerns about *zina* (or reproduction outside of wedlock). Indeed, at least one popular Lebanese Shia cleric, as well as Ayatollah Khamene'i in Iran, have condoned the idea of human cloning (Clarke 2009; Clarke and Inhorn 2011). Nonetheless, other Muslim religious leaders continue to debate the pros and cons of reproductive cloning, and no authorities, either Sunni or Shia, have come forward to openly encourage cloning for infertile Muslim couples. However, their opinions, particularly in the Shia world, may evolve over time, with potentially profound implications for infertile Muslim couples.

These new-millennial technological developments in the Muslim Middle East clearly require empirical investigation. ARTs and Muslims' attitudes toward them provide a compelling nexus for the study of what might be called "Islamic technoscience in practice." Little is currently known about Islam and technoscience, if technoscience is defined broadly as the interconnectedness between science and technology through "epistemological, institutional, and cultural discursive practices" (Lotfalian 2004: 1). As noted in *Islam, Technoscientific Identities, and the Culture of Curiosity,* there is a glaring lacuna in the literature on science and technology in cross-cultural perspective, particularly from the Islamic world, where, according to Lotfalian (2004: 6), there are "really only two strains of relevant work"—one on the Islamic medieval sciences and the other on philosophical arguments for civilizational differences between Islamic and Western science and technology (the so-called clash of civilizations thesis). This dearth of relevant scholarship clearly applies to the cross-cultural study of ARTs. For example, in the seminal volume on *Third Party Assisted Conception Across Cultures: Social, Legal and Ethical Perspectives* (Blyth and Landau 2004), not a single Muslim society is represented among the thirteen country case studies.

Clearly, the time has come to examine the globalization of ARTs to diverse Islamic contexts, particularly given the rapid technological development and globalization of these biotechnologies. Currently, there are about a dozen researchers—nearly all of them included in this volume—who are engaging in empirical studies of ARTs in the Islamic world. Their studies point to interesting variations in both the Islamic jurisprudence and the cultural responses to ARTs, particularly between the two major branches of Islam, but also between Muslim countries, between secular and religious forces within countries, and among cosectarians living in different settings (for example, Shia Muslims in Iran versus Lebanon).

Islamic Legal Thought and ARTs: Marriage, Morality, and Clinical Conundrums

Islamic religious leaders have played a prominent role in the legitimization of ARTs for overcoming infertility (Clarke 2008, 2009; Inhorn 2003, 2005, 2006a; Serour 1996, 2008; Tremayne 2005, 2006, 2009). Since the emergence of ARTs in the 1980s, leading Muslim scholars have focused on theorizing the impact and ramifications of ARTs on reproduction, family, and kinship, which are considered foundational, sacrosanct institutions and the guiding principle of human social organization. These scholars returned to early Islamic texts, in order to examine and better understand the basis upon which kinship and family relations are formed. Initially, both Sunni and Shia scholars shared the view that the treatment of infertility and use of ARTs should take place only between a married couple, and that no third party should be involved in this process. The rationale behind this argument was the protection of the purity of lineage (*nasab*), which the intrusion of a third party would destroy and which would lead to biological and social confusion (Inhorn 2003; Clarke 2009). The effects on kinship and family relations, and the consequent social disorder, were considered profound.

However, religious leaders' interpretations of the Islamic texts have not been monolithic. Differences of opinion have emerged among the four Sunni legal schools (*madhhabs*), and on basic principles, such as what constitutes lineage, or who can be considered the legitimate parent or child in a family. Likewise, Shia leaders have not been unanimous in their views and remain divided in their interpretations and verdicts on the extent to which the ARTs can be applied. Some Shia scholars remain closer in their deliberations to the conclusions of the Sunni *madhhab*s, for example, than to Shia religious leaders such as Ayatollah Khamene'i in Iran. Furthermore, differences exist among the Shia clergy in Iran, where 90 percent of the total population of 70 million is Shia.

According to some Shia clerics, third-party donation is legitimate and does not breach any religious rules. However, the majority of Sunni scholars, IVF practitioners, and patients follow the original fatwas declaring third-party donation to be religiously forbidden. As a result, a gap has developed between the main Sunni and Shia interpretations of lineage, kinship, and family relations. Whereas today, the majority of Shia resort to most forms of ARTs, including third-party donation and surrogacy, a religious ban on third-party donation exists for Sunni Muslims. In short, the permission of third-party donation for Shia Muslims versus the prohibition for Sunni Muslims has divided the Muslim world into two opposite factions— the major dichotomy highlighted in this volume.

In Section I, entitled "Islamic Legal Thought and ARTs: Marriage, Morality, and Clinical Conundrums," the authors examine and highlight the differences in approach, interpretation, and application between the two major branches of Sunni and Shia Islam, as well as within each branch. Contributors to this section examine the fundamental principles in Islam that concern procreation and marriage, and ask how reproduction has been understood and interpreted in both historical and contemporary contexts by religious leaders. The chapters in this section focus on the intricate legal discussions surrounding the establishment of children's lineage (*nasab*) from ancient to contemporary times, and, ultimately, what this means for the children born from ARTs. The authors compare the different legal reasoning used by Sunni and Shia religious authorities, showing how different understandings of legitimate marriage, procreation, sexuality, adultery, paternity, lineage, and the "need" for children, both on the individual level and on the level of social reproduction, are understood. All of the contributors to the first section clearly challenge the idea that Islam is a rigid religion, which has no built-in mechanisms for adjusting to modernity. Indeed, these authors show that Muslim authorities are engaged in comprehensive ethical and legal debates and arguments about the importance of reproduction, the "need" and "right" to have children, and the rights of children themselves. These debates have involved the classical texts, as well as consideration of the contemporary plight of infertile couples and the ARTs available to them. Through the use of these ARTs, Islam, in general, has provided solutions to cope with reproductive suffering.

As Thomas Eich argues in chapter 1, "Constructing Kinship in Sunni Islamic Legal Texts," the reason for the rejection by contemporary Sunni scholars of heterologous insemination (by a third-party donor) is that only marriage can contribute the legal framework for licit procreation. This link would be disrupted through sperm or egg donation, which would carry elements of illegal fornication (*zina*). Children resulting from *zina* do not have legally relevant genealogical links to their biological fathers. Against this background of contemporary religious legal debate, Eich analyzes Islamic legal discussions between the four Sunni legal schools within their historical context. He illustrates how the definition of "marriage" has differed between these four schools, and how the importance of sexual intercourse for defining marriage has varied greatly. He concludes that, based on such differences, biological considerations have played different roles in defining what would actually constitute a child born out of wedlock.

In chapter 2, "Islamic Jurisprudence (*Fiqh*) and Assisted Reproduction: Establishing Limits to Avoid Social Disorders," Sandra Houot expands the discussion of ARTs to examine the debates surrounding a number of modern reproductive technologies (e.g., contraception, abortion). Muslim scholars have used concepts from traditional *fiqh*, such as *darura* (necessity) and *maslaha* (common or public interest), as tools to justify the necessity of these fertility interventions. Houot argues that the notion of *maslaha* is one of the main tools used in ethical debates in Islam. It has also been used extensively in contemporary debates by Islamic jurists to allow the application of ARTs. Based on her analysis of the fundamental symbolic values of filiation (*nasab*) and parenthood, Houot argues that assisted reproduction fits well in the Islamic value system, which has adapted to modern practices.

In addition to *maslaha*, Farouk Mahmoud shows in chapter 3, "Controversies in Islamic Evaluation of Assisted Reproductive Technologies," that other conceptual tools such as *istihsan*—seeking an equitable and just solution—are also used as a way to accommodate modern biotechnologies for the greater good of the public. His chapter reviews a large number of ARTs and related reproductive practices, examining both their accommodation by Islamic jurists, as well as the controversies that have erupted as a result of the Sunni-Shia dichotomy described above. As both an ART scholar and practitioner, Mahmoud focuses on the clinical dilemmas posed by the Islamic debates. For example, is it permitted to discard excess embryos? Should siblings be allowed to donate gametes, embryos, or uteruses as surrogates? Should PGD be used for sex selection? And, in the future, will it be allowable to transplant ovaries and uteruses? Mahmoud surveys the opinions of both Shia and Sunni scholars in his chapter, and also discusses practical dilemmas for IVF physicians treating Muslim patients. His chapter is especially useful in this regard.

In general, Section I of this book will appeal most to those interested in the intricacies of Islamic legal thought and jurisprudence. It is less anthropological than theological; it looks to Islamic history and to differences in Sunni and Shia legal reasoning to discern contemporary normative approaches to ARTs. In this regard, it provides a legal background for the complex social realities portrayed in Sections II and III of this volume. It also introduces important terms in Arabic and Persian (used in Iran), which will be emphasized throughout the volume and which are defined in the "Glossary of Arabic, Persian, and Turkish Terms" at the beginning of this volume.

From Sperm Donation to Stem Cells: The Iranian ART Revolution

Section II of this volume focuses on the special case of Iran, which, since the sixteenth century, has been the global epicenter of Shia Islam. To understand the "Iranian ART revolution" (Abbasi-Shavazi et al. 2008), it is necessary to examine three fundamental aspects of Shia Islam: (1) the Shia concept of the Imamate, in which political authority and religious excellence are seen as inherited through the line of descendants from the Prophet Muhammad's daughter and her husband 'Ali, the Prophet's cousin; (2) the nineteenth-century development of the concept of "sources of emulation" (*marja' al-taqlid*), or Shia religious scholars who are to be followed for their learnedness; and (3) the Shia emphasis on independent reasoning (*ijtihad*) to find new answers to arising problems (Clarke 2006b).

Unlike their Sunni counterparts, Shia scholars remain reluctant to engage in formal collective *ijtihad* deliberations on issues of global importance. Instead, they rely on individualistic independent reasoning, which has led to a diversity of opinions among Shia *marja'*s, who are not necessarily in agreement with one other, and who, in fact, take opposing views on the interpretation of the Qur'an. Historically, such developments have led to the senior *marja'*s forming their own groups of followers. In addition, the great scope of opinions has led to considerable "flexibility" for the Shia *marja'*s in al-

lowing the introduction of scientific and other innovations. It is the
individualistic practice of *ijtihad* that has paved the way for the Shia
to engage dynamically with most forms of biotechnology. However,
it has also led to the Sunni-Shia dichotomy described above.

Initially, both Sunni and Shia religious authorities restricted the
use of ARTs to married couples, thereby excluding the use of a wide
range of possibilities that are available to overcome infertility (see
Mahmoud and Inhorn et al., this volume). However, by the beginning of the new millennium, the Iranian Shia had found solutions
within the religious rules that allowed the use of all forms of ARTs,
including most importantly third-party donation. Lebanese Shia
communities soon followed suit, albeit in moderation (see Inhorn et
al., this volume; Clarke 2009). To be able to apply third-party donation, the Shia in Iran extended the definition of marriage to include
"temporary marriage," a form of marriage that is practiced by Shia
only (Haeri 1989; Tremayne 2009). They did so by allowing a donor
to become a legitimate, although temporary, spouse, thereby donating an egg or sperm within the bounds of legal marriage (Tremayne,
this volume; Inhorn 2003; Clarke 2006b; Tremayne 2006, 2009).
Several Iranian religious leaders engaged in further debates on other
forms of third-party donation, and, as a result, embryo donation was
legally approved, followed by surrogacy on the same grounds (Garmaroudi Naef, this volume). Such approval has most recently been
extended to allow stem cell research in Iran (Saniei, this volume),
and has been applied for other forms of biotechnology as well, including organ donation and transgender surgery. Indeed, the Shia of
Iran have gone much farther in embracing all forms of third-party
donation than most Western Christian countries, as demonstrated
by chapter 8 in this volume.

To understand the reasons for and the speed by which such "liberal" (Clarke 2009) decisions have been made and accepted into
practice in Iran, it is essential to realize that decisions are ultimately
made by the legislative councils—themselves part of Iran's theocratic regime, made up of political as well as the religious leaders.
These councils' decisions become "official," but those who do not
wish to use them can turn to their own *marja'* without the worry of
breaking any rules. For example, as shown in both chapters 6 and 7,
the approval of third-party donation was the result of many years
of intensive debate among several *marja*'s. Finally, the endorsement
of the supreme religious leader, Ayatollah Ali Hussein Khamene'i,
gave third-party donation "official" legitimacy in 1999. However,
approval or disapproval by Ayatollah Khamene'i does not mean

that all Shia leaders are in agreement with him. Quite the contrary! While the Sunni seem to speak with one voice against third-party donation (see Inhorn et al., this volume), no definitive, universal conclusion has been reached among the Shia jurisprudents to justify the use of third-party reproductive assistance. Indeed, the Shia religious leaders are deeply divided among themselves on this and other divine matters. Due to the fundamental structure of Shia jurisprudence, there may never be a consensus among the Shia about whether or not third-party donation should be permitted.

Herein lies the key to the flexibility of Shia practice: it allows supporters to adhere to the views of one or another *marja'* as they see fit, allowing for their own metaphysical and cosmological understandings of what constitutes procreation and proper kinship relations, regardless of the "official" version. Through such liberties offered by the diversity of opinions among the Shia leaders, the users of third-party donation (i.e., doctors and patients) have been able to exercise a great degree of agency and control over actual clinical practices, including who can serve as a donor, thereby reinforcing independent understandings of what constitutes kinship and relatedness (Garmaroudi Naef, this volume; Tremayne 2009).

Section II of this volume, "From Sperm Donation to Stem Cells: The Iranian ART Revolution," examines the legitimization of third-party donation in Iran from legal, religious, and ethical aspects, and the impact of the "flexible practice" of third-party reproductive assistance on kinship, family, and gender relations. In deciding on the legitimacy of various ARTs, religious leaders do not necessarily act alone; instead, they engage with other specialists in Islamic law, medicine, psychology, and various disciplines to explore the legal and bioethical ramifications of these biotechnologies on society, the family, marriage, and the children born as a result of ARTs.

In chapter 4, "More than Fatwas: Ethical Decision Making in Iranian Fertility Clinics," Robert Tappan raises serious questions about the bioethics of Shia "flexibility" in clinical settings in Iran. He argues that while Islamic law, presented as fatwas, or legal opinions of Islamic scholars, plays a key role in Islamic bioethics, the assertion that "Islamic bioethics" is synonymous with fatwas does not bear out in Iranian fertility clinics. There, clinicians and ethical committees consider a wide range of sources, not limited to fatwas, and including civil law, Western bioethical notions, and *ijtihad*. These efforts, in Tappan's view, are part of the wider articulation of Islamic bioethics that includes, or goes beyond, mere reference to Islamic law. Yet, based on his reading of the Islamic legal scholar, Abdulaziz

Sachedina, Tappan argues that Iranian clinicians and jurists have both failed to unfold deeper, more foundational grounds for Islamic bioethics, and for the application of important theological, ethical, and legal principles. For example, the rights of the child born from third-party donation must be considered, but child rights and rights of the unborn are rarely invoked in clinical discussions, based on Tappan's ethnographic research in Iranian ART clinics.

The justification for allowing the use of third-party donation in Iran has been to ensure the stability and happiness of the family through the birth of children, thereby reducing the suffering among infertile couples (see Garmaroudi Naef, this volume). Indeed, the focus throughout these Shia jurisprudential debates has remained on the family, which is considered the foundation of society. Nonetheless, the dynamic array of ART donor practices allowed in Iran has opened the way for myriad bioethical, legal, and personal dilemmas, which can turn into a minefield. In chapter 5, "The 'Down Side' of Gamete Donation: Challenging 'Happy Family' Rhetoric in Iran," Soraya Tremayne shows how three parties—lawmakers, physicians, and patients, each with their own agendas—may not always be equipped to deal with the complex ethical and interpersonal problems that are generated by ARTs. In fact, religious texts and religious authorities cannot always solve the contemporary dilemmas arising from third-party donation. In cases of male infertility in particular, Iranian men may "secretly" resort to donor sperm rather than be seen as infertile. By doing so, they take an opportunity provided by ARTs to reinforce the values of procreation and doing one's duty to the social group. However, in her poignant chapter based on refugee-asylum cases in the United Kingdom, Tremayne shows how Iranian women who have been coaxed or coerced into accepting third-party gamete donation (both sperm and egg) may suffer horrible consequences, including emotional and physical abuse, abandonment, and divorce. Their donor children, too, may suffer in a multitude of ways, including being used as "pawns" by bitter husbands who regret their initial decisions to go forward with gamete donation. In short, despite the "happy family" rhetoric used to rationalize third-party donation by religious leaders and clinicians in Iran, there is a "down side"—and a very dark one indeed—as shown in the case studies in this chapter.

In chapter 6, "Gestational Surrogacy in Iran: Uterine Kinship in Shia Thought and Practice," Shirin Garmaroudi Naef analyzes the legitimizations of yet another new ART practice in Iran. The case of surrogacy provides the perfect example of the malleability of reli-

gious arguments through *ijtihad*. In explaining the reasoning behind
the approval of surrogacy by Iranian religious authorities—not only
of surrogacy, but of surrogacy between siblings of both sexes—Garmaroudi Naef shows that Shia scholars have built their argument
around the notion of physical contact. Namely, surrogacy does not
entail physical contact (i.e., sex) between the two parties, and therefore no illicit act takes place in reproduction through such procedures. Garmaroudi Naef confirms that the basis for the endorsement
of surrogacy was the interpretation by some senior religious scholars
of what constitutes kinship. They judged that surrogacy between
siblings does not break any rules of adultery or incest. But, as she
points out, there are a considerable number of equally senior Shia
authorities who have produced a counterargument for such practices, and some have even rejected them vehemently. In the midst of
these surrogacy debates, Garmaroudi Naef focuses on the way that
Iranian surrogates themselves—some of whom are siblings of the
infertile individual they are helping—attempt to transform surrogacy from a controversial issue into a normative way of overcoming
infertility. Garmaroudi Naef's rich ethnographic data suggest that
earlier anthropological theories of Islam and "blood" kinship need
to take into account notions of "uterine kinship" in Shia thought
and practice.

The final chapter of this section, chapter 7 on "Human Embryonic Stem Cell Research in Iran: The Significance of the Islamic
Context," by Mansooreh Saniei, explores the local moral and ethical arguments upon which stem cell research has been endorsed
in Iran. The Iranian religious rulers, in their mutual role as political leaders, have eagerly engaged in debates with secular experts
on matters regarding science and technology, and are responsible
for, inter alia, social planning and public health. Such a position
has led to the understanding and legitimizing of many new health
technologies, which are otherwise viewed as unacceptable according to traditional Islamic values. As is clear from Saniei's chapter,
the endorsement of stem cell research has not been taken lightly or
in isolation, but comes from a genuine concern for health and overcoming complex medical problems. Having been faced with various
health crises ranging from overpopulation to a postwar generation
of disabled men, Iranian religious leaders have resorted to the traditional Islamic concepts of *maslaha* and *istihsan* to legitimize stem cell
research. Saniei argues that through endorsing stem cell research,
senior Iranian religious leaders promise a return of the "golden age,"
in which Iran will be at the forefront of scientific innovations. In-

deed, Shia Iran has taken the lead in stem cell research among the Middle Eastern Muslim countries, although, as the chapter shows, other Sunni Muslim countries may eventually follow.

While there is no denying that humanitarian, moral, and ethical motivations are driving forces behind the endorsements and legitimization of stem cell technologies, the political reasons cannot be overlooked. For example, Iran won the United Nations Population Award in 1998 by bringing down its population rates in a dramatic fashion. This occurred because religious leaders had come to realize that the country was headed toward a population explosion. They saw overpopulation as a threat to the ideology upon which they had come to power—namely, the promise to help the poor and to provide basic health and educational services. Thus, they took effective action to reduce population growth (Hoodfar 1995; Tremayne 2004). As with population, Iran's religious rulers continue to argue that a Muslim country should not be forced to rely on the West for its health technologies, including therapeutic stem cells.

Islamic Biopolitics and the "Modern" Nation-State: Comparative Case Studies of ART

Lest readers be left with the impression that ARTs are practiced only in Shia Iran, it is important to note that the Sunni countries—namely, Egypt, Jordan, and Saudi Arabia—were the first to introduce IVF to the Muslim world in 1986 and that Turkey, a Sunni-majority country, has the highest number of clinics in the region (>100). In fact, Sunni Islamic countries can be characterized as "ART-friendly"; an ART industry is thriving across the Middle East, and most South Asian and Southeast Asian Muslim countries can also boast of a flourishing ART sector. (Muslim Africa is the exception to this rule.)

However, it is important to reiterate that third-party donation is effectively banned across the Sunni Muslim world. With the exception of Iran and Lebanon (which has followed the Iranian lead), no other single Muslim-majority country allows the practice of third-party donation, either by law or fatwa decree. The strength of this religious ban is impressive, considering that it has "held" since 1980, when the first pro-IVF, antidonation fatwa was issued at Al Azhar University in Cairo, Egypt. Most Sunni IVF practitioners and their patients continue to support the third-party ban for a variety of religious and moral reasons. Those who do not must cross international borders as "reproductive tourists," usually in secrecy. However, "cracks" in the ban are beginning to unfold in places like Turkey and Lebanon. This suggests that Islamic biopolitics can change over time, especially in "secular" and "multisectarian" societies within the Islamic world. In every society, politics, religion, and culture intermingle to define both the possibilities for, and the "arenas of constraint" on, ART practice (Inhorn 2003).

Section III, entitled "Islamic Biopolitics and the 'Modern' Nation-State: Comparative Case Studies of ART," focuses on the wider implications of ARTs on culture, politics, and religion in a variety of Middle Eastern and Mediterranean countries where secular and religious debates on the application of ARTs are being carried out. This section highlights the role of the state (or lack thereof) in regulating ARTs, and how states and political parties may use ARTs to highlight their own "modernity." It also includes a comparative perspective on ARTs by juxtaposing the Catholic Church and Sunni Islam; various Muslim and Christian sects living (and using ARTs) within the same country; and secular and religious attitudes toward ARTs within Turkey, a supposedly "secular but Muslim" Middle Eastern country with a booming ART industry.

In chapter 8, "Third-Party Reproductive Assistance around the Mediterranean: Comparing Sunni Egypt, Catholic Italy, and Multisectarian Lebanon," Marcia C. Inhorn, Pasquale Patrizio, and Gamal I. Serour undertake an unlikely comparison of three Mediterranean societies, one Sunni Muslim, one Roman Catholic Christian, and one multisectarian (with eighteen officially recognized religious sects). The authors begin in the Sunni Muslim world, providing comprehensive coverage of Egypt and the third-party donation ban that has remained in full force in all Sunni-dominant countries. Against such a backdrop, the chapter moves to Italy, which used to be on the forefront of third-party donation practices, but has joined the Sunni world in banning donor technologies as the result of a 2004 Vatican-inspired law. Perhaps unexpectedly, multisectarian Lebanon—partly Christian, mostly Muslim, with a large Shia population—has ended up being the most "permissive" of the three nations with regard to third-party donation. Following the Iranian lead, Shia IVF practitioners introduced donor technologies, which were also welcomed by the Christian IVF physicians in the country. Although most Sunni IVF doctors and patients remain firmly against such practices, Lebanon has become a hub for "reproductive tourism," primarily of Sunni Muslims from other Middle Eastern countries where donor gametes and technologies are unavailable. This chapter provides the perfect example of a situation whereby the agency of users—both physicians and patients—comes to shape the practice of ARTs amid considerable religious diversity. In this chapter, the similarities between Sunni Egypt and Catholic Italy are shown to be closer than between the Sunni and Shia Muslim populations within two Middle Eastern countries. The authors conclude that the unique multiconfessional nature of Lebanese society has led to a lack of religious and political consensus, and hence, to a degree of permissiveness toward all forms of reproductive assistance not found in more religiously unified countries of the Mediterranean.

Morgan Clarke's chapter 9, "Islamic Bioethics and Religious Politics in Lebanon: On Hizbullah and ARTs," zeroes in on Lebanon, particularly the Iranian-backed Hizbullah political party, whose clerical elites favor a "contemporary" vision of Islamic law, which makes room for ARTs and third-party donation. Clarke interweaves biomedical with religious and political discourses, suggesting that a focus on religious opinion alone is not sufficient for an accurate understanding of what an "Islamic bioethics" might be—either as an independent phenomenon in its own right, or as the object of Western academic fascination. As Clarke shows for Lebanon's Hizbullah, which follows the Iranian lead, religious-legal positions are situated within wider intellectual and political projects; thus, the possibility of isolating bioethics as a distinct institution and practice implies a particular assembly of relations of authority, the topography of which, in the Middle East, is more varied than is sometimes implied. Worldwide, medical knowledge has been growing as one of the main sources of authoritative knowledge. Clarke explores how senior Hizbullah leaders in Lebanon, in their anxiety to demonstrate their "modernity" (see also Deeb 2006), are giving recognition to biomedical practices such as third-party donation, partly as a demonstration of their own authority and wisdom.

The inextricable links between reproduction and state policy are showcased in the final chapter, chapter 10 by Zeynep Gürtin on "Assisted Reproduction in Secular Turkey: Regulation, Rhetoric, and the Role of Religion." In Turkey, a Sunni Muslim country that prides itself on being a secular state, ARTs are flourishing. Gürtin's discussion revolves around the practice of ARTs in Turkey, which receives support from both the secular state and religious institutions and which is growing dramatically among married Turkish couples. The extensive coverage by the media and other forms of public endorsement confirm both the popularity and the acceptance of ARTs, giving them an "uncontroversial" character. Despite the idealized synchrony between cultural sensibilities, civic law, and religious prescriptions, Gürtin opens up yet another hitherto unexplored aspect of the ARTs: namely, that the secular Turkish state is seemingly anxious to draw the line between religion and culture in the legitimization of ARTs, and to accord more weight to the cultural aspects of such approval. Gürtin points out that although it may not be practically possible to disaggregate "culture" from "religion," within the secular politics of Turkey the latter is unacceptable as a causal explanation for state regulation of donor technologies. However, the Turkish state *does* forbid third-party donation, as in all other Sunni countries, thereby forcing Turkish couples to travel to neighboring Cyprus for donor gametes. Indeed, in March 2010, Turkey became the first country in the world to enact a law banning cross-border reproductive travel of its citizens seeking third-party reproductive assistance (Gürtin 2011). Although this law is more symbolic than enforceable, it demonstrates how these discourses about Islam, secularism, and culture may be used and understood rather differently by internal and external commentators, but pertain to sensitive questions about Turkey's identity and international affiliation as a "democratic," "secular," "democratizing," but also "Muslim" society.

Conclusion: ARTs in Action—The Emerging Issues

As shown by all of the contributors to this volume, Islam considers procreation to be one of the most important pillars of society; thus, the duty of each Muslim is to reproduce and ensure the perpetuity of his or her social group. Given Islam's pronatalism and the many biotechnological innovations to overcome infertility, Muslim religious leaders willingly engage in debates to make ARTs possible for infertile couples without breaching any religious rules. In doing so, they resort to some of the key conceptual tools available to Islamic jurisprudents, such as "necessity," "public interest," and "seeking a just and equitable solution." As such, they help to make it possible for infertile Muslim couples to benefit from ARTs.

This volume also highlights the ways in which infertile Muslims are engaging with ARTs, and the difficult reproductive choices they make. In most Muslim countries, deeply rooted religious beliefs remain an important—perhaps *the* most important—determining factor in the reproductive decisions of infertile couples. Most couples resort to ARTs only if they can fit these technologies into cultural and religious understandings of reproduction. Faced with the choice of having a baby they desperately want or breaking what they believe to be the religious rules, most Muslim couples will give up on treatment and go without a child (Inhorn 2003, 2006).

Yet, the ART "revolution" in Iran has opened up new "local moral worlds" hitherto unseen (Kleinman 1995). Garmaroudi Naef's ethnographic study of surrogacy in Iran points to the fact that whenever possible, infertile couples resort to their siblings or other close relatives for surrogacy, throwing into question notions of consanguinity and incest. Tremayne's chapter on the aftermath of third-party donation in Iran—where it has been practiced for more than ten years, with hundreds if not thousands of donor children born—suggests that an assessment of the long-term impact on families is in order. Her findings raise several questions regarding the unforeseen consequences of the use of donor technologies. Although third-party donation has been embraced in Iran through Islamic ethical debates, Islam may be inadequate in solving the complex human dilemmas emerging from donation, which the religious rulings and interpretations could not have predicted.

One of the most overlooked aspects of ART ethics involves the rights of the child, as discussed at length by Robert Tappan in this volume. The Iranian asylum cases discussed in Tremayne's chapter reveal that donor children may not be as cherished as anticipated, and may become pawns in the hands of parents, especially fathers. The study reveals the differences in outcome for cases of third-party donation, depending upon whether the infertile party is the wife or the husband. The chilling findings show a broadening gap in gender relations, an increase in violence from infertile men towards their fertile wives, the frequent cases of rejection of donor children, especially those resulting from sperm donation, and the overall unflinching attitude of society toward women and children, who are blamed for deviating from social norms. The fact that one of the major ART research institutes in Iran has recorded many such cases and hopes to initiate a study on domestic violence—with the help of both editors of this volume—bespeaks the importance of this issue. The future of donor children in the Muslim world is an uncertain one, which is why, even in "permissive" Lebanon, most men reject the idea altogether, stating that a donor child "won't be my son" (Inhorn 2006b, 2012).

Finally, an interesting observation emerges from this collection. The general understanding of contemporary religious authorities and the Muslim public is that lineage (*nasab*) means biological belonging of the offspring to their parents. Recent ethnographic research confirms this in a variety of Muslim contexts (Clarke 2009; Inhorn 2003, 2006a; Tremayne 2009). The Sunni religious authorities have banned third-party donation on this basis—namely, that it will confuse lineage. However, as Eich demonstrates in this volume, in establishing lineage, the four different *madhhab*s in Sunni Islam have traditionally defined lineage in a number of ways, through elaborate arguments and different bases. For example, the Hanafis link lineage to the existence of a marriage contract and not to sexual intercourse between the spouses. Therefore, any child born six months after marriage is considered to belong to the husband. Eich further examines whether classical Islamic texts have considered lineage as being "biological" or "social." Eich's description of what constitutes lineage in Sunni Islam links strikingly well with the situation of contemporary Shia men in Tremayne's study. Namely, to maintain their rightful position as fathers and to reproduce their social group, some Iranian Shia men are prepared to forgo their firm belief in "biological" descent and resort to "social" fatherhood of a donor child, as long as this can be done in secrecy.

In some respects, then, the purported Sunni-Shia dichotomy, which we have laid out in this volume, may be overstated. We can conclude that the Sunni and the Shia share one belief: namely, that human reproduction and the need to preserve one's social group are paramount. When it comes to social reproduction—or the belief that having children and perpetuating kinship structures into the future is important—there is little difference between the Sunni and the Shia, even though they are now achieving biological reproduction through different biotechnological means. In both cases, they are being "assisted" by their religious leaders, whose role in the introduction, permission, innovation, and expansion of ARTs in the Islamic world cannot be overstated. Indeed, when it comes to ARTs, Islam has proved to be a facilitating factor, especially when compared to certain major forms of Christianity such as Catholicism. The role of Islam in promoting most forms of ART defies East-West stereotypes, and suggests that additional study of Islam and technoscience is imperative in the new millennium.

References

Abbasi-Shavazi, Mohammad Jalal, Marcia C. Inhorn, Hajiieh Bibi Razeghi-Nasrabad, and Ghasem Toloo. 2008. "'The Iranian ART Revolution': Infertility, Assisted Reproductive Technology, and Third-Party Donation in the Islamic Republic of Iran." *JMEWS (Journal of Middle East Women's Studies)* 4(2): 1–28.

Blank, Robert. 1998. "Regulation of Donor Insemination." In *Donor Insemination: International Social Science Perspectives*, ed. Ken Daniels and Erica Haimes. Cambridge: Cambridge University Press, 131–50.

Blyth, Eric, and Ruth Landau, eds. 2004. *Third Party Assisted Conception across Cultures: Social, Legal and Ethical Perspectives*. London: Jessica Kingsley.

Braverman, Andrea M. 2001. "Exploring Ovum Donors' Motivations and Needs." *American Journal of Bioethics* 1: 16–17.

Brockopp, Jonathan E., ed. 2003. *Islamic Ethics of Life: Abortion, War, and Euthanasia*. Columbia: University of South Carolina Press.

Brockopp, Jonathan E., and Thomas Eich, eds. 2008. *Muslim Medical Ethics: From Theory to Practice*. Columbia: University of South Carolina Press.

Carmeli, Yoram S., and Daphna Birenbaum-Carmeli. 2000. "Ritualizing the 'Natural Family': Secrecy in Israeli Donor Insemination." *Science as Culture* 9: 301–24.

Clarke, Morgan. 2006a. "Islam, Kinship and New Reproductive Technology." *Anthropology Today* 22(5): 17–20.

———. 2006b. "Shiite Perspectives on Kinship and New Reproductive Technologies." *ISIM Review* 17: 26–27.

———. 2008. "New Kinship, Islam and the Liberal Tradition: Sexual Morality and New Reproductive Technology in Lebanon". *Journal of the Royal Anthropological Institute* 14 (1): 153-69

———. 2009. *Islam and New Kinship: Reproductive Technologies and the Shariah in Lebanon*. New York and Oxford: Berghahn Books.

Clarke, Morgan, and Marcia C. Inhorn. 2011. "Mutuality and Immediacy between *Marja'* and *Muqallid:* Evidence from Male IVF Patients in Shi'i Lebanon." *International Journal of Middle East Studies* 43: 409–427.

Cohen, Lawrence. 2002. "The Other Kidney: Biopolitics beyond Recognition." In *Commodifying Bodies*, ed. Nancy Scheper-Hughes and Loic Wacquant. London: Sage, 9–29.

Deeb, Lara. 2006. *An Enchanted Modern: Gender and Public Piety in Shi'i Lebanon*. Princeton, NJ: Princeton University Press.

Deech, Ruth. 2003. "Reproductive Tourism in Europe: Infertility and Human Rights." *Global Governance* 9: 425–32.

Franklin, Sarah. 1996. *Embodied Progress: A Cultural Account of Assisted Conception*. London: Routledge.

Gürtin, Zeynep. 2011. "Banning Reproductive Travel: Turkey's ART Legislation and Third-party Assisted Reproduction." *Reproductive BioMedicine Online* 23: 555–64.

Haeri, Shahla. 1989. *Law of Desire: Temporary Marriage in Shi'i Islam*. Syracuse: Syracuse University Press.

Hoodfar, Homa. 1995. "Population Policy and Gender Equity in Post-Revolutionary Iran." In *Family, Gender and Population in the Middle East: Policies in Context*, ed. Carla Makhlouf. Cairo: American University of Cairo Press.

Inhorn, Marcia C. 1994. *Quest for Conception: Gender, Infertility, and Egyptian Medical Traditions.* Philadelphia: University of Pennsylvania Press.

———. 2003. *Local Babies, Global Science: Gender, Religion, and In Vitro Fertilization in Egypt.* New York: Routledge.

———. 2005. "*Fatwa*s and ARTs: IVF and Gamete Donation in Sunni v. Shi'a Islam." *Journal of Gender, Race & Justice* 9: 291–317.

———. 2006a. "Making Muslim Babies: IVF and Gamete Donation in Sunni versus Shia Islam." *Culture, Medicine and Psychiatry* 30(4): 427–50.

———. 2006b. "'He Won't Be My Son': Middle Eastern Muslim Men's Discourses of Adoption and Gamete Donation." *Medical Anthropology Quarterly* 20: 94–120.

_____. 2012. *The New Arab Man: Emergent Masculinities, Technologies, and Islam in the Middle East.* Princeton, NJ: Princeton University Press.

Kahn, Susan Martha. 2000. *Reproducing Jews: A Cultural Account of Assisted Conception in Israel.* Durham, NC: Duke University Press.

Kirkman, Maggie. 2003. "Egg and Embryo Donation and the Meaning of Motherhood." *Women & Health* 38: 1–18.

Kleinman, Arthur. 1995. *Writing at the Margin: Discourse between Anthropology and Medicine.* Berkeley: University of California Press.

Konrad, Monica. 1998. "Ova Donation and Symbols of Substance: Some Variations on the Theme of Sex, Gender and the Partible Body." *Journal of the Royal Anthropological Institute* 4: 643–67.

Lorber, Judith. 1989. "Choice, Gift, or Patriarchal Bargain? Women's Consent to *In Vitro* Fertilization in Male Infertility." *Hypatia* 4: 23–36.

Lotfalian, Mazyar. 2004. *Islam, Technoscientific Identities, and the Culture of Curiosity.* Dallas: University Press of America.

Moosa, Ebrahim. 2003. "Human Cloning in Muslim Ethics." *Voices across Boundaries* (Fall): 23–26.

Musallam, Bassim F. 1986. *Sex and Society in Islam: Birth Control before the Nineteenth Century.* Cambridge: Cambridge University Press.

Pollock, Anne. 2003. "Complicating Power in High-Tech Reproduction: Narratives of Anonymous Paid Egg Donors." *Journal of Medical Humanities* 24: 241–63.

Serour, Gamal I. 1996. "Bioethics in Reproductive Health: A Muslim's Perspective." *Middle East Fertility Society Journal* 1: 30–35.

———. 2008. "Islamic Perspectives in Human Reproduction." *Reproductive BioMedicine Online* 17(Suppl. 3): 34–38.

Serour, Gamal I., and Bernard M. Dickens. 2001. "Assisted Reproduction Developments in the Islamic World." *International Journal of Gynecology & Obstetrics* 74: 187–93.

Shanley, Mary Lyndon. 2002. "Collaboration and Commodification in Assisted Procreation: Reflections on an Open Market and Anonymous Donation in Human Sperm and Eggs." *Law & Society Review* 36: 257–83.

Storrow, Richard F. 2005. "Quests for Conception: Fertility Tourists, Globalization, and Feminist Legal Theory." *Hastings Law Journal* 57: 295–330.

Thompson, Charis M. 2005. *Making Parents: The Ontological Choreography of Reproductive Technologies.* Cambridge, MA: MIT Press.

Tremayne, Soraya. 2004. "'And Never the Twain Shall Meet': Reproductive Health Policies in the Islamic Republic of Iran". *Reproductive Agency, Medicine and the State: Cultural Transformations in Childbearing.* ed. Maya Unnithan-Kumar. New York and Oxford: Berghahn Books

———. 2005. "The Moral, Ethical and Legal Implications of Egg, Sperm and Embryo Donation in Iran." Paper presented at the International Conference on Reproductive Disruptions: Childlessness, Adoption, and Other Reproductive Complexities, 19 May, in University of Michigan, Ann Arbor.

———. 2006. "Not All Muslims Are Luddites." *Anthropology Today* 22(93): 1–2.

———. 2009. "Law, Ethics and Donor Technologies in Shia Iran." In *Assisting Reproduction, Testing Genes: Global Encounters with New Biotechnologies,* ed. Daphna Birenbaum-Carmeli and Marcia C. Inhorn. New York and Oxford: Berghahn Books.

Van der Ploeg, Irma. 1995. "Hermaphrodite Patients: In Vitro Fertilization and the Transformation of Male Infertility." *Science, Technology, & Human Values*: 460–81.

Part I

Islamic Legal Thought and ARTs
Marriage, Morality, and Clinical Conundrums

PART I INTRODUCTION

Frank Griffel

Let me begin this introduction to Islam and assisted reproductive technologies by looking somewhat generally at the way in which Islamic law deals with legal issues surrounding marriage and procreation. The guiding principle in almost all of the individual rules of sharia around such subjects as marriage, divorce, or inheritance is to allow a clear and unambiguous identification of a person's father. Islamic family law is first of all patrilineal family law. If, as a student of Islamic law, one ever feels unsure as to which ruling applies to a certain case of family law, it is always a good guess to choose that one which creates the most certainty about the identity of the father. At any given time period, women are only allowed to have sex with one man, which is a rule that men are not bound to. Women must wait for as long as it takes to show the effects of a pregnancy before they can remarry, while men are not restricted by any waiting period. This strong sense of patrilineality is clearly a part of Islam and stood at times in contrast to the customary law of some pre-Islamic societies.

For some Islamic societies Islamization meant the transition from matrilineality to patrilineality. In certain West African countries, for instance, rulership passed along matrilineal lines, meaning it passes from a male ruler, not to his son, but to his nephew, i.e., the son of his sister. The reason for this was, of course, the uncertainty of any given father-son relationship in a premodern society without the possibility of DNA evidence. While there is always some element of uncertainty in the identity of one's father, there can be hardly any uncertainty about who one's mother is. Matrilineality establishes family rights along the biological relationship of a mother to her sons and daughters. We can think of a strong matrilineal society where one's closest relatives are the mother and after her all the children she gave birth to, i.e., one's siblings and possibly half-siblings, while the biological father has no established rights over his children.

In Islamic law that would be, of course, unthinkable. Given that we always know a person's mother, there must be a certain order to her sexual relations that allows the establishment of who the father is. Like most legal systems in premodern Western countries, Islamic law chose the pattern of time frames. If the mother is married, all the children that she bears during marriage and during the nine months after a possible divorce are considered children of her husband, no matter what opinion one might have about the biological father. Given the natural limitations in any premodern society, classical Islamic law aims at creating *an order* that always allows the establishment of the identity of a single father, and this is what is meant by *nasab*. It is implied that this father by *nasab* need not be the biological father. It seems almost that in premodern sharia there is no concept of a biological father. A man could claim any children born by his married wives and his slaves as his own—even if he knew he was not the biological father.

This principle is valid for all four schools of law, and the Hanbalis of the thirteenth and fourteenth centuries make no exception. Thomas Eich, in his illuminating chapter on "Constructing Kinship in Sunni Islamic Legal Texts," says that Ibn Taymiyya and Ibn Qayyim al-Jawziyya "went a step further and stated explicitly that a child born out of wedlock could be attached to his or her biological father if there was no *firash*, i.e., if the woman was neither married nor a slave who had been penetrated licitly." Ibn Taymiyya's and Ibn Qayyim's "biological" criterion applies only to women who are not in a legal sexual relationship to a man. If they were, biology would again be overruled by the legal rights of their husband or, in the case of slaves, their owner. But what does "biological criterion" mean here? Ibn Taymiyya and Ibn Qayyim had no way of knowing with certainty who fathered the offspring of an unmarried woman. As far as I know, all four schools accept in such cases that the father or the mother, ideally both, identify the father—a system that does not necessarily lead to establishing the "biological" father.

Eich is right to point out that the Hanbalis of the thirteenth and fourteenth century do change the rules about incestuous relationships and consider biological father-daughter relationships where other schools would still apply the sometimes fictional husband-offspring relationship dictated by the law. It is unclear whether this has been triggered by an increasing awareness of biology. Rather, it may be due to the literalism of the Hanbali school, who take the words "your daughters" in the legal sources more seriously than the other schools.

Sandra Houot looks at the contemporary period, particularly at the rulings of the legal body connected to the Islamic World League and the Syrian jurist Muhammad Sa'id al-Buti (1929–), who is a Hanafi. Al-Buti brings in *maslaha*, an important legal category that, broadly speaking, did not exist before the eleventh century. While *maslaha* is not considered one of the four sources of Islamic law, it nevertheless assumes the role of a source of law after the twelfth and thirteenth centuries. In the modern period it becomes a very important source of law and is often seen as a vehicle for legal change. Creating offspring is one of the five "necessities" that, according to al-Ghazzali, *maslaha* must serve. However, it is unlikely that a consideration of *maslaha* would overrule other objections against, for instance, the use of sperm or egg donors. One should not forget that for Muslim jurists of the classical period, *maslaha* means to safeguard not the creation of any children, but only those who have sound *nasab*. Once we know with certainty that children are not in blood relationships with one of their parents, there is no sound *nasab*, and one can no longer invoke the principle of *maslaha*.

Farouk Mahmoud's chapter brings up the question of the flexibility of Islamic law. Here, Sunni Islamic scholars tend to apply the strategy of staying clear from the fence: if there are doubts about the legality of a practice, better be on the safe side and declare it illicit. One should not forget that for believing Muslims the stakes are high: it is an eternity either spent in heaven or in hell. Thus, it is unlikely that Sunni Muslim scholars will easily come around to the point of view of their Shia counterparts, who have allowed third-party assisted conception. For one, Sunnis have always polemicized against the practice of *mut'a* (a fixed term contract of temporary marriage in Shia Islam) as legitimizing prostitution. Second, clarity about one's *nasab* is an important principle in Islamic law that the jurists cannot easily throw overboard. One's *nasab*, here the paternal lineage, is part and parcel of a Muslim's identity. Declaring it inferior to the relationship one has to the person that takes care of one's upbringing is not all that easy, neither for a society that has put so much stress on *nasab*, nor for the individuals who would be affected by such a change.

Chapter 1

CONSTRUCTING KINSHIP IN
SUNNI ISLAMIC LEGAL TEXTS[1]

Thomas Eich

About 85 to 90 percent of the over 1 billion Muslims today are Sunnis, approximately 10 percent Shia and a small percentage followers of other denominations, with the Sunni-Shia divide going back to a religious-political schism during the first decades of Islamic history in the seventh century. Islamic law (sharia) has developed as a reflection on the correct application of rulings and principles laid down in a set of texts to a historically changing social and political reality. All Muslims agree that one of these texts is the Qur'an, which they believe to have been fixed during the seventh century as the text we know today. Sunnis and Shia differ considerably about the second textual source of Islamic law, which is the collection of authoritative statements and the recorded exemplary deeds of the Prophet and a group of other people of early Islamic history. Because of their differing assessments of the first decades of that history, the Sunnis and Shia differ as to who these other people are and who was a trustworthy transmitter of the words and deeds of the Prophet. The Sunnis accept especially pious contemporaries of Muhammad and several rulers who followed him as political leaders of the Muslim community after his death. The Shia view many from this group as nonexemplary and developed the so-called Imamate concept in which political authority and religious excellence were inherited through the line of descendants from the mar-

riage between Muhammad's daughter Fatima and his cousin 'Alī
b. Abī Ōālib (d.661). These charismatic leaders were called imams.
According to the concept of history of the largest Shia group there
were twelve infallible imams, the twelfth imam being labeled as
"hidden," because he did not die but waits in a hidden place until the
end of the world approaches. A decisive person in the development
of Twelver Shia legal discourse was the sixth imam, Ja'far al-Sádiq
(d.765), who collected many authoritative sayings. Because of the
overarching importance of Ja'far al-Sádiq for Twelver Shia jurisprudence (*fiqh*), it is sometimes labeled as "the *madhhab* (legal school)
of Ja'far" (for example, in Article Twelve of the Iranian constitution).
For most of their history Shia were a minority and did not control
political power. This situation changed for the Iranian region after
1500, when the country was converted to Shiism due to political
measures. During the nineteenth century the concept of *marja'iya*
was put into practice according to which there is a small group of
highly qualified religious scholars who should be chosen as models
of emulation (*marja' al-taqlid*). One of these *marja'*s was Grand Ayatollah Khomeini, for example. This concept led to the emergence of
groups of worldwide followers of *marja'*s among the Shia, which are
set apart from each other depending on which *marja'* they choose
to emulate.

In Sunni Islam, so-called legal schools (*madhhab*s) developed
roughly during the first five hundred years of Islamic history. Four
have survived until today and have shaped most of Islamic legal
history: the Hanafis (named after Abu Hanifa [d.767]), the Malikis
(named after Malik b. Anas [d.795]), the Shafi'is (named after Muhammad b. Idris al-Shafi'i [d.820]) and the Hanbalis (named after
Ahmad b. Hanbal [d.855]). These schools differ in their legal methodology as well as in their views on particular legal issues, as will
be illustrated in this chapter. (For a useful overview of Shiism, see
Momen 1987; for interpretations of early Islamic legal history from
different perspectives, see, e.g., Coulson 1964 and Johansen 1999:
1–72.)

For most of its history, Islamic law functioned without a hierarchical and centralized structure. Of course, there were important centers of learning at different places in different times, but
there were always several of them and none could claim to stand
above all the others. This situation changed during the twentieth
century in two respects. First, the genesis of modern nation-states
led to the establishment of an Islamic religious state hierarchy in
all Muslim majority countries. Often these are so called "fatwa of-

fices" (for an exemplary study see Skovgaard-Petersen 1997). Fatwas are legal opinions, which do not have a binding character, their
guiding authority among the people depending heavily on the person or institution issuing the fatwa. Second, since the 1970s the
two major Islamic international organizations—the Muslim World
League and the Organization of Islamic Conferences—have set up
so-called Islamic *Fiqh* Academies (IFAs, *majma' al-fiqh(i) al-islami*),
which organize annual conferences in order to discuss "the challenges of our time" from the Islamic legal point of view (Schulze
1990). At these conferences eminent Sunni and Shia legal experts—
mostly from Arab countries and Iran (but in theory from all over
the world)—meet. Over the last years the international institutions
have increased their authority over the public, which correlates
with a loss of authority on the side of the national institutions. In
part this loss of authority is caused by the close identification of the
latter with the country's respective political regimes, whose authority is increasingly being questioned.

All of these institutions (and many individual scholars, of course)
discuss medical innovations among other things, and therefore also
address issues of reproductive medicine. When it comes to assisted
reproductive technologies (ARTs), a concept of fundamental importance is *nasab* (lineage). Historically speaking, *nasab* was primarily
linked to procreation through licit intercourse and only to biology to
a secondary degree in Islamic law. Of course, this was a result of legal procedural reasoning, i.e., it was impossible to establish whether
a child had been created from a particular man's sperm. Here I de-
liberately avoid phrases such as "establishing the *real* father" or
"whether the child was *his.*" Kinship relations and their meanings
are always socially constructed. In this process biology or genetics form one possible way to establish kinship, but even if genetics
are granted a decisive role, as is the case in today's Europe and the
United States, the actual meanings of "hard data" on the DNA level
can still differ considerably between societies (see, for example, Ottenheimer 1996). Also, caution is imperative in order not to project
back on historical sources the contemporary axiom to label a child's
biological father as its "real father," which would inevitably lead to
the inherent assumption that a kinship concept that did or still does
not grant exclusively decisive importance to genetics would be a
"wrong concept." Rather, in a time when genetic testing was not
an option, giving genetics a legally binding role was simply not a
socially meaningful option. In Arabic Sunni Islamic legal discourse,
the differentiation between the "social" and the "biological" father,

for example—as it might be labeled today—has been rendered for centuries by distinguishing between the "legal" (*shar'i*) and the "linguistic" (*lughawi*) meaning of a term. Islamic *fiqh* is ready to grant that a child born out of wedlock is termed "the man's child" in common language usage. However, because it was created through illicit sex (*zina*), it is legally speaking not his child. In contemporary legal texts the same terminology is commonly used, and in some instances the distinction is rendered as "biological vs. legal fatherhood" ('Awadi and Gendi 2000: II, 999f). *Zina* is defined as primarily heterosexual intercourse without a legitimizing legal framework, which was historically speaking constituted by a marriage bond or a master-slave relationship. Two subcategories to these legitimizing frameworks are the "defective marriage" (*nikah fasid*), in which one or several elements of the legally correct wedding procedure was lacking (such as, e.g., the consent of the legal guardian [*wali*]), and "intercourse in doubt" (*wat' bi-shabh*), i.e., when two people erroneously assumed to act within a legitimizing framework. In these instances the perpetrators were not punished for *zina*, and a child resulting from that intercourse would legally be treated as licitly conceived (if the two established a legitimizing framework properly).

Establishing a *nasab* affects the child's as well as the mother's status. The child acquires rights to inheritance as well as sustenance. In addition, if the mother is a slave and the child receives a *nasab* to her free master, the child is also considered free. The mother in turn acquires sustenance rights from her husband to a certain degree, and if she is a slave and her child is recognized to be her master's, her status changes to *umm walad*, i.e., she cannot be sold anymore and will be freed automatically at her master's death. Conversely, none of this materializes if a child does not have a *nasab* to his or her father, who is by definition the "social" or "legal" father within a sharia framework. For this reason, establishing a *nasab* is usually discussed in connection with these legal issues (for overviews of Islamic lineage and inheritance law see Coulson 1971 and Powers 1990).

In Sunni law a person's *nasab* to his or her mother is established automatically through pregnancy and birth, whereas Shia *fiqh* considers motherhood a social status achieved through a legal act (Kohlberg 1985). This explains among other things the marked differences between the two on oocyte donation and surrogacy. Fatherhood has always been perceived as a status established through a legal axiom or act in both legal traditions. In other words, Muslim jurists always knew that the "biological" and "social" father were possibly not the same person, but since they did not have the means to prove that, biology did not play an overarching role in their basic definition of fatherhood and legal ways to establish it. Today genetic testing and every other aspect of contemporary reproductive medicine have become available in Muslim majority countries. Consequently, the debate among Islamic jurists has changed from asking "*What* is a father?" to "*Who* is the father?" just as in any other jurisprudential discourse debating issues of contemporary reproductive medicine.

In this chapter, I want to draw a differentiated picture of how kinship ties are constructed in early Sunni Islamic legal discourse until roughly the fourteenth century. This is done to illustrate that there is not one single Sunni-Islamic way of this construction, once the legal terminology and especially the reasoning behind it are analyzed more closely. I will show that even when the representatives of the different *madhhabs* use the same terminology, they do not necessarily mean the same things. This is partly caused by the fact that when two legal schools arrive at the same ruling, the assumptions preceding it and/or the methodology used for arriving at it might differ completely. Therefore the wider implications of a legal ruling, statement, or axiom can differ considerably although they might seem to be identical at first sight. The final section will relate these findings to the contemporary debate.

I will analyze the reasoning behind the *madhhabs'* positions on two questions relating to *zina*. First, does *zina* cause marriage prohibitions for the male fornicator towards his daughter born out of wedlock? Second, can a *nasab* be established in spite of *zina*? The Hanafis responded to the first question positively and to the second negatively, the Shafi'is and largely the Malikis answered both questions to the negative, whereas later Hanbalis from the thirteenth and fourteenth century replied positively for both of them. They can be summarized in the following overview of positions according to Sunni legal schools.

TABLE 1.1: Overview of positions according to Sunni legal schools

	Hanafis	*Shafi'is and Malikis*	*Hanbalis*
Does *zina* cause marriage prohibitions?	yes	no	yes
Does *zina* establish a *nasab*?	no	no	yes

These differences are caused by a variety of reasons. Among these I will highlight two larger complexes. The first relates to the interpretation of a particular passage in the Qur'an and mainly illustrates how the legal schools discussed the first abovementioned question. The second complex is linked to several decisions by Muhammad and relates primarily to the second question.

Part I: Qur'anic exegesis

Qur'an 4:22–23 reads in the Arberry translation:

> And do not marry women that your fathers married (*lā tankiḥu ma nakaḥa ābā'ukum min al-nisā'*), unless it be a thing of the past; surely that is indecent and hateful, an evil way. (22) Forbidden to you are your mothers and daughters, your sisters, your aunts paternal and maternal, your brother's daughters, your sister's daughters, your mothers who have given suck to you, your suckling sisters, your wives' mothers, your stepdaughters who are in your care being born of your wives (*min nisā'ikum*) you have been in to (*dakhaltum bi-hinna*)—but if you have not yet been in to them it is no fault in you—and the spouses of your sons who are of your loins, and that you should take to you two sisters together, unless it be a thing of the past; God is All-forgiving, All-compassionate (23).

These verses describe the transitory situation during the first decades of Islam, when several pre-Islamic (*jahili*) forms of establishing kinship had been abolished. They specify the group of women who are forbidden for a man to marry. Among them are women with whom the fathers of the future husbands have had *nikah*. The exact meanings of this term became hotly contested during the first centuries of Islamic legal thought. Did *nikah* mean that the fathers had only had a marriage contract with the respective women or that they had also had sex with them? As I will show, this issue of terminology was directly related to the question whether a male fornicator is allowed to marry his biological daughter born out of wedlock.

Linguistics

Fundamental for the exegetical discussion about the term *nikah* is the jurists' differentiation between two possible meanings of a term, the literal (*haqiqa*) and metaphorical one (*majaz*). In Islamic legal discourse it is commonly assumed that Qur'anic terms ought to be interpreted to denote their literal meaning, unless there is textual evidence that the metaphorical should apply (Hallaq 1997: 42f; Heinrichs 1992: 258–70). In the case of the term *nikah*, the legal scholars generally agreed that *nikah* has a double meaning: marital intercourse and marital contract, because linguistically it simply meant "uniting between two things" (jam') (Jaṣṣāṣ 1928: II, 136; Ibn al-'Arabī 1957: I, 198, 369; Harrās 1974–76: II, 216). The question was, which of the two possible meanings was the literal one and which the metaphorical? The Hanafis and Shafi'is showed the most pronounced differences on this issue.

The Shafi'is stated that, for example, in another Qur'anic passage (Q 33:49), *nikah* clearly meant a contract without intercourse: "O believers, when you marry (*nakahtum*) believing women and then divorce them before you touch them …" (Māwardī 1994: IX, 216; Harrās 1974–76: II, 216). Therefore, for the Shafi'is the literal meaning of the term *nikah* was the marriage contract rather than consummation.

The Hanafis also mentioned the usage of *nikah* in Q 33:49 but did not take this as a text passage specifying the term in general. Rather, they insisted that generally speaking *nikah* could have both meanings, which were to be subsumed under "uniting between two things." Uniting in reality took place through intercourse and not speech, i.e., the contract. Therefore the literal meaning of *nikah* was sexual intercourse, and the term had to be applied to the marriage contract metaphorically, "because the contract is the reason for arriving at sexual intercourse" (Jaṣṣāṣ 1928: II, 136).

Therefore, the Shafi'is stated that the marriage prohibitions from Q 4:22 had to apply already after a marriage contract, whereas the Hanafis argued that a combination of marriage contract and consummation was necessary. This means that both positions were not mutually exclusive. Rather, the legal act of marriage was viewed as a process consisting of several steps. They differed as to whether the Qur'anic ruling of marriage prohibitions should be linked to the beginning of that act (so said the Shafi'is) or its end (the Hanafis) (Ibn al-'Arabī 1957: I, 198).

Now, although the Hanafis had argued that in Q 4:22 *nikah* meant the combination of marriage contract and consummation, they had to put the emphasis on the intercourse and thus made it the causa legis (*'illa*) for the prohibition spelled out in that verse. This led to the question of whether *zina* would have the same legal consequences in this respect as licit intercourse. The Hanafis answered to the positive:

> God's speech "And marry not women whom your fathers married" has made it obligatory to forbid marrying a woman for a man, if his

father or somebody else [from his close relatives] has had illicit intercourse with her. This term comprises [this meaning] on the literal level, so it must be applied here. ... This is proven by God's speech 'and your step-daughters under your guardianship, born of your wives whom you have penetrated *(dakhaltum bi-hinna)*'[2] (Q.4:23) [The verb *dakhaltum bi-hinna* is derived from the infinitive form *Dukhūl bi-hā*, which] is a term for sexual intercourse. It is general pertaining to all forms of intercourse, be it allowed or prohibited, marriage or fornication. This means that the daughter becomes prohibited [for marriage] because of an intercourse, which he had with her mother before he married her. This is because of God's speech 'whom you have penetrated *(dakhaltum bi-hinna)*'.

In this passage the Hanafi scholar Jaṣṣāṣ (d. 981) makes the exegetical argument that in Q 4:22–23 *nikah* must mean "marital intercourse" with an emphasis on intercourse, which is indicated by the use of the term *dukhul* in that same passage. From this he concludes that the reason for the marriage prohibition spelled out here must be the intercourse in general, because *dukhul* is not restricted to "licit intercourse." Jaṣṣāṣ further substantiates his exegetical argument by searching for the common basis of several sharia rulings about marriage prohibitions, which he finds to lie in sexual intercourse. For example, if a man and a woman have intercourse in doubt, i.e., they erroneously assume marriage, the daughter of the woman would become prohibited for the man to marry although there was no correct *nikah* contract, when he had sex with the daughter's mother. Therefore the reason for the prohibition cannot lie in the existence of a proper legitimizing framework for sex but in the fact that it had been actual intercourse. From this Jaṣṣāṣ concludes that the marriage prohibitions in Q 4:22–23 are not restricted to *nikah* and therefore must be applied to *zina*, too (Jaṣṣāṣ 1928: II, 138).

The Shafi'is disagreed, refuting both arguments. First, according to them, in Q 4:22 *nikah* clearly meant the marriage contract only. Among other things *dukhul* in Q 4:23 did not refer to sexual intercourse in general but only to marital sex, because it took the grammatical object "your wives" *(nisa'akum)* in that verse and thus could only refer to marital intercourse (Harrās 1974–76: II, 217). Therefore Jaṣṣāṣ's conclusion would be erroneous that intercourse and not only the contract would be the legal cause for the marriage prohibition linked to *nikah*. Second, to them the unifying principle of the several forms of sexual intercourse apart from *zina* (i.e., *nikah*, *nikah fasid* [intercourse in doubt, licit sex with a slave]) was not that it was intercourse, but that the children born out of this intercourse actually had a *nasab* to their biological fathers whereas the children born out of wedlock did not (Māwardī 1994: IX, 215).

To this latter argument, Jaṣṣāṣ countered that the *nasab* was of no significance here:

> If somebody concludes a *nikāḥ* contract with a woman, the establishing of a *nasab* is already linked to the *nikah* contract [even] before the intercourse has taken place. Even if she gives birth to a child before [the first] penetration but six months after the contract has been concluded, [the husband] has obligations towards the child. And prohibition of [marrying] the [wife's] daughter is not linked to the contract [before penetration of the mother]. ... Consequently we know that the establishing of a *nasab* has no significance in this. What has to be taken into account is nothing but the intercourse. (1928: II, 138).

Here Jaṣṣāṣ refers to a specific Hanafi concept, which is not shared by other schools, that a *nasab* is established by only two formal criteria: the date of the marriage contract and the date of birth. The other schools add a third criterion: that the spouses had or at least possibly had sex with each other. This means that for Jaṣṣāṣ the establishing of a *nasab* was not a possibly unifying element between the several forms of sex, because to him sex was not a necessary criterion to establish a *nasab*. Rather, the unifying element between the various forms of intercourse was the fact that it had been sex.

The Shafi'is's major argument was a Prophetic saying (hadith): The messenger of God was asked about a man, who commits *zina* with a woman and then wants to marry her or her daughter. He said: "The prohibited does not prohibit the allowed (*lā yuharrim al-ḥarām al-ḥalāl*). [Only] what happened in *nikah* causes the prohibition" (Qurṭubī 1967: V, 115).

The philosophical question behind this dictum *la yuharrim al-haram al-halal* was whether *haram* (prohibited) and *halal* (permitted) could overlap or were always and in every aspect set apart from each other. The Shafi'is argued for the latter view. For them *zina* and *nikah* could not have the same ruling. It was not conceivable that the marriage prohibitions spelled out in Q 4:23 were a punishment, because they were linked to *nikah*, the legitimate framework for intimacy between the sexes. Consequently these marriage prohibitions were a grace from God, who had given humankind two kinship principles to organize their societies: *nasab* and marriage ties, as stated in the Qur'an (Q 25:54). If the same prohibitions would follow *zina*, they had to be considered a punishment. The same ruling could not be considered benevolent in one case and a punishment in the other. Therefore, *nikah* and *zina* could not take the same ruling. (Shafi'i 1903–8: V, 136ff; Māwārdī 1994: IX, 217f; Harrās 1974–76: II, 220–24) In addition, *nikah* and *zina* had to be considered opposites. In terms of legal methodology, the Shafi'is argued, it was not possible to build analogical reasoning on opposing starting points (Māwārdī 1994: IX, 214f).

The Hanafis countered, first, that many versions of that hadith did not match the standards of hadith criticism. Second, in those versions that did match these standards, it was not clear if Muhammad's dictum really applied to intercourse. Third, the meaning of the hadith was not general, but had to be restricted to the particular context in which Muhammad had said this sentence (Jaṣṣāṣ 928, II: 139–41).

The differences in opinion about the precise legal meaning of *nikah* and the exact legal applicability of the axiom *la yuharrim al-haram al-halal* explains why the Hanafis state that a man is not allowed to marry the daughter of a woman he had illicit intercourse with, whereas the Shafi'is posit the opposite. Both apply this general rule also on the case of the daughter born out of wedlock (*bint al-zina*), who was "created out of the man's sperm." Therefore the Shafi'is allow—though with disapproval—a fornicator to marry his biological daughter born out of wedlock, because there is no *nasab* between the two that would forbid a marriage (Māwārdī 1994: IX, 218; Harrās 1974–76: II, 269; Schacht 1952: 107). The Hanafis apply their rule that *zina* creates marriage prohibitions. Although the *bint al-zina* is legally speaking not his daughter, she is forbidden for the fornicator to marry because all daughters of the woman he had illicit sex with are forbidden to him.

Part II: Muhammad's Decisions

After addressing the question of marriage prohibitions relating to *zina*, which is largely linked to differing interpretations of Q 4:23, I will now turn to the question of whether a *nasab* can be established in spite of *zina*, a question usually discussed with reference to several decisions of Muhammad.

In the lifetime of Muhammad, 'Utba b. Abī Waqqās swore to his brother Sa'd that "the son of the female slave of Zam'a is from me." Later on Sa'd approached this son and called him his brother, trying to integrate him into his family this way. This was opposed by 'Abd b. Zam'a, who also called him his brother, "son of my father's slave, born to his *firash.*" The term *firash* (lit. "bed") is a broader concept than *nikah,* because it is not restricted to marriage but also comprises intercourse with a slave. The two men went to the Prophet, who ruled that 'Abd b. Zam'a's claim was correct, because "the child belongs to the *firash* and the fornicator gets the stone" (*al-walad li-l-firāsh wa li-l-'āhir al-ḥajar*). This means that the female slave had become *firash* to Zam'a, because he had had sex with her at least once. 'Utba had had sex with the same slave without Zam'a's consent, i.e., illicitly. The Prophet then added in the direction of Sauda bint Zam'a, "veil yourself towards him [i.e., the son in question]" (e.g., Bājī 1912–13: VI, 4f). The story can be illustrated in the following way.

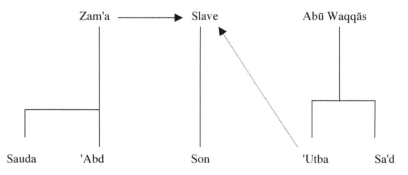

ILLUSTRATION 1.1. The story of Zam'a's slave
Lines indicate undisputed "blood relationship," and the arrow indicates licit sex, while the dotted arrow indicates illicit intercourse.

The broader framework of this story is the abolition of several pre-Islamic, *jahili* forms to establish kin relationships, especially *di'wa* in which the *nasab* link was changed from one father to another by mere claim and mutual consent (on the *di'wa* in early Islamic history see Rubin 1993). In Islamic legal discussions the *al-walad li-l-firash* dictum became the foundation for the rule that a child born out of wedlock could by no means have a *nasab* to his/her biological father. If the mother was married or a slave who had had sex with her master, the child would in a first step automatically be linked to this person but under certain circumstances the man could refuse it. If this husband's or master's plea succeeded, the child could still not be linked to his/her biological father as long as he admitted that it had been created through an act of *zina.* Rather the two fornicators (or at least one of them) had to make statements that they had acted in the erroneous but true belief that their intercourse was licit (e.g., Sarakhsī 1986: pt. XVI, 154–61).

The Issue of Similarity

In the story just mentioned, the Prophet's order towards Sauda to veil herself seemed surprising given the fact that Muhammad had apparently just decided that the respective man had to be considered to be Sauda's (half-)brother, i.e., a part of her family. The veil should only be necessary if he were a stranger. In the story, which was transmitted by Muhammad's wife 'Ā'isha, the explanation was given "because of the [physical] similarities with 'Utba [i.e., the representative from the other family] which he noticed." It is interesting to see how the different schools reacted to this part of the story.

Shafi'i stated first that the story was about establishing a *nasab*, i.e., that the person in question actually was Sauda's half-brother. Then he argued that the Prophet's order towards Sauda had nothing to do with physical similarities with Sa'd, but was caused by her elevated status as one of the Prophet's wives (Ibn al-'Arabī 1992: III, 917). For Shafi'i this was the most reasonable explanation, because he promoted the legal maxim to minimize inductive reasoning, which would have been the case had similarity been the basis for the Prophet's ruling. This did not mean that Shafi'i was sure that Zam'a was the person's biological father. He just stated that this did not matter, neither in the question of Sauda's veiling nor in the establishment of a *nasab*. He bolstered his position with a quote from the second caliph 'Umar, who had stated explicitly that in case biological fatherhood (lit. "the semen," *nutfa*) and *firash* differed, the legal ruling had to be made according to the latter (Muzanī 1903–8: VII, 305f).

The Hanafis and also the Malikis argued differently. They doubted that the Prophet had verified a *nasab* here, because he had only said to 'Abd b. Zama, "He is yours" (*huwa laka*). He did not say, "He is your brother." So it was argued that in this story Muhammad had made a ruling about inheritance rather than *nasab* relations. It was also stated that the explanation that the Prophet ordered Sauda to veil herself "because of the similarities he saw between her and Sa'd" was not Prophetic speech but the interpretation of the story's first transmitter, 'Ā'isha (Ibn al-'Arabī 1992: III, 918; Sarakhsī 1986: pt: XVII, 101; Óaḥāwī 1967: III, 114ff). Finally, it was argued that similarity could not be the issue here, because in another story Muhammad had explicitly ruled out similarity as a yardstick for arriving at a legal ruling. In that story, a man wants to refuse a child because it is black. Muhammad draws an analogy to camel breeding where camels sometimes do not resemble their parent generation and thus refuses the man's request (Óaḥāwī 1967: III, 116).

There was a third story, which was commonly referred to in the discussion about similarity as a basis for a legal decision. Hilāl b. Umāyya had suspicions that his wife was not pregnant from him but from illicit intercourse with Sharīk b. Sahma. So he practiced *li'an*, i.e., he declared that the child was not his and by implication his wife was divorced because she had committed adultery. The Prophet said they should wait until the wife gave birth to the child. If it showed certain characteristics (especially black hair), Hilāl's statement should be refused; if the child had red hair, it should be considered to be Sharīk b. Sahma's. The child had red hair, so the *li'an* procedure was considered to be correct.[3] Muhammad clearly made similarity the basis for a ruling here. However, it must be pointed out that this story was not understood to imply that the child had a *nasab* to Sharīk b. Sahma. Rather it was restricted to negating the child a *nasab* to Hilāl (Ibn al-'Arabī 1992: III, 918; Bājī 1912–13: VI, 10).

Although the Hanafis, Shafi'is, and Malikis differed considerably on the role of similarity in the legal process of establishing or negating a *nasab*, their debates never questioned the legal maxim that a child born out of wedlock cannot have a *nasab* to his biological father as long as it is stated that the child was created through an act of *zina*, which the two fornicators committed knowingly and willingly.

Hanbali Legal Reasoning

So far, the analysis of primarily the Hanafi and Shafi'i (and to a lesser degree the Maliki) positions has drawn on materials that were mostly written until the twelfth century CE, i.e., during the first six centuries of Islamic history. I will now turn to the writings of three towering Hanbali legal scholars from the twelfth to fourteenth centuries: Ibn Qudāma (d. 1223), Ibn Taymiyya (d. 1328) and Ibn al-Qayyim (d. 1350). Although their *madhhab*'s eponymous founder Ahmad b. Hanbal had already died in 855, the Hanbalis were "latecomers" among the Sunni legal schools, becoming well established significantly later than the others, which was to a large extent the result of the work of the three abovementioned scholars. On the two questions relating to *zina* discussed in this chapter—Does *zina* cause marriage prohibitions for the male fornicator towards his daughter born out of wedlock? And can a *nasab* be established in spite of *zina*?—almost no argument the Hanbalis used was entirely new, as will be seen. However, the way they arranged, weighed, and used the arguments formed a significant contrast to the reasoning of the other *madhhab*s as we have encountered them so far.

The Hanbalis argued, first, that the term *nikah* in Q 4:22 meant marital intercourse. After expressing the marriage prohibition for those with whom the fathers had *nikah*, the verse went on to state, "It was shameful" (*innahu kāna fāḥishatan*). The term *fahisha* in comparable Qur'anic contexts usually refers to sexual intercourse. So the Hanbalis argued that *nikah* meant marital intercourse, but the causa legis (*'illa*) was that it was intercourse. For this reason *zina* had to cause the same marriage prohibitions as did *nikah* (Ibn Qudāma 1999: IX, 526f). From this the question arose as to whether there was a difference between vaginal and anal sex in this respect. Ahmad b. Hanbal (d. 855) had opined that the two were on the same level, because he and others interpreted the Qur'anic term "to penetrate" (*dakhala*) from Q 4:23 exclusively to be defined physically. For this reason the marriage prohibitions linked to vaginal *zina* also covered anal penetration and thus applied to homosexual intercourse as well (Qurṭubī 1967: V, 116). Here later Hanbalis such as Ibn Qudāma (d. 1223) disagreed, stating that women penetrated anally were not included in the Qur'anic verse and therefore Q 4:24 had to apply, which stated that all categories of women who were not mentioned in the verse could be married. In order to make this argument Ibn Qudāma had to establish why vaginal penetration would integrate women into one of these categories whereas anal penetration would not: "The [vaginal] intercourse with the wife makes her a part (*sabab li-l-ba'ḍiya*). The dower is obligatory then, the *nasab* is attached to it, the woman becomes *firash* through it and rulings become manifest, which do not materialize through anal sex" (Ibn Qudāma 1999: IX, 528f).

As becomes clear from this and a following passage, where he discusses whether necrophilia and intercourse with a sexually immature girl cause marriage prohibitions, Ibn Qudāma uses the term *ba'diya* to express the idea that the woman can technically become pregnant through intercourse, which is, in this instance, only the case for penetration of the vagina and not the anus (Ibn Qudāma 1999: IX, 530). This reasoning ties in with the Hanbalis' concept of marriage, which is almost exclusively defined as the legal framework for procreation and does not view the creation of an interpersonal emotional bond as an additional and equal goal of marriage as the Malikis do, for example (Ibn al-'Arabī 1992: II, 697; Scalenghe 2004/5; see also Shafi'i 1903–8: V, 136).

This can also be seen in Ibn Taymiyya's opinion that a *firash* is only established through actual intercourse, which contrasts with the Shafi'is and Malikis, who accepted the possibility of intercourse, and the Hanafis, who linked the *firash* to the marriage contract (Ibn al-Qayyim 1950: IV, 115).

In this context Ibn Qudāma approaches the question of whether a man is allowed to marry his biological daughter born out of wedlock. After mentioning the position of Shafi'i and Malik that such a marriage could be allowed, Ibn Qudāma's rejoinder reads as follows:

> We have God's speech "Your mothers and daughters were forbidden to you." She is his daughter, because she is a woman created of his semen. This is a reality, which is no different whether [the sexual act and consequently the semen] was allowed or forbidden. This is indicated by the Prophet's words towards the woman of Hilāl b. Umāyya: "Look at him," i.e., her son. "If she gives birth to him and he has these characteristics, he belongs to Sharīk b. Sahma," i.e., the fornicator.

> Because she is created out of his semen, she resembles a woman, who was created through intercourse in doubt, and because she is a part of him. Therefore she is not allowed to him, just like his daughter from a marriage. The fact that some rulings [about her status] are different does not negate that she is his daughter. (1999: IX, 529f)

Although Ibn Qudāma arrives at the same ruling as the Hanafis that a man is not allowed to marry his biological daughter born out of wedlock, the reasons he gives for his opinion differ completely. For the Hanafis, until the tenth century the fact that the biological daughter is among other things created from the man's semen was of absolutely no importance in their legal reasoning, whereas for Ibn Qudāma this is the pivotal point. For the Hanbalis she has thus to be subsumed to the Qur'anic passage, "Forbidden to you are your mothers and daughters" (Q 4:23). For them "the verse covers all that this term ["daughters" (*banat*)] encompasses be it literally (*ḥaqīqatan*) or metaphorically (*majazan*)," as Ibn Taymiyya put it (1961–66: XXXII, 135).

As simple as this statement might look, it constitutes a fundamental methodological difference to the Hanafi and especially the Shafi'i reasoning that has been analyzed so far, because they followed the principle that a term cannot signify its literal and metaphorical meanings at the same time (Sarakhsī 1986: pt. XXX, 290f; Harrās 1974–76: II, 216; Heinrichs 1992: 269). To bolster his view, Ibn Taymiyya first posited that the fact that a daughter born out of wedlock has no sustenance and inheritance rights towards her biological father does

not necessarily imply that she is not his daughter. Rather, the terminology in Q 4:23 about marriage prohibitions is much more general
than the terms used, for example, in Q 4:11 spelling out inheritance
rules (see also Sarakhsī 1986: pt. XXX, 290ff; for an opposing Shafi'i
view see Māwardī 1994: IX, 219). Therefore, a woman to whom Q
4:11 does not apply can be subsumed under Q 4:23. In addition, Ibn
Taymiyya interprets the story of Zam'a to indicate that Muhammad
made the slave woman's son Sauda's brother in one particular aspect relating to *nasab*, i.e., the inheritance laws, but not in another as
indicated by the veiling order (Ibn Taymiyya 1961–66: XXXII, 135–
37). Therefore, Ibn Taymiyya argues, being considered as a daughter
does not always have to come with a complete set of rulings such as
inheritance. Although she is not a daughter in the legal sense of the
term, the marriage prohibition has to apply.

This is also born out by an argumentum a fortiori relating to milk-
kinship. The passage "Forbidden to you are … your mothers who
have given suck to you, your suckling sisters" in Q 4:23 set up the
principle that breastfeeding establishes marriage prohibitions. Most
legal scholars agreed that the wet-nurse's husband was forbidden
to marry the breastfeeding daughter arguing that the milk was the
result of a pregnancy, which in turn resulted from the husband's semen (Giladi 1999: 79–81; Jaṣṣāṣ 1928: II, 153; for a dissenting view
see Harrās 1974–76: II, 235f). If such an indirect contact with the
man's semen already established marriage prohibitions, being created from that semen should result in the same ruling even more so,
Ibn Taymiyya argued (1961–66: XXXII, 136, 139).

Therefore the terms "son" (*ibn*) and "daughter" (*bint*) in Q 4:23
would be so general that they encompassed anybody related to a
person, even the "milk daughter" (*bint min al-rida'*). This was also
indicated by the passage "Forbidden to you are … the spouses of
your sons who are of your loins" in Q 4:23, which was commonly
understood to relate to the story of Muhammad's foster-son Zayd,
who divorced his wife Zaynab so that Muhammad could marry her.
In his time, Zayd was commonly addressed as "Zayd son of (*ibn*) Muhammad." Consequently, the marriage prohibitions of Q 4:23 would
have made a marriage between Zaynab and Muhammad impossible;
therefore, argued the exegetes, the verse specified "sons who are of
your loins" (*abnā' min aṣlābikum*) and thus explicitly ruled out the
case of Zayd and Zaynab. Ibn Taymiyya concluded from this that
the terms "son" and "daughter" in Q 4:23 were very general, otherwise the specification for Zayd's case would not have been necessary
(1961–66: XXXII, 136, 139).

Semen in the Legal Definition of "Son" and "Daughter"

I would argue that Ibn Qudāma's and Ibn Taymiyya's views that a fornicator is forbidden to marry his daughter born out of wedlock because "she is created of his semen" reflect a development in Islamic legal discourse that probably occurred during the tenth and eleventh century CE, i.e., fourth and fifth century AH. The structure of the two Hanbalis' arguments indicates that semen is given increased importance in the legal definition of the terms *ibn* (son) and *bint* (daughter). Semen had played no role whatsoever in defining these terms in Shafi'i and Hanafi legal texts of at least the first three centuries of Islamic history. The Hanafis did not even make marital intercourse a condition for ascribing a child to a marriage as long as it was born at least six months after the contract had been concluded. The Shafi'is did make possible intercourse a condition, but stated explicitly that in determining the child's status as son or daughter the *firash* was the decisive criterion, not the semen. Because of the lack of a *firash* in *zina*, the Shafi'is allowed a fornicator to marry his daughter born out of wedlock—though they viewed it as reprehensible (*makruh*). On the other hand, the Hanafis forbade such a marriage, but as previously shown this was not because they saw any specific "semen-based" relation between the two parties. Rather they applied the rule that any of the woman's daughters fell under the marriage prohibitions of Q 4:23.

This situation obviously changed in the fifth Islamic century (eleventh century CE). In one of his writings the Shafi'i scholar Abū l-Hasan al-Māwardī (d.1058) recorded the following on the Hanafi position in this specific question:

> Abū Ḥanīfa said: It is forbidden for the fornicator to marry her [i.e., his daughter born out of wedlock]. His followers disagreed on the reason for this prohibition. The earlier ones (*al-mutaqaddimūn*) said: Because she is the daughter of a woman he had *zinā* with. Consequently the prohibition rulings relating to marriage ties apply to her ... The later ones (*al-muta'akhkhirūn*) said: She is forbidden, because she is his daughter, created out of his semen ... As a proof they referred to God's speech: "Forbidden to you are your mothers and daughters." She is his daughter, because the Arabs (*al-'arab*) term her as "daughter" and the marriage contract does not play any role in this. (Māwardī 1994: IX, 218)

In Islamic legal history the term *mutaqaddimun* signifies the scholars who lived during the first three centuries whereas *muta'akhkhirun* characterizes those who came afterwards (Melchert 2003: 294). This means that the Hanafis kept their position on this question but after the third century changed their reasons for doing so. This would testify to a changed position regarding semen in their thinking about the definition of the terms "son" and "daughter" in that time.

An additional example comes from the Malikis. There were conflicting statements from their eponymous founder Malik b. Anas (d. 795). In the Muwatta, which they considered to be authored by Malik himself, he was recorded to have opined that zina does not cause marriage prohibitions. In the Mudawwana, which the Malikis ascribed to Saḥnūn b. Saʿīd (d. 854) and therefore in their view was the more indirect and later source, he was reported to have ruled to the opposite—though without giving any reasons for this. For example, the eminent Maliki jurist al-Qāḍī Ibn al-ʾArabī (d.1148) solved the tension between the two statements by declaring the first one to be correct, largely replicating the Shafiʿi line of argumentation evolving along the *al-ḥarām lā yuharrim al-ḥalāl* dictum (Ibn al-ʾArabī 1992: II, 703f). About a century later Abū ʿAbdallāh al-Qurṭubī (d.1273) added interesting material to this discussion when he came to the second opinion expressed in the Mudawwana. Al-Qurṭubī states that this view would be based on a story told by the Prophet Muhammad about the pious hermit Jurayj among the Israelites. A prostitute tried to seduce him without success and then had sex with a shepherd who tended a flock of sheep nearby Jurayj's hermitage. She became pregnant and claimed that Jurayj was the father. As a result the Israelites insulted Jurayj and destroyed his housing. When asked for their reasons they accused him of having committed *zina* with the prostitute, who had now given birth to a baby boy. Jurayj approached the boy in his cradle and asked him who his father was. The boy answered: "I am the son [*ibn*] of the shepherd." After this miracle the Israelites apologized to Jurayj (Ibn Kathīr 2003: III, 38). This whole story received authoritativeness within the Islamic framework, because it was the Prophet Muhammad himself who told it. For al-Qurṭubī this story had become a reference Malikis typically referred to when they wanted to opt for Mālik's opinion expressed in the Mudawwana that *zina* creates marriage prohibitions. For them the story of Jurayj served as a precedence that the term "son" (and conversely "daughter") could be applied to describe the position of a child born out of wedlock vis-à-vis its biological father. Al-Qurṭubī proceeds: "And it is also concluded from this that the woman who results from the semen of *zina* is not allowed for the man who committed *zina* with her mother. And this is widely accepted [*mashhur*]" (Qurṭubī 1967: V, 115).

But like the Shafi'is, Qurṭubī is quick to argue that it is allowed for a man to marry his biological daughter born out of wedlock, because the marriage prohibitions follow the *nasab* as a God-given principle organizing society, and there is no *nasab* between the two. The story of Jurayj in which Muhammad had implicitly established a *nasab* from *zina* would constitute an exception (Qurṭubī 1967: V, 114f).

Among the analyzed materials, this passage of al-Qurṭubī is the first to mention a linkage between the legal issue of marriage prohibitions following *zina* and the story of Jurayj. That Ibn al-'Arabī about a century earlier does not mention it does not necessarily mean that this link did not yet exist, but at least it indicates that it had not become a typical point of reference in that debate. I would thus argue that after the ninth century CE the idea that semen might be given more importance in defining fatherhood than before gained ground. Afterwards, possibly during the twelfth and thirteenth centuries, the story of Jurayj was introduced into the debate to provide religiously authoritative linguistic precedence for the term *ibn* being applied to a child born out of wedlock.[4]

Ibn Taymiyya's conceptual framework of the terms *ibn* and *bint* expressed in his discussion about marriage prohibitions also led him to state that a child born out of wedlock could be attached to his or her biological father if there was no *firash*. He argued that the *al-walad li-l-firash* dictum could not be applied to unmarried women, because they were not *firash* (Ibn Taymiyya 1988: 64f). Ibn al-Qayyim provided an additional argument:

> The father is one of the two [i.e., the male and female] fornicators. So if [the child] is attached to his mother, has a *nasab* to her, they both inherit from each other, and also the *nasab* between him and her relatives is established, although she conceived him in *zinā*, and it is found that the child is from the semen of the two fornicators [i.e., the man and the woman] and they both had a share in him, and they agree that he is their child, so what could keep us from attaching him to his father if nobody else claims him? ...

> And Jurayj said to the young man, whose mother had committed *zinā* with the shepherd: Who is your father, young man? He answered: such and such, the shepherd. (Ibn al-Qayyim 1950: pt. IV, 119)

It is important to note the difference between Ibn al-Qayyim's, and, for example, the Hanafi's concept of establishing fatherhood in such a situation. Whereas the Hanafis would introduce the condition that at least one of the sex partners has to claim that he or she

erroneously assumed the existence of a legitimizing legal framework
(Sarakhsī 1986: XVI, 154–61), Ibn al-Qayyim does not make fatherhood depend upon such a statement anymore and speaks explicitly
of *zina*.[5] On the other hand, his wording of this passage is careful
to avoid the expression "establishing the *nasab*" (*thubūt al-nasab*);
rather, he uses the term *luhuq / istilhaq* ("attaching"). This is an important distinction for the inheritance issues involved, which Ibn
al-Qayyim addresses immediately after his quoted statement. He argues that a child, after having been attached to his father this way,
only has rights in inheritance issues following this point in time.
Any inheritance case settled before the *istilhaq*, in which the child
would have had rights to receive a share, shall remain settled (Ibn
al-Qayyim 1950: pt. IV, 119f).

The Contemporary Debate

Why is all this important? Because in countries of Sunni Muslim
majority populations, status law is heavily influenced by the sharia
and the issue of children born out of wedlock acquiring a *nasab* is
usually regulated along the broad lines laid down by the Malikis,
Shafi'is, and Hanafis, not the Hanbalis of the twelfth to fourteenth
centuries. Since, for example, acquiring citizenship is linked to establishing a *nasab* to a man, children born out of wedlock without
such a *nasab* are denied citizenship and as a consequence access to
public schooling. In addition, they and their mothers have no sustenance rights whatsoever.

    Under historical conditions even Ibn al-Qayyim's view quoted
above would not have changed this situation a lot, since it is clear
that the child could not be attached to its father, if he refused. In the
classical Islamic legal sources it was never the question whether a
man could be sued for fulfilling his obligations as a father against his
will, because it was impossible to prove fatherhood beyond doubt.
Historically speaking, the man's testimony and the clear and un-
equivocal evidence could never collide, since physical similarity was
never considered to constitute such evidence as shown above. As
a consequence, applying Ibn al-Qayyim's reasoning to legal practice would still have depended completely on the man's testimony.
This, of course, has changed because of the technical possibilities of
genetic testing. Therefore, referring to Ibn al-Qayyim's fourteenth-
century reasoning under the significantly altered contemporary conditions gives his words an entirely new dimension.

This became clear in 1998, when the Islamic Organization of Medical Sciences (IOMS) in Kuwait devoted its annual meeting to "Genetics, genetic engineering, the human genome, and genetic therapy—an Islamic view." The meeting's fifth session was devoted to "Islamic legal aspects of the genetic fingerprint and in how far it can serve to establish or negate childship (*bunuwa*)." After enumerating the traditional legal principles establishing childship in Sunni Islam—among others *al-walad li-l-firash* and *istilhaq* ('Awaḍī and Gendī 2000: I, 397–401, 412–15, 446–50, 471)—the four papers delivered by Islamic legal scholars during the session devoted most space to the question of negating a *nasab* through *li'an*, the procedure in which a husband publicly declares that a child is not his, which includes divorcing his wife. In the closing statement and recommendations of the conference, a final word about the role of genetic testing in establishing or negating a *nasab* was postponed: "The IOMS agreed that a panel of specialist jurists and scientists be called to discuss the matter and make the appropriate recommendations" (see the IOMS homepage, islamset.com).

During the discussion following the presentation of the four papers, Ra'fat 'Uthmān, the former dean of the Faculty of Shariah and Law and Professor for Comparative Fiqh at Al Azhar University, mentioned Ibn al-Qayyim's position on the *walad al-zina*, which he obviously had just remembered. Several scholars seconded 'Uthmān while others refused this view by arguing that the Prophetic saying "the child belongs to the *firash*" would be a general formulation, i.e., there could be no exceptions from it. 'Uthmān was also criticized by a Moroccan scholar for raising the issue, because it would encourage young people to have illicit relations ('Awaḍī and Gendī 2000: I, 504–6, 508f, 521). Later on Ra'fat 'Uthmān delivered a long statement in which he made three points. First, he argued that one should trust the reliability of modern technologies such as genetic testing and genetics at large. In certain cases modern genetic knowledge might even contribute to doubting some recorded rulings of early Islamic authorities ('Awaḍī and Gendī 2000: I, 527). Second, the possibility of genetic testing does not support the principle of *al-walad li-l-firash*. Third, *al-walad li-l-firash* is not a general principle, because the second caliph 'Umar had attached children from the Jāhiliya period preceding Islam, who according to Islamic standards had been born out of wedlock, to their biological fathers[6] ('Awaḍī and Gendī 2000: I, 526–28).

Afterwards 'Uthmān devoted a whole paper to the issue, which he presented initially at Islamic legal conferences in Europe in 2004, in particular the second conference of the Assembly of Muslim Jurists of America held in Copenhagen. The key authority for his paper was Ibn al-Qayyim with his argumentation quoted above, and 'Uthmān reiterated that the *al-walad li-l-firash* dictum should not be applied to unmarried women. He added the following argument: *al-walad li-l-firash wa li-l-ʿāhir al-ḥajar* was intended to punish the fornicator by not ascribing the child to him. However, if the child was denied a *nasab* to his or her (biological) father, he or she would be punished for somebody else's illicit act ('Uthmān 2008). This means that 'Uthmān very cautiously introduces the notion of children's rights into this Islamic legal debate. So far, his view is undoubtedly a minority view among the contemporary legal scholars. However, his argumentation shows how modern technological possibilities significantly change the implications of Ibn al-Qayyim's ruling, which rested on two major pillars: first, that both sex partners contributed physically through bodily substances to the new child; and second, that the father admitted that it was his child. Because modern possibilities of genetic testing were lacking for most of Islamic history, it was not possible that these pillars could contradict each other, because the first could not be proven. This has changed and therefore the structure of the whole argument becomes modified in 'Uthmān's contemporary reasoning: now, the proofs generated by genetic testing might possibly overrule a man's refusal of a child in order to secure the child's rights. The final recommendations of the Copenhagen conference were largely in accordance with 'Uthmān's ideas and reiterated the perspective of children's rights, though the recommendations stated explicitly that this should only apply to countries where Muslims are a minority.[7]

Children's rights were also the key argument in Tunisia, where two laws (no. 75 from 28/10/1998 and no. 51 from 7/7/2003) introduced genetic testing as a means to prove fatherhood—against the opposition of the "religious camp." The laws could pass parliament only because many MPs abstained from voting.[8] Also, in 2008 Egypt passed legislation enhancing the rights of children born out of wedlock after a public campaign against female genital mutilation, which among other things focused on the notion of children's rights (Bentlage 2009: 37). However, one should be cautious to detect a general trend here: the Mudawwana in Morocco, the much hailed and praised legal reform work in status law from 2004, which did a lot to enhance the legal position of women, has been criticized for not having touched the question of children born out of wedlock (Bargach 2005).

Conclusion

In this chapter I have scrutinized the changing ways in which Sunni legal schools have constructed kinship by analyzing the link between their respective concepts of illicit intercourse, marriage, procreation, and marriage prohibitions. I have argued that even when the representatives of the different schools use the same terminology for making the apparently same legal ruling, they do not necessarily mean the same things. This is caused by the differing assumptions preceding the ruling and/or because the methodology used for arriving at it might differ completely. Whereas the jurists of the first five centuries of Islamic history (until the twelfth century CE) gave overarching importance to the issue of whether the child had—legally speaking—been conceived licitly, Hanbali jurists of the twelfth to the fourteenth centuries gave more weight to the question of the physical contribution to the creation of the new child. Before the invention of modern tools of diagnosis, even in this view it remained clear that a child could not be attached to its father, if he refused. This situation has changed through the technical possibilities of genetic testing. In the contemporary debate the Hanbali view has developed some influence, though it remains far from becoming the dominant position, as demonstrated by the fact that the recent Moroccan reform of status law has avoided addressing the issue of children born out of wedlock.

In conclusion, I would argue that Islamic legal statements or rulings about issues related to kinship have to be contextualized in two ways. First, they must be put into perspective in terms of the way in which broader legal concepts are linked to specific issues. For example, in order to figure out the exact meaning of the term "daughter" (*bint*) for the several Sunni legal schools, it is necessary to understand their differing opinions on the term *nikah*, which indicates the conclusion of a marriage contract for some or (probable) sexual intercourse for others. Second, sharia rulings need to be contextualized historically. For example, changes in technological circumstances impact heavily on the social implications of a certain ruling. Therefore even a contemporary verbatim quote of a ruling formulated in the fourteenth century CE has significantly different implications today than it did six hundred years ago. With these two contextualizations the decisive nuances of legal change become visible and a more differentiated picture can substitute for essentialist, static statements on "the Islamic way" of constructing kinship.

Notes

1. Unfortunately the publication of the edited volume of Pierre Bonte, Enric Porqueres et Jérôme Wilgaux (éds), *L'argument de la filiation aux fondements des sociétés méditerranéennes et européennes*, Paris, MSH 2011 came
   to my knowledge after finishing the final draft of this chapter; thus, the
   substantial contributions of Corrine Fortier and Mohammed Benkheira
   could not be integrated into the writing of this chapter.
2. In the English Qur'an translations this is often translated as "to whom
   you have gone in."
3. For two slightly differing versions of this story see Muzanī 1903–8, VII:
   305f.
4. Mohammed Benkheira, *L'amour de la loi. Essai sur la normativité en Islam*,
   (Paris, 1997), esp. p. 350–54 analyzes the Hanbali and Shafi'i views on
   marriage prohibitions towards the daughter born out of wedlock on the
   basis of thirteenth- and fourteenth-century sources and therefore views
   Islamic law in this particular issue as static. The diachronic approach of
   the present chapter adds the dimension of legal change to the analysis. I
   thank Sandra Huout for referring me to Benkheira's inspiring book.
5. Based on the historical sources used for this chapter, I obviously disagree
   here with the generalizing statement in Frank Griffel's introduction that
   "all four schools accept in such cases that the father or the mother, ideally both, identify the father."
6. The third argument had also been advanced by Ibn Taymiyya 1998: 64f.
7. See the assembly's website at http://www.amjaonline.com/ar_d_details
   .php?id=109.
8. Interview with Bechir Hamza, Comité national d'éthique médicale, Tu-
   nis, April 2004.

References

'Awaḍī, 'Abd ar-Raḥmān al-, and Aḥmad Rajā'ī al-Gendī, eds. 2000. Ru'ya
   islāmiyya bi-ba'ḍ al-mushkilāt al-ṭibbiyya al-mu'āṣira. Thabat kāmil li-
   a'māl nadwat: "al-Wirātha wa l-handasa al-wirāthiyya wa l-jīnūm al-
   basharī wa-l-'ilāj al-jīnī—ru'ya islāmiyya" al-mun'aqada fī-l-Kuwait
   fī-l-fitra min 23–25 Jumāda al-Āhkara 1419 h al-muwāfiq 13–15 Uktu-
   bir 1998 m. 2 vols. Kuwait: Islamic Organization of Medical Sciences.
Bājī, Abū-l-Walīd Sulaimān al-. 1912–13. Kitāb Muntaqā—sharḥ al-Muwaṭṭa'.
   7 vols. Cairo: Maṭba'at Dār al-Sa'āda.
Bargach, Jamila. 2005. "An Ambiguous Discourse of Rights: The 2004 Family Law Reform in Morocco." *Hawwa* 3(2): 245–66.
Benkheira, Mohammed. 1997. L'amour de la loi. Essai sur la normativité en
   Islam. Paris: Presses universitaires de France.
Bentlage, Björn. 2009. "Der Abtreibungsdiskurs in Ägypten." In *Reproduk-*

tionsmedizin bei Muslimen: säkulare und religiöse Ethiken im Widerstreit, ed. Thomas Eich. http://tobias-lib.ub.uni-tuebingen.de/volltexte/2009/3785 /pdf/Tagung_Islamische_Medizinethik_2008.pdf.

Bonte, Pierre, Enric Porqueres, and Jérôme Wilgaux, eds 2011, L'argument de la filiation aux fondements des sociétés méditerranéennes et européennes, Paris: MSH.

Coulson, Noël J. 1964. *A History of Islamic Law*. Edinburgh: Edinburgh University Press.

———. 1971. *Succession in the Muslim Family*. Cambridge: Cambridge University Press.

Giladi, Avner. 1996. *Infants, Parents and Wet Nurses: Medieval Islamic Views on Breastfeeding and their Social Implications*. Leiden: Brill.

Hallaq, Wael B. 1997. *A History of Islamic Legal Theories*. Cambridge: Cambridge University Press.

Harrās, 'Imād al-Dīn b. Muḥammad al-Óabarī Ilkiya al-. 1974–76. *Aḥkām al-Qur'ān*. 4 vols. Cairo: Maṭba'at Íassān.

Heinrichs, Wolfhart. 1992. "Contacts between Scriptural Hermeneutics and Literary Theory in Islam: The Case of Majâz," *Zeitschrift für Geschichte der arabisch-islamischen Wissenschaften* 7: 253–84.

Ibn al-'Arabī, Abū Bakr Muḥammad b. 'Abd Allāh. 1957. *Ahkām al-Qur'an*. 4 vols. Cairo: Maṭba'at 'Īsā al-Bābī al-Íalabī.

———. 1992. *Kitāb al-Qabas fī sharḥ Muwaṭṭa' Mālik b. Anas*. 3 vols. Beirut: Dār al-Gharb al-Islāmī.

Ibn al-Qayyim, Abū 'Abd Allāh Muḥammad. 1950. *Zād al-Ma'ād fī hadī khayr al-'Ibād Muḥammad Khātim al-nabīyīn wa Imām al-mursalīn*. 2 vols. in 4 pts. Cairo: Maṭba'at Muṣṭafā al-Bābī al-Íalabī.

Ibn Kathīr, Ismā'īl b. 'Umar. 2003. *al-Bidāya wa-l-nihāya*. 20 vols. Riyad: n.p.

Ibn Qudāma, 'Abd Allāh b. Aḥmad. 1999. *al-Mughnī*. 15 vols. Riyad: Dār al-'Ālam al-Kutub.

Ibn Taymiyya, Aḥmad b. 'Abd al-Íalīm. 1961–66. *Majmū' fatāwā Shaykh al-Islām Aḥmad b. Taymiyya*. 37 vols. Riyad: Maṭābi' al-Riyāḍ.

———. 1988. *Fatāwā al-zawāj wa 'ishrat al-nisā'*. Cairo: Maktabat al-turāṯ al-islāmī.

Jaṣṣāṣ, Abū Bakr Aḥmad b. 'Alī al-Rāzī al-. 1928. *Aḥkām al-Qur'ān*. 3 vols. Cairo: al-Maṭba'a al-Bāhiya al-Miṣriya.

Johansen, Baber. 1999. *Contingency in a Sacred Law: Legal and Ethical Norms in the Muslim Fiqh*. Leiden: Brill.

Kohlberg, Etan. 1985. "The Position of the Walad Ziná in Imámí Shī'ism." *Bulletin of the School of Oriental and African Studies* 48(2): 237–66.

Māwardī, Abū l-Íasan 'Alī b. Muḥammad al-. 1994. *al-Hāwī al-kabīr fī fiqh madhhab al-Imām al-Shāfi'ī wa huwa sharḥ mukhtaṣar al-Muzanī*. 19 vols. Beirut: Dār al-Kutub al-'Ilmiya.

Melchert, Christopher. 2003. "The Early History of Islamic Law." In *Method and Theory in the Study of Islamic Origins*, ed. Herbert Berg. Leiden: Brill, 294–324.

Momen, Moojan. 1987. *An Introduction to Shi'i Islam: The History and Doctrines of Twelver Shi'ism.* New Haven, CT: Yale University Press.

Muzanī, Ismāʿīl b. Yaḥyā al-. 1903–8. *Ikhtilāf al-ḥadīth lahu bi-Riwāyāt al-Rabīʿ.* 7 vols. Cairo: al-Maṭbaʿa al-kubrā al-amīriya. (printed on the margins of Shāfiʿī 1903–8)

Óaḥāwī, Abū Jaʿfar Aḥmad b. Muḥammad al-. 1967. *Sharḥ maʿānī al-āthār.* 4 vols. Cairo: Maṭbaʿat al-Anwār al-Muḥammadiya.

Ottenheimer, Martin. 1996. *Forbidden Relatives: The American Myth of Cousin Marriage.* Urbana: University of Illinois Press.

Powers, David S. 1990. "The Islamic Inheritance System: A Socio-Historical Approach." In *Islamic Family Law,* ed. Chibli Mallat and Jane Connors. London: Graham & Trotman.

Qurṭubī, Abū ʿAbd Allāh Muḥammad b. Aḥmad al-Anṣārī al-. 1967. *al-Jāmiʿ li-Aḥkām al-Qurʾān.* 20 vols. Cairo: Dār al-Kātib al-ʿArabī.

Rubin, Uri. 1993. "'al-Walad li-l-Firâsh'—On the Islamic Campaign against 'Zina'." *Studia Islamica* 78: 5–26.

Sarakhsī, Bakr Muḥammad b. Aḥmad al-. 1986. *Kitāb al-mabṣūt.* 16 vols. in 32 pts. Beirut: Dār al-Maʿrifa.

Scalenghe, Sara. 2004/5. "The Deaf in Ottoman Syria, 16th–18th Centuries." *Arab Studies Journal* 12(2)/13(1): 10–25.

Schacht, Joseph. 1952. "Adultary [sic] as an Impediment to Marriage in Islamic and in Canon Law." *Revue Internationale des Droits de l'antiquité* 2nd series, I: 105–23

Schulze, Reinhard. 1990. *Islamischer Internationalismus im 20. Jahrhundert: Untersuchungen zur Geschichte der Islamischen Weltliga.* Leiden: Brill.

Shāfiʿī, Muḥammad b. Idrīs al-. 1903–8. *Kitāb al-Umm fī furūʿ al-fiqh.* 7 vols. Cairo: al-Maṭbaʿa al-kubrā al-amīriya.

Skovgaard-Petersen, Jakob. 1997. *Defining Islam for the Egyptian State: Muftis and Fatwas of the Dar al-Ifta.* Leiden: Brill.

ʿUthmān, Raʾfat. 2008. "Vaterschaft aus unehelichem Geschlechtsverkehr." In *Moderne Medizin und Islamische Ethik. Biowissenschaften in der muslimischen Rechtstradition,* ed. and trans. Thomas Eich. Freiburg i. Brsg.: Herder, 71–79.

Chapter 2

ISLAMIC JURISPRUDENCE (*FIQH*) AND ASSISTED REPRODUCTION
ESTABLISHING LIMITS TO AVOID SOCIAL DISORDER

Sandra Houot

Introduction

M edically assisted conception is often a primary focus of bioethical debates, despite the fact that practices remain fairly
limited. The ethics of these invasive, "artificial" manipulations of the
body are often questioned, especially when crossing cultural divid-
ing lines. Beyond the normative dimensions attached to the medical
practice of assisted reproduction itself, the field of Islamic jurisprudence (*fiqh*) confronts the reflexive ethics of assisted reproduction.
Indeed, it can be argued that the effects of medically assisted conception on the human condition engage the most fundamental values,
such as the status of the embryo and the meanings of parenthood
and lineage.

To explore issues of medically assisted procreation in the Islamic
sphere, our focus here is on contemporary Islamic *fiqh*. We shall
measure the contributions of the Qur'an and the Sunna to Islamic
legal theory, and then examine how these elements influence current positions of *fiqh* towards assisted reproduction. In particular,
we will be focusing on one of the main subsidiary legal principles of
fiqh, maslaha (common interest/public interest), which is, "the most
important vehicle to extend and adapt the revealed law to changed

circumstances and to retain its relevance to Islamic society" (Opwis 2007: 66, 79).

From this point of view, the corpus of Islamic law has very practical implications for assisted reproduction. Using the framework of the fatwa as a focal point from which to identify debates within contemporary Islamic society, we will illustrate how the field of assisted reproduction allows for an advanced exploration into the sphere of Islamic jurisprudence. Subsequently, this will allow us to highlight the complexities of what is at stake in this bioethical debate surrounding assisted reproduction in the Islamic context.

The major primary Islamic sources on the ethical dimensions of assisted reproduction are issued today by contemporary authorities of Islamic jurisprudence, such as the Islamic Jurisprudence Council (Majlis al-majma' al-fiqhī) (Islamic World League/Rābi at al-'ālam al-islāmī) created in 1977[1] and the International Academy of Islamic Jurisprudence (Majma' al-fiqh al-islāmī al-duwalī)[2], inaugurated in 1983 (The Organisation of Islamic Conference/ Munazzama al-mu'tamar al-islāmī)[3]. These organizations structure discourses on bioethical questions whose implications regulate and resonate within the Muslim sphere. Another related institutional authority, the European Council for Fatwa and Research (ECFR), which was established in March 1997 in Dublin, has the goal of shaping Islamic jurisprudence to fit into a Western context.[4]

As well as examining institutional authorities, this chapter also addresses the individual delivery of fatwas regarding assisted reproduction by reviewing a popular medical journal, *Ṭabībuka*[5], written by an authority of the Sunni leadership, the Syrian Sa'īd Ramadān al-Būtī, who was born in 1929.[6] These three resources (the Academies of Islamic Jurisprudence, the European Council for Fatwa and Research, and Sa'īd Ramadān al-Būtī's fatwas) take part in the plurality of voices that compose the bioethical debate on assisted reproduction in the world of Islamic jurisprudence. As such, this chapter will focus on different interpretations of *fiqh* that address situations of *darura* (necessity); this semantic framework will then provide a means for exploring assisted reproduction. Further, both "artificial" and traditional forms of parenthood and lineage will be explored.

Treatment of Infertility in *Fiqh*

Confronted with questions stemming from biomedical developments, *fiqh* consequently explores and elucidates bioethical thought that, in turn, impacts biomedical experimentation. Rather than being predefined on established principles of a normative morality, the intellectual activity of the interpretation of Islamic jurisprudence reflects the downstream experience of adaptation. As such, *fiqh* supports some legal tools, and particularly subsidiary legal principles, that take into account contextual morality. In the following, I will examine pragmatic solutions to medically assisted conception that have emerged from *fiqh*.

The Need (Haja) *for a Child*

The members of the Council of the Academy of Islamic Jurisprudence of the World Islamic League, who held a meeting in Mecca in 1985, agreed, "For a married woman who cannot procreate, a need for a child is considered a justified aim" (al-Būtī 1992a). Contrary to desire (*raghba*), the meaning of *haja* (need) was agreed upon as having moral significance and seen as a right of the parents.

The notion of *haja* induces a context of exception, which is, in this particular case, infertility. "The majority of the Muslim jurists agree upon the need for a married man in expectation of child and his wife to be able to procreate, considering the intention and considering the project, her treatment is authorized by means of an approved method: artificial insemination" (al-Hawārī 2006: 171). Thus, according to *fiqh,* infertility primarily concerns the wife. Sperm have traditionally been considered to be fertile; therefore, the wife is often viewed as the person responsible for the couple's infertility. The case of the following testimony from a man, in the grip of infertility and asking for a fatwa, shows a similar position.

> I have been married for ten years, however my wife did not procreate, so we consulted a specialist for advice. Medicines recommended were taken in vain. It makes me nervous, especially when my wife informs me about the coming of her menstruation. Afflicted, she is saddened for me and for her. She is always by my side to console me and relieve me, by asking God to entrust us with a child to whom we can look forward. I do not know honorable *cheikh* how to solve this problem. I feel that the law is robbing us by depriving us of what we wish for most in this existence. I know that as time continues the situation is getting worse and worse. Although no doctor has diagnosed the infertility of my wife, it meant for me that it was a small problem requiring a medication to stimulate ovulation. (al-Būtī 1997).

The medically unexplained infertility amplifies the couple's anxiety, while the body of the woman becomes a laboratory for experimentation. While it is not confirmed in this case that it is actually the woman who is infertile, the technique for ovarian stimulation inaugurates the initial step of assisted reproduction. The lack of a child is thus transformed into a medical hardship for the woman.

Besides the infertile couple's feeling of being stigmatized by social pressure, the absence of a child can also be interpreted as a lack of virility. Sometimes associated with this is the feeling of being cursed. Further, the experience of infertility takes away from the couple the possibility of *nasab*. Offspring, viewed in sharia as the fourth fundamental value to be protected,[7] constitutes a key point of the present ethical debates around assisted reproduction, which is often based on *maslaha*.

Maslaha: *Contextualizing Ethics*

The notion of *maslaha* is deducted from what the law "did not establish by a formal text, the nullity or the liceity" (Laoust 1970: 167). This concept was introduced by the Maliki school and completed by Abū Ishāq al-Shātibī[8] (d.790/1388), a Maliki jurist (Abū Zahra 1952); it signifies, "the consideration of needs and necessities of the moment," and, more widely, consideration of the general interest (Khadduri 1993: 727–28). It is Abū Ḥāmid al-Ghazzālī (d.505/1111) who dedicated the concept of *maslaha* as the "ultimate purpose of Sharia."[9] As such, *maslaha* demonstrates a dynamic framework that allows adaptation of sharia "to real situation [*wāqiʿ*]" (al-Qaradāwī 2007: 89).

Maslaha's use of the criterion of suitability breaks with an interpretation that would see Islamic law as only an idealized, disembodied model. Moreover, *maslaha* assumes a reflexive field via its contextualization, with its different forms and levels illustrating an ethical complexity. So, we now return back to this concept of *maslaha* in order to better understand the ethical issues surrounding medically assisted conception in Islamic jurisprudence. Responding to a request for legal advice from an infertile couple, the Syrian *mufti* al-Būtī proposes an alternative: "You can act only by two recognized and legal manners: the one is that you unite with a second woman by having been assured that you are not the cause of the infertility. The other is to have recourse, and is designated by a test-tube baby; the solution is authorized only in unique cases of necessities."[10]

This legal advice demands that the fertility of the husband be medically diagnosed. Then, if the husband knows that he is fertile, he can engage in a second marriage. The secondary marriage is presented as a framework in which to have legitimate children by affiliating them to a group, in the case that the first wife is infertile. The choice of a test-tube baby or, more generally, assisted reproduction, is the second means of reproducing that al-Būtī indicates is allowed for an infertile couple. This method is, however, limited to the context of necessity.

But how are these necessities defined? According to al-Ghazzalī's categorization, the purpose (*maqsud*) of sharia is to secure the five essential elements/principles of human existence, namely, "religion, life, offspring, intellect, and property"[11] (al-Būtī 1992b: 110). These elements become known in legal writings as *al-darurat, al-daruriyyat al-khamsa* (essential necessities) (al-Būtī 2001). According to *maslaha*, the essential necessities needed to transgress scriptural sources are: Qur'an, Sunna, and *ijma'* (consensus).

Assisted reproduction clearly inaugurates a new means for giving birth to a child that separates the sexual act from reproduction. It is a complex topic that demands further exploration from bioethicists (see Tappan, this volume), in order to ascertain the contexts of necessity under which assisted reproduction is allowed.

Medical "Artificialization" of Fertilization

"Intraconjugal artificial insemination," which demands that the husband "draw the sperm" and "deposit it in the womb" of his wife (al-Hawārī 2006: 172), is not in itself an object of debate for Islamic jurisprudence. Contrary to this is in vitro fertilization (IVF), which requires "the taking of an oocyte," which is inseminated and cultivated "in a test tube by a certified technique" (al-Hawārī 2006: 172). As an embryo, it will finally be inserted, via the vagina, into the womb for a possible impregnation.

In vitro cultures of oocytes and sperm cells separate the traditionally intransgressible link between a sexual act and childbirth. For this reason, the Catholic Church has outlawed IVF (Leroy 1995). The church attempts to justify its interdiction by stating that it prefers the method of adoption. Muslim leadership, in contrast, allows IVF "in the situations of exceptional [*istithna'iyya*] necessity" (al-Būtī 1984: 133).

Darurat (necessities), which establish the first level of the hierarchy of values, instigates a standpoint of moral consequentialism. In questions about reproduction by the method of test-tube babies, Sa'īd Ramadān al-Būtī answers: "A method which consists in procreating by the process of the test-tube child is authorized in situations of necessity, within particular links between the couple. We shall not discuss this subject any further."[12]

The character of this consultative opinion underlies ethical issues that stress fundamental values: the origin of life, relationships and heredity. The Syrian *mufti* al-Būtī legally justifies his posture by utilizing the concepts of permissibility (*ibaha*) and sacredness (*hurma*) (1984: 132). It is around these two principles of Islamic jurisprudence that IVF oscillates, "An opened gate to the pretext to justify numerous interdicts, among which, the most dangerous: beginning with the confusion of descent [*ikhtilat al-ansab*]."[13] Al-Būtī's mention of the concept of *nasab*, the third measure to be protected according to the purpose of the law, situates the debate over assisted reproduction at the level of lineage. It illustrates that the interests in tension are "the right of the fetus [*haqq al-janin*]" and "the right of the parents [*haqq al-abawayn*]" (al-Būtī 1988: 38).

The Right of the Fetus

Bioethical reasoning produced by Islamic jurisprudence regarding medically assisted conception is based on the concept of the common interest, which is associated with "the obligation of the restriction of regulating determinants of the overriding necessities" (al-Būtī 1988: 38). Dealing with the notion of *huquq* (rights), it has drawn a complex of derived sacred principles, oscillating between "the sacred right to life, and human dignity, the highest right" (al-Būtī 1988: 38), with right to life being defined as an extension of God's right. In ethical terms, conflicts of interest arise from a tension that Islamic jurisprudence translates in terms of "the right of the parent" and "the right of the fetus" (al-Būtī 1992a).

Some argue that the right of the fetus prevails over the right of the parent. This integralist position is advocated by a minority of rigorist *'ulama* who are proponents of the absolute welfare of life. This stance "forbids any means to block the reproduction or to postpone the period of the pregnancy. ... This act belongs to the meaning of the infanticide [lit. "of being buried alive," (*wa'dā*)]" (al-Būtī 1988: 38).[14]

The example of being "buried alive" extends from pre-Islamic custom in *al-Jahiliyya* (the period of ignorance). This ancient custom was used as an argument by the Andalusian theologian, Ibn Ḥazm (d. 456/1064) to forbid this practice of infanticide. The suggestive power of this analogy, in particular, was adopted by a rigorist minority of the religious authorities to support its point of view against contraception.

In contrast, the mainstream thinking of the Sunni orthodoxy authorizes contraceptive pills and intrauterine devices or coils.[15] Both contraceptive methods, which separate sexuality from reproduction, necessitate an interpretation of the relative status of the embryo. It is advisable to look to *maslaha* in order to understand here how the rights of the embryo and the parents are in tension. These rights are argued to be absolute or relative under the circumstances, by virtue of the legal precept: "the necessities are measured according to their own scale [*al-darurat tuqaddaru bi qadriha*]."[16]

In Islamic *fiqh*, the inviolable right to life is stressed in order to protect the future interest of the child and usually prevails over the interests of the parent. Concerning assisted reproduction, the superior interest is that of the fetus, which also holds true in the debate on abortion (which is defined as a "detestable act with licit character)"[17] (Majma' al-Fiqh al-islāmī al-duwalī 1988).

However, this position does take into account the possible physical and psychological distress of the mother, and in situations where her life is threatened, others place her health over that of the fetus. This was justified by al-Būtī, in the name of Islamic law: "To save the mother, we grant to her life to sacrifice the embryo that we do not know and to whom we are not attached. Nevertheless this motive does not possess the slightest value in the balance of the absolute justice" (1988: 104). This solution, which detaches us from the fetus, distinguishes the biological human life from the status of a human person, and subsequently brings up many ethical questions.

With the spirit of free individual examination, ethics reports upon the complexity of human relations and its experiences. Its tentative efforts examine human vulnerability and finitude, while insisting upon, in relation to *maslaha*, the necessity of regulation. Islamic jurisprudence's description of embryogenesis is drawn on a continuum, conferring with the scriptural source on which it bases itself regarding the discussion about the legal status of the embryo. "Verily your creation is on this wise. The constituents of one of you are collected for forty days in his mother's womb in the form of blood (*nutfa*), after which it becomes a clot of blood (*'alaqa*) in another period of forty days. Then it becomes a lump of flesh (*mudgha*) and forty days later Allāh sends His angel to it with instructions concerning four things, so the angel writes down his livelihood"[18] (Aldeeb 1994: 42–52; Matraji 1993).

An evolutionary approach to the embryonic life distinguishes between the conditions of biological possibility and spiritual animation. If *nutfa* becomes connected with the concept of fertilization, *'alaqa* concerns the stage of nidation (when an embryo is implanted into the endometrium of the uterus), during the second week. As for *mudgha,* it defines the embryo from the end of the fourth week. At the end of the vital process spirit *(ruh)* has animated the human being, so enclosing the evolutionary completion of the embryo. As mentioned by Dalil Boubakeur, "This perfection implies a fulfillment of its potentialities: physical, physiological, spiritual, intellectual. ... The quranic assertion of a perfect creation can mean for the observer that it is unsurpassed and unsurpassable in all that is created"[19] (1996: 299).

Contrary to the vitalist position, this *continuum* does not regard the embryo as requiring absolute protection from the inextricable link connecting human nature with genetic inheritance. Tensions between the interests of the couple and that of the embryo operate in a relational context, following the case of abortion. This extends to the definition of embryogenesis, which presents the embryo as an item of ethical complexity and defines the embryo as the key factor in ethical discussions of assisted reproduction.

Anticipating Damage to Embryo and Child

Elements of ethical indecision are present in the many breaks in the continuum of embryogenesis. This can be seen in the fusion of reproductive cells in the "artificial" conditions of a test tube, as they are inserted at the stage of the embryo into the womb of the mother. Questions regarding conception outside the female body and the possible impacts of "the experimentation" prompted al-Būtī to state that the problem at stake lies in the "repercussions of this practice on the fetus after its birth, as in the importance of the damage attached to its cause [*sabab*]" (al-Būtī 1988: 133).

We cannot assert, before the transfer of the embryo, the safety of the environment of the test tube's synthetic culture. In such a case, there are fears both for the child later learning that he was conceived outside of his mother's body, as well as the potential for the child to have physical abnormalities. Nevertheless, there is no process in place that allows an individual originating from IVF to claim reparations for such damages, as al-Būtī notes when he states, "Even if the meeting (parental gametes) takes place in a plastic box (al-Būtī 1988: 133) ... the test tube baby, from a legal point of view, is incontestable."[20]

Being prenatal, the embryo nevertheless has a specific human reality that the mention of the notion "cause," understood by al-Būtī as a metaphysical principle, focuses upon. In other words, the "fetal condition" (Boltanski 2004) results from a continuous "creation," which is separate from the rules of the medical experience. This limitation of biomedical autonomy refers to a moral position that is articulated around the theological model of the divine creation. The chain of causes and effects is intrinsically connected to the distinctive status of the first cause, which indicates the presence of the divine figure. It is here expressed in the Qur'anic occurrence: "He possesses the keys of the mystery that only He knows perfectly."[21]

As one of the clinical procedures taking place during pregnancy, prenatal diagnosis and its technical capacity to choose the sex of the child was the object of a decision in November 2007. Given by the Council of the Academy of Islamic Jurisprudence of the World Islamic League, it relies on verse 57–59, of the Sura XVI, *Bee*.[22] In response to the pre-Islamic custom of infanticide, the council's decision supports a law opposing sex discrimination (or sex-selective abortion).

The premature determination of the sex, which can occur as early as twelve weeks, is considered morally unacceptable. Moreover, this method underlines the paradox of what it means to be a parent: it provides the possibility of giving birth to a child, but involves the potential to interfere with the evolution of the child. This is forbidden with the exception of hereditary illnesses that only prenatal screening can reveal.

This posture raises the question of hubris with the religious authorities. To face it, deontological ethics is needed to take part in the moral regulation of reproduction. Medical ethics, in the case in question, allows a deontologization of the revealed law by moving the debate away from a transcendental level and towards ethical issues. In addition, with its diagnostic and clinical skills, the medical corps is transformed and presented as an agent possessing moral expertise. Thus, requests to establish ethical committees within hospitals translate as cases of preventive intervention.

Predictive and preventive, the ethical issues attached to prenatal diagnosis[23] join those of the debate on therapeutic abortion—both of these oscillate between a relative and an absolute value regarding the status of the embryo. "The only recognized categorical imperative" writes the vice-chancellor of the Mosque of Paris and doctor Dalil Boubakeur, "is bound to the survival of the mother or to feto-embryonic certain lethality."[24] The example of prenatal diagnosis systematically directed to detect somatic abnormalities, such as trisomy 21 (the primary cause of Down Syndrome), is thus understood as a drift of active eugenics, which violates God's project.

The Controversy of Extra Embryos

The embryo's existence questions the role of human responsibility in the genesis of life. This topic is dealt with in a fatwa delivered by the European Council for Fatwa and Research. The mother of a child conceived by IVF immigrated to Great Britain and asked for a ruling about the future of nine overproduced embryos, which, after a cycle of IVF, underwent a cryogenic preservation by liquid nitrogen. The council's response was:

> Can she implant some of the embryos to her uterus and leave the others frozen, with the health authorities in Britain, bearing in mind that the family will almost certainly not return to Britain? Or should she dispose of them?

> The lady may implant any of these embryos in her uterus as long as she is still the wife of the man from whom the sperm was taken. But if she is separated from him through death, divorce or the like and thus is no longer under the bond of marriage with him, it will be unlawful to implant any of them and she should destroy them or what remains of them.

> In case the wife leaves Britain, and she thinks she will come to this country again to implant one of the embryos, she is permitted to keep the embryos frozen until then for that purpose. But if she thinks that she will not (or most probably will not) return, it will be unlawful to leave them behind, and she or her husband should destroy them.

> In all cases, we find nothing against destroying them, whether the lady will or will not return. However, with the probability of not returning, it is not permissible to leave them, but they must be got rid of. (Majlis al-urūbbī li-l-iftā'wa-l-buḥūth 2002: 119–20)

Produced "artificially" during IVF, the extra embryos are preserved in liquid nitrogen. In the above legal advice, the embryo is at the disposal of the parents. This interpretation, moreover, goes against the recommendations emitted by the International Academy of Jurisprudence, which intends to uphold the right of the fetus.

The creation of embryos is kept to a minimum to avoid creating extra embryos and thus running the risk of their exploitation by third parties. We can hypothesize, then, that the time frame for freezing embryos, which varies from five to ten years, further distances the embryo from the processes of fertilization and gestation. Instead, they are turned into a material, a disposable thing. If we agree that the purpose of IVF is to create life, in spite of infertility, this situation seems, at best, paradoxical.

The abandonment of embryos, moreover, brings to light the position of Islamic jurisprudence experts who believe that the anticipation of a potential social disorder (*fitna*) prevails over the emotional attachment of the couple to their desire to be parents. They argue that extra embryos should be destroyed, lest they later create social upheaval. There is no mention, among these legal experts, of the use of the extra embryos for research and freezing, which would avoid the dangers of repeated ovarian stimulations. This practice of freezing embryos is seen as analogous to adoption, which is legally forbidden.

This procedure of freezing embryos, declares al-Būtī, stems only from "the personal right [*haqq shakhsī*]," by contrast with "the right of society [*haqq al-mujtama'*]" (1992a). Perpetuating the freezing of embryos with no time constraints, and then later transplanting them, could also be problematic in that it may skip over generations. Even worse, the transplantation of an embryo under a renewed shape created by biotechnology puts the traditional rules in danger that help organize "the family ties [*silat al-rahim*]"[25] (al-Hawārī 2006: 172) and, more broadly, lineage. Thus, the freezing procedure is perceived as an "immoral action."[26]

The position that IVF is incompatible with the family model becomes centered around "a confusion of the lineages,"[27] and it depends upon "a disjunction between the links of blood and lineage which are to be considered in their inseparable and their incorporated characters, such the arena of the family system, concerning the effects [which will have repercussions] on the personality of the child if he comes aware of the truth."[28] The trajectory of the fetus, it is argued, would not be more than a prolonged life defined by the trauma of being born out of wedlock.

Further, the introduction of a third party shows itself incompatible with the Islamic legal family model, as far as the "the heterologous artificial insemination [*al-talqīh al-sinā'ī al-musammā*]" or "the surrogate mother [*al-umm al-hādina*]"[29] goes. It highlights procedures of reproduction that have been traditionally associated with adultery. The jurists also confirm the existence of potential problems that may be assumed by nongenetic parents. Besides the fact that third-party donation or surrogacy separates reproduction from the period of gestation, it also creates disjunction between reproduction and parenthood. It questions the legal foundation of the maternal institution, which the jurists view as anchored in the reality of the process of giving birth and not in that of the genes. In this case, it is argued that the surrogate mother, and not the genetic mother, would function as the social mother.

Paternal and Adoptive Lineage

Contrary to maternity, which is proven by gestation, the subject of proving paternity is more complex. Scriptural sources like prophetic hadīths show particular arrangements that form the paternal lineage.[30] The gray zone between biological and social paternity, which is elucidated by *fiqh*, becomes a place of tension. In particular, an interpretation by Shafīʿī scholar Fakr al-Dīn al-Razī (1149/543–1209/606), states that "lineage is attested by the Law," (Benkheira 1997: 352)[31] unlike paternity, which is traditionally interpreted by Islamic jurists as "a fiction, a metaphor" (Benkheira 1997: 352). The uncertainty of the function of the father may be traditionally likened to the material impossibility of proof of paternity. In return, "Whoever claims to be the son of a person other than his father, and he knows that person is not his father, then Paradise will be forbidden for him."[32] Besides sealing the justifiable union, *nikah* prevents a child from being born out of wedlock and dedicates "the first legitimacy of the children to create ipso facto to their membership in a group" (Héritier 1994: 257).

This is further expanded upon in the Qur'anic occurrences, 4 and 5 of the Sura XXXIII, The Coalition,[33] which gave evidence of the abolition of adoption during the fifth year of the Hijra (Powers 2009). Adoption (*tabanni*)[34] is regarded in the Islamic sphere as a subversive institution that threatens the family order, from the point of view of succession and links of alliance. In a continuation on the interdiction on adoption, IVF with a donor, following the example of the surrogate mother, questions the impossible erasure of the biological parents and the origin of the child. Techniques of reproduction that necessitate a third person confirm the separation between the biological and the parental links, and each one introduces potential causes of social disorder.

Conclusion

The potentially damaging effects of assisted reproductive technologies (ARTs) to the family order and to lineage help to shed light on the complexity of positions towards ARTs in the Islamic sphere. The discursive sources borrowed from the universe of *fiqh* testify to its capacity to neutralize by "arrangements" the interests in tension, or to block innovations when a potential social disorder appears.

Auxiliary tools of Islamic legal theory and their contribution to finding solutions to the conflicts of interests demonstrate how, in the face of sometimes dire human consequences ensuing from assisted reproduction, ethics is discussed, debated, and articulated. Situated in a context of articulation of the norm and lived experiences, the expertise of the contemporary Islamic jurists stresses the complexities that are inherently bound to childbirth. Abortion, in this respect, can be viewed as a subject that allows us to think more deeply about the social dimensions of the body and its reproductive capacities. The procedure of freezing embryos and its symbolic impacts testifies to the visibility of differentiated positions between the interests of the child and the parent.

In this respect, the new medical procedures of reproduction shift meanings previously considered intransgressible. By way of dealing with reproduction, the forms of parenthood and lineage affect the practices of social systems. The construction of reasoning that comprises Islamic jurisprudence assures the regulation of divergent interests. Its capacity to form mental representations and to make understandable the human world is made difficult both by IVF as well as by gestational surrogacy. Further, the question of paternal lineage, traditionally assumed by *fiqh*, is questioned by the concept of adoption. Perceived as a subversion of the conditions of lineage, such a practice is objected to on the pretext of the "biological truth of the lineage" (Tort 1992: 282–86).

The sphere of Islamic jurisprudence highlights a reflexive field around assisted reproduction. As shown in this chapter, it attempts to avoid the potential pitfalls and social disorders that might arise from the use of ARTs. Via contextualized ethics, the dynamics of its legal tools take place within larger bioethical debates surrounding the beginning of life, the status of the embryo and fetus, the rights of children and their parents, the legality of sex selection and abortion, and the permissibility of third-party assisted reproduction and surrogacy. These are key ethical complexities in the twenty-first century, of which the Islamic authorities are deeply aware.

Notes

1. http://www.themwl.org/Home.aspx?l=ar. This organization belongs to the World Islamic League (Rābi at al-'ālam al-islāmī) which was created in 1962 at Mekkah.
2. http://www.fiqhacademy.org.sa/.
3. This was founded at Jeddah in 1969, but its name was changed on June 28, 2011 to the Organization of Islamic Cooperation (Munazzama al-Ta'āwūn al-islāmī).

4. http://www.e-cfr.org.
5. *Ṭabībuka. Majalla sihhiyya 'ilmiyya ijtimā'iyya* [Your doctor, the scientific and social journal of health], Beirut. Created in 1956 by the Syrian doctor Sabrī al-Kabbanī, this monthly review of popular medicine reports scientific and medical advances for the common people.
6. On this matter I refer back to my doctoral thesis, "*Sens et médiation. Contribution du magistère du cheikh syrien, Sa'īd Ramadān al Būtī à une compréhension de l'islam contemporain.*" It will be published in 2013 with French editions Geuthner.
7. In addition, and according to this hierarchical order: religion (*dīn*), life (*nafs*), intellect (*'aql*) and offspring (*māl*).
8. The concept of *maslaha* was initially forged by Mālik b. Anas (d.179/795), the founder of the Maliki *madhhab*. According to al-Shātibī, al-Juwaynī (d.478/1085) he would have been the first one to draw the attention to this concept.
9. Concerning this concept, we refer to the synthetic article committed by Felicitas Opwis, 2007, "The Concept of *Maslahah*," 62–82.
10. Al-Būtī, *Tabībuka*, Febuary 1998.
11. Ibid., 287. For the contemporary period, this classification (*dīn, nafs, nasl/nasab, 'aql,* and *māl*) is resumed by Sa'īd Ramadān al-Būtī.
12. Al-Būtī, *Tabībuka*, April 1998.
13. Ibid.,132.
14. According to the prophetic hadīth narrated by Ghudāma bint Wahb, sister of 'Ukkāsha. Ahmad Ibn Hanbal, *Musnad*, ch. XIV "Musnad al-qabā'il (*la tradition des tribus*)," hadīth h26176, http://www.al-eman.com/hadeeth: "O Messenger of Allah (SAW) I have a slave girl and I practice '*azl* with her. I do not want her to get pregnant but I desire what men desire. The Jews say that '*azl* is the minor live burial of children (*dhalika al-wā'd al-khafī'*). He said: "The Jews have lied. If Allah wanted to create a child you could not stop Him." This hadith refers to verse 8 of sura LXXXI, The Overthrowing, "when the female infant buried alive is asked."
15. Al-Būti, *Tabībuka*, February 1994.
16. Ibid., April 1990.
17. It means that the abortive act, following the example of contraceptive use, must be held remote from what is considered as forbidden. As, for example, the temporal limit, abortion is accepted in the first six weeks of amenorrhea.
18. Hadīth narrated by 'Abd Allāh b. Mas'ūd. *Sahīh Muslim, Kitāb al-qadr* [The book of destiny], ch. 1, "Kayfa-l-khalq al-adamī fī batn ummihi wa kitabuhu rizqihi wa ajlihi wa 'amalihi wa shaqāwatihi wa sa'ādatihi" [The growth of a child in the womb of a mother and his destiny in regard to his livelihood, his deeds, both good and evil], n°4781. http://hadith.al-islam.com. English translation by Abdul Hamid Siddiqi, Book 033, n°6390. Centre for Religion and Civic Culture, Centre for Muslim-Jewish Engagement, http://www.usc.edu. The occurrences of the

quranic passages that approach the question of creation are present in suras XXII, The Pilgrimage, 5; XXV, The Criterion, 5; XXIII, The Believers, 12–14; XXXII, The Prostration, 7–9; XXXV, The Originator, 11; XL, The Forgiver, 67; LXXV, The Resurrection, 36–39.

19. Sura XCV, The Fir, 4.
20. Al-Būtī, *Tabībuka*, December 1996.
21. Sura VI, The Cattle, 59.
22. "And they assign daughters for Allah—Glory be to Him!—and for themselves what they desire. When news is brought to one of them, of [the birth of] a female [child], his face darkens, and he is filled with inward grief! With shame does he hide himself from his people, because of the bad news he has had! Shall he retain it on [sufferance and] contempt, or bury it in the dust? Ah! what an evil [choice] they decide on?"
23. Experimental frame that composes the commonplace sonography or the amniocentesis with sometimes a sampling of blood or fetal cells.
24. Dalil Boubakeur, "Diagnostic prénatal," http://www.mosquee-de-paris .net.
25. This is mentioned in the European context of the diasporic right, which brings up the idea that sexual relations should remain confined in the religious sacrament, which is the only source of filiation.
26. Al-Būtī, *Tabībuka*, September 1996.
27. Ibid.
28. Ibid.
29. This is for "gestational surrogacy" or "altruistic surrogacy."
30. "A bedouin came to Allah's Apostle and said, "My wife has delivered a black boy, and I suspect that he is not my child." Allah's Apostle said to him, "Have you got camels?" The bedouin said, "Yes." The Prophet said, "What color are they?" The bedouin said, "They are red." The Prophet said, "Are any of them Grey?" He said, "There are Grey ones among them." The Prophet said, "Whence do you think this color came to them?" The bedouin said, "O Allah's Apostle! It resulted from hereditary disposition." The Prophet said, "And this [i.e., your child] has inherited his color from his ancestors." The Prophet did not allow him to deny his paternity of the child." Hadīth narrated by Abū Hurayra, Sahīh Bukhārī, Kitāb al-i'tisām bi-l-kitāb wa-l-Sunna [Holding fast to the Qur'ān and Sunnah], "Man shabbah aslān ma'lūmān bi aslin mubīnin qad bayyana Allāh hukmahumā" [Of the one who assimilates a determined thing to another evident thing on the principle of which God gave his opinion], n°6770, http://hadith.al-islam.com. English translation by M. Muhsin Khan, vol. 9, book 92, 417, Center for Muslim-Jewish Engagement, University of Southern California, http://www.usc.edu.
31. *Al-tafsīr al-kābir*, Beirut, n.d, vol. 16, 10, 28.
32. Hadīth narrated by Sa'd ibn Abī Waqqas, Bukhārī, *Sahīh*, Kitāb al-farā'id [Law and inheritance], "*Man ad'ākhān wa ibn akh*" (Whoever claims to be the son of a person other than his father), n°6268, http://hadith

.al-islam.com. English translation by M. Muhsin Khan, vol. 8, book 80, n°758. Centre for Religion and Civic Culture, Centre for Muslim-Jewish Engagement, http://www.usc.edu.

33. "Allah hath not assigned unto any man two hearts within his body, nor hath He made your wives whom ye declare (to be your mothers) your mothers, nor hath He made those whom ye claim (to be your sons) your sons. This is but a saying of your mouths. But Allah saith the truth and He showeth the way. Proclaim their real parentage. That will be more equitable in the sight of Allah. And if ye know not their fathers, then (they are) your brethren in the faith." It is advisable to return on the context of the Revelation that shows, in 605, the adoption by the Prophet of a Syrian, Zayd b. Hāritha al-Kalbī. He was the first male adult to become Muslim. He was also the husband of a young lady, Zaynab, whom the Prophet Muhammad, after the separation of his adopted son and his daughter-in-law, would marry after a moral crisis. The present verse introduces the abolition of the filiation by adoption, and the union of the Prophet with his ex-daughter-in-law is allowed. "So when Zayd had performed that necessary formality [of divorce] from her, We gave her unto thee in marriage, so that there may be no sin for believers in respect of wives of their adopted sons, when the latter have performed the necessary formality [of release] from them. The commandment of Allah must be fulfilled." Sura XXXIII, The Coalition, verse 37.

34. The status of the abandoned child who is assumed by the Islamic *fiqh*, through the lexical item "*kafāla*," confirms a legal category to mean "the care." It is, also, similar to the Western right to delegate authority.

References

Abū Zahra, Muhammad. 1952. *Mālik*. Cairo: Maktabat al-Anjlū al-misriyya.

Aldeeb, S. A. S. 1994. "Les Musulmans face aux droits de l'homme, Religion." *Droit et Politique* (étude et documents). Bochum: Winkler.

Benkheira, Mohammed H. 1997. *L'Amour de la loi, essai sur la normativité en islâm*. Paris: Presses Universitaires de France.

Boltanski, Luc. 2004. *La Condition foetale. Une sociologie de l'avortement et de l'engendrement*. Paris: Gallimard.

Boubakeur, Dalil. 1996. "L'Embryon dans l'Islam." In *L'Embryon humain: approche multidisciplinaire*, ed. Brigitte Feuillet-Le Mintier. Paris: Économica, 297–301.

Būtī, Sa'īd Ramadān al-. 1984. *Al-Islām, maldh kull al-mujtama' Majma'āt al-insāniyya limādhā...? Wa kayfa ?* [Islam: Shelter for all the human societies. Why...? How...?], Damascus: Dār al-Fikr.

―――. 1988. *Mas'alat tahdīd al-nasl, wiqāya wa 'ilāj* [The question of the birth limitation, prevention and treatment]. Damascus: Maktabat al-Fārābī.

————. 1990–2000. *Ṭabībuka. Majalla sihhiyya 'ilmiyya ijtimā'iyya* [*Your doctor, the scientific and social journal of health*]. Beirut.

————.1992a. Conference, *Atfāl al-anābīb* [Test-tube babies], Damascus: Dār al-Hāfiz [audio-recording].

————. 1992b. *Dawābit al-maslaha fī-l-Shariah al-islāmiyya* [The regulating determinants of *maslaha* in the Islamic *sharī'a*]. Damascus: Dār al-muttahida.

————. 1997. *Tabībuka. Majalla sihhiyya 'ilmiyya ijtimā'iyya* [Your doctor, the scientific and social journal of health]. Beirut.

————. 2001. *Alā Tarīq al-'Awda ilā-l-Islām* [Return towards the Islam way]. Damascus: Dār al-Fikr.

Hawārī (al-), Muhammad. 2006. "Asas binā' al-usrī fī-l-Islām" [The Foundations of the family building in Islām]. In *Al-Majalla al-'ilmiyya li-l-majlis al-urūbbī li-l-iftā'wa-l-buhūth* [The scientific review of the European Council for Fatwā and Research (ECFR)], http://www.e-cfr.org, vol. 7, 119–72.

Héritier, Francoise. 1994. *Les deux soeurs et leur mère, anthropologie de l'inceste.* Paris: Odile Jacob.

Khadduri, Madjid. 1993. "Maṣlaḥa." In *Encyclopédie de l'Islam,* Leyde: E. J. Brill, Paris: G. P. Maisonneuve, vol. 6, 727–29.

Laoust, Henri. 1970. *La Politique de Ghazalî.* Paris: Geuthner.

Leroy, Fernand. 1995. "Fivette." In *Les mots de la bioéthique,* ed. Gilbert Hottois and Marie-Hélène Parizeau. Bruxelles: De Boeck, 240–44.

Majma' al-Fiqh al-islāmī al-duwalī (The International Academy of Jurisprudence). 1988. *"Tahdīd al-nasl wa tanzīmihi* [The birth limitation and its control],"Munazzama al-Ta'āwūn al-islāmī (The Organisation of islamic Cooperation), fifth session, Jedda, 6–11 February, vol. 1, 168–94.

Majlis al-urūbbī li-l-iftā' wa-l-buhūth (European Council for Fatwa and Research), 2002. *Qarārāt wa Fatāwā* [Resolutions and consultative advices, Dublin]. Cairo: Dār al-tawzī' wa-l-nashr al-islāmiyya, 2 vols.

Matraji, Muhammed. 1993. *Sahīh Muslim* (corrected and revised by Amira Zrein Matraji). Beirut: Dār al-Fikr. 8 vols.

Opwis, Felicitas. 2007. "The Concept of *Maslaha.*" In *Shari'a Islamic Law in the Contemporary Context,* ed. Abbas Amanat and Frank Griffel. Stanford, CA: Stanford University Press, 62–82.

Powers, David S. 2009. *Muḥammad Is Not the Father of Any of Your Men: The Making of the Last Prophet.* New York: University of Pennsylvania Press.

Qaradāwī (al-), Yūsuf. 2007. "Al-'alāqa bayn al-dīn wa-l-siyāsa 'ind al-islāmiyyīn wa-l-'ilmāniyyīn" [The relation between the religion and the politics according to the Muslims and the secularists). In *Al-majalla al-'ilmiyya li-l-majlis al-urūbbī li-l-iftā'wa-l-buhūth* [The scientific review of the European Council for Fatwa and Research (ECFR)], http://www.e-cfr.org, vol. 6, 227–55.

Rābitat al-'ālam al-islāmī (The World Islamic League). 2007. *Akhbār al-'ālam al-islāmī* [Information of the Islamic world], 12 November, Mecca.

Tort, Patrick.1992. *Le désir froid, procréation artificielle et crise des repères symboliques.* Paris: La Découverte.

Chapter 3

CONTROVERSIES IN
ISLAMIC EVALUATION OF
ASSISTED REPRODUCTIVE TECHNOLOGIES

Farouk Mahmoud

Introduction

Of the 50–80 million infertile people worldwide, more than half are Muslims (Serour 1993), and there is a high incidence of tubal and male infertility reported in the Middle East (Serour et al. 1991; Inhorn 2003). The reason for this is not entirely clear. Muslim societies are strongly family oriented and pronatal in line with the Qur'anic verses[1] and the Prophet Muhammad's high regard for pro-creation.[2] The social status, dignity, and self-esteem of the Muslim woman is closely related to her procreative potential (Serour 1995), reflecting the marital, social, and cultural implications of infertility. Prophet Muhammad advocated seeking treatment for ailments, and since the appropriate treatment for tubal and severe male infertility is IVF, the concept of assisted reproductive technologies (ARTs) has been welcomed among most Muslim cultures as a pragmatic pathway to alleviate their infertility. For Muslims, ARTs must be sharia[3] compliant; however, divergences between and among Sunni and Shia Muslims have led to controversies in sharia evaluation. My study explores the bases of divergences among Muslim communities and the consequent controversies that have posed a sharia dilemma in ART practice.

Research Methodology

This chapter is based on a critical review of current English literature on Islamic perspectives of ARTs along with a research component that consisted of a mainly qualitative, semistructured survey of Islamic scholars, ART physicians, and infertile couples. The main locations for the multisite study were Cairo, Egypt, and Yazd, Iran, both conservative heartlands of Sunnis and Shia respectively, in addition to the Vindana IVF Centre, Colombo, Sri Lanka, and the University Hospital, Coventry, United Kingdom. The project included a six-week fellowship at the ART Center at Al Azhar University, Cairo, and two weeks each in Yazd and the International Islamic University, Kuala Lumpur, Malaysia. ART specialists (n = 34) from thirteen Muslim countries were surveyed, some by personal interview (n = 6) and the rest by an e-mailed questionnaire (n = 28). The sample of Islamic scholars and infertile couples is tabulated below in Table 3.1.

TABLE 3.1. Centers and numbers of scholars and infertile couples

Location	Sunni scholars	Shia scholars	Infertile couples
Al Azhar ART	6		75
Malaysia	3		
Sri Lanka	1		10
United Kingdom	4	2	5
Iran		4	86
Total	14	6	176

The study also included personal interviews with eminent scholars from other religious denominations, anthropologists, scientists, embryologists, stem cell technologists, ART physicians, and counselors.

For Muslims, ARTs must conform to sharia. Therefore, the evaluation of sharia, both in terms of how it is expressed in Islamic debates on ARTs as well as how it shapes clinical debates, constitutes a vital component for addressing the role of ARTs for Muslims. This chapter comprises two sections; in the first section I explore Islamic debates surrounding ARTs, while the second is a discussion of the clinical impacts of the Islamic debates on ARTs. In both sections I have intercalated my personal observations alongside unresolved controversies and also my comments as an IVF physician.

Islamic Debates Surrounding ARTs

Sharia and Fiqh

The evaluation of sharia compliance is a complex field that involves weaving through the maze of hermeneutics of Islamic scripture, consisting of the Qur'an and hadith, which constitute the primary sources of sharia and the cornerstone of Islamic law.

While divine proscriptions from the Qur'an or hadith are generally considered inviolable, most Islamic jurists make a distinction between injunctions that cover worship (*'ibadat*) as immutable and social transactions (*mu'amalat*) as amenable to change to cater to the needs of society.

> "O you who believe obey God and obey the Messenger, and those of you who are in authority; and if you have a dispute concerning any matter refer it to God and to the Messenger." (Qur'an, al-Nisa 4:58)

According to Hashim Kamali (2006a), the Qur'anic verse above provides the textual authority for all the principle sources of the sharia, namely, the revelations from God (Qur'an), the divinely inspired sayings, actions and tacit approvals of Prophet Muhammad (hadith), consensus or agreement (*ijma'*) of all Islamic jurists and drawing an analogy from the Qur'an or hadith (*qiyas*), which together constitute the principle sources or roots of sharia (*usul al-fiqh*). Where these do not suffice, their deliberations are augmented by scholarly hermeneutics and erudite extrapolation or reasoned judgment by Islamic jurists referred to as *ijtihad*. Apart from *usul al-fiqh*, jurists of Islam utilize other useful adjuncts or principles of *fiqh*, which consist of the essence of sharia (*maqasid al-sharia*[4]), goals and higher objectives (*maqasid*) of Allah (Kamali 2006), public benefit (*maslaha*), juristic preference (*istihsan*[5]), blocking the means to a later harm (*sadd al-dhara'i'*), legal stratagem to overcome sharia rules (*hiyal*) and legal maxims (*qawa'id al-fiqh*[6]) to formulate their fatwas. The sum total of the jurists' deliberations constitute a human construct of legal theories over the past 1,400 years that has evolved into the corpus of *fiqh*.

Mujtahid, Ijtihad, *and Fatwas*

The essential triad in evaluating sharia compatibility consists of the *mujtahid*,[7] *ijtihad*,[8] and fatwas.[9] *Ijtihad* is the most powerful instrument employed by orthodoxy and modernists, both Sunni and Shia, for formulating fatwas. Neither the Qur'an nor the hadith provide any direct quotes on ARTs, and where the Qur'an and the hadith do not suffice, Islamic jurists (*fuqaha*) utilize *ijtihad*, providing, as Yale anthropologist Marcia Inhorn puts it, an "Islamically correct" solution to the many contemporary issues for which an answer is not readily available (see Tappan, this volume, for a discussion of Islamic bioethics).

Collective *ijtihad*, compared with individual *ijtihad*, is more robust, enriched by the expertise of participants from other appropriate disciplines and capable of examining the special nuances and intricacies of ARTs, which are ineluctably intertwined with sharia evaluation of ARTs. Muftis and *marja'i* (Shia scholars chosen for their knowledge, piety and competence) are undoubtedly proficient in Islamic jurisprudence, but they cannot be expected to be well informed with the subtleties and complexities of ART or other disciplines as well. The Sunni infrastructure entertains both independent and collective *ijtihad*, the latter comprising sharia councils, *fiqh* academies, and other collective assemblies that are manned by experts from many disciplines.

The Shia claim more experience with *ijtihad*,[10] and certainly their *ijtihad* is bolder, as well as innovative and pragmatic; however, they do not have a multidisciplinary consultative assembly practicing collective *ijtihad*. For Shia, "The religious duty incumbent upon each Shia believer to follow the rulings of one high-ranking Shia scholar, or *marja' al-taqlid* leads to a plurality of religious rulings" (Tappan, this volume). Ayatollah Fadlallah's initial call for the reformation of the institution of the *marja' al-taqlid*, the authoritative "source of emulation" for Shia laymen, has not materialized (Clarke, this volume). Despite this, in practice, the *marja'i*,[11] like independent Sunni muftis,[12] do consult experts and have lengthy engagements with medical forums and secular experts (Tremayne 2009). In Iran, the National Ethical Guidelines for Biomedical Research compiled in 2005 by experts in religion, law, ethics, medicine, and related fields of science, which led to state approval for stem cell research and cloning for therapeutic purposes (Zahedi and Larijani 2008) is an example of collective *ijtihad*.

For all Muslims, next to divine texts, fatwas constitute the most important component of contemporary literature on Islamic perspectives of ARTs. Though authoritative, fatwas are not legally binding unless backed by government statute, and an infertile couple could opt for the fatwa of their choosing; for example, Sunnis could adopt a ruling from a different Sunni legal school (*madhhab*). Moreover, they could theoretically go across the Sunni-Shia divide and "borrow" a doctrine from the Shia Jafari *madhhab*, adopting the concept of *takhayyur*[13] (Coulson 1994), if that is more to their liking. Finally, they could transgress the sharia boundary and employ prohibited ARTs, facing the consequences in the hereafter (*akhira*). The state, by its power of *siyasa sharia*,[14] reserves the right to overturn any fatwa it deems inimical to Islam or Muslim society. For example, in 2003 the Iranian Parliament, on the advice of the Guardian Council of spiritual leaders, overturned the fatwa of Ayatollah Khamene'i, the spiritual leader of Iran, which permitted extramarital conception and sperm donation, including its use posthumously (Tremayne 2009).

Phrasing of the question is important, and fatwas must be assessed in the context and particular circumstance in which they were issued. This would explain some fatwas that appear to be at odds with conventional norms.[15] The fatwa should delineate the religious and ethical reasoning behind the rulings and be issued on a value scale of five (*akham al-khamsa*[16]). In 1980, Shaykh Jad al-Haq, the leading cleric at Al-Azhar University, issued his historic fatwa on ARTs. This was the first fatwa on ARTs to be issued for the Muslim world, both Sunni and Shia. The essentials of the fatwa consisted of:

- The protection of sanctity of life—Qur'an 17:33[17]

- Conception within marriage—Qur'an 25:54[18]

- No confusion of family lineage—Qur'an 33:4–5[19] and Qur'an 25:54

- No mixing of genealogy—Qur'an 33:4–5 and Qur'an 25:54 and

- Gestational carrier to be designated as the mother—Qur'an 58:2[20] and Hadith[21]

All Muslims followed Shaykh Jad al-Haq's fatwa until Ayatollah Khamene'i, fatwa in 1999, after which the Shia diverged on issues of *mut'a* (temporary or flexible) marriage (Al-Hakim 2005), third-party assistance, and conception outside marriage. To understand this divergence, it is pertinent to note that unlike the Sunnis of Ash'ari inspiration (Traditionalists), the Shia along with the Sunni

Mu'tazila (who together constitute the Rationalists described below), claim that humanity was endowed with *'aql* (intellect) and hence able to differentiate right from wrong, thus leading the way for innovative *ijtihad*.

Though Muslim jurists are beginning to appreciate the significance of bioethics, its neglect in sharia deliberations (Sachedena 2009a), and on ARTs has been highlighted by Tappan (this volume), who states that fatwas in Iran do not seem to encompass the full scope and range of moral concern in bioethics for clinical decision making.

Schisms among Muslims

Sunni and Shia and Traditionalism and Rationalism constitute two major divisions in the Muslim community. As stated in the following epithet by the illustrious contemporary Shia scholar, Seyyed Hossein Nasr: "*Shi'ism* is not a heterodox sect and *Sunnism* and *Shi'ism* are both orthodox interpretations of the Islamic revelation and constitute two different perspectives of Islam" (Nasr 1994).

The orthodox Traditionalists of Ash'ari inspiration,[22] who constitute the vast majority of Sunni Muslims, declared that human actions were predetermined, that the Qur'an was eternal and that humanity was not capable of deciding what was right and what was wrong. In the early eighth century, Mu'tazilism (Rationalism) made a foray into Islam with metaphysical inquiries and along with the Shia formed the Rationalists, who maintained that life was not predetermined, that the Qur'an was created, and that humanity was gifted with intellect, giving them the ability to distinguish right from wrong. This distinction paved the way for the latter to formulate fatwas even without the "backing" of scriptural sources. The Rationalist ("Modernist") scholars[23] have emphasized the need for accurate interpretation (*tafsir*)[24] and explanation of the inner meaning (*ta'wil*)[25] of the Qur'an and the need for an engagement with the full spectrum of Islamic thought and practices (Safi 2003). According to them the authenticity of the Prophet's Sunna (hadith, plural *ahadith*), which has been shrouded since its inception, needs clarification. Also, in matters of law, the *ahadith* should be restricted to his prophetic mission, which are of divine inspiration and therefore free from error (Rahman 1979). Currently six Sunni compendia of *ahadith* are extant, *Sahih Bukhari* and *Sahih Muslim* being considered the most reliable. The Shia recognize only part of the Sunni *ahadith* as authentic, and unlike the Sunnis, whose hadith ceased with the death of the Prophet, the *ahadith* of the Ithna-Ash'ari Shia continued up to their twelfth imam, who, being direct descendants of the Prophet, are deemed infallible. The Jafari legal school represents Shia jurisprudence, and they compiled their own *ahadith* comprising four volumes.

Investigation of the interplay between the dynamic changes in Islamic perspectives and the cutting edge of ART demonstrates diverse contexts in the Islamic world and considerable variation in the way in which Islamic scholars perceive which ARTs are and are not permitted by sharia. This is due to divergences in sharia interpretation between and among the mainstream Sunni and the less populous Shia and has led to controversies in the sharia status of ARTs.

The Shia jurists, like their Sunni counterparts, base their fatwas mainly on scriptural texts but lean significantly towards *ijtihad*, reflecting Shia enthusiasm to direct the new technologies towards diagnostic and therapeutic goals. Recent liberal fatwas originating from the Ithna-Ash'ari Shia[26] quarters in Iran and Ayatollah Fadlallah in Lebanon show significant deviations from the classical Sunni view. While these Shia scholars were dynamic and keen on examining the avenues available for a solution, their pragmatic *ijtihad* and their recent rulings on ART issues have led to a paradigm shift from conventional marriage to *mut'a* arrangement and finally to conception outside marriage. The legitimacy of these fatwas and other pragmatic, yet nevertheless unconventional, innovations of the Shia remain controversial. The Shia scene shows that some of their religious rulings may be dictated by consumer demand and driven by service-provider enthusiasm, with ART specialists interpreting Islamic rules quite differently from the scholars, leading to many variances in clinical practice (Tremayne 2009). Ambiguity and pluralistic rulings with their attendant legal hair splitting are not conducive to providing clear answers for questions posed by the uninformed infertile couple, nor is it easy for the physician to choose a pathway that is deemed sharia compatible.

Clinical Impacts of the Islamic Debates on ARTs

Islamic controversies arising from divergences in sharia interpretation, particularly among and between the Sunni and Shia, do have an effect on the clinical practice of ARTs among Muslims, and consequent pluralistic rulings have led to confusion among medical professionals and infertile couples. Critical clinical issues of fetal reduction, termination of early pregnancy, discarding of embryos, embryo research, and third-party assistance in conception (sperm-egg-embryo donation and surrogacy), preimplantation genetic diagnosis, and other controversies which are directly impacted by the Islamic debates over ARTs are discussed below.

Embryo Reduction, Abortion, and Research

Sanctity of the fetus, when life begins and when personhood is conferred, are important in deliberations on embryo reduction and abortion. Muslims, while accepting that life begins at fertilization, grade its value on gestational age and consider ensoulment at 120 days[27] as a watershed, after which the fetus assumes the status of a human. The distinction between preimplantation and implanted embryo has important connotations for the status of the embryo, the former bearing only a potential for life while the latter is already a growing fetus.

Embryo reduction was introduced to reduce complications to the mother, enhance fetal survival, and prevent the risk of extremely severe prematurity with all its attendant complications.[28] The incidence of high-order multiple pregnancies is fast declining, the transfer of multiple embryos having being replaced by single- or two-embryo transfer. In this study the response to embryo reduction from infertile couples, both Sunni and Shia, was variable with 60 percent of Sunni and 35 percent of Shia infertile couples agreeing to embryo reduction, the rest declaring that they were unwilling to "kill some of their babies." An important consideration to note here is that when couples have to pay substantial sums for ART, they opt to maximize its returns and prefer a multiple pregnancy despite its attendant complications.

Further, in this survey all scholars, both Sunni and Shia, approved of termination of a pregnancy if continuation poses a threat to the life of the mother, based on the Qur'anic verse 6:145[29] and the Islamic principle that the mother's life is more important than the fetus. Abortion for other indications is, however, controversial. In justifiable cases, the concessionary alternative of *ruksa*[30] to override strict sharia rule (*azeema*) permits jurists to justify abortion, with scholars again utilizing the Qur'anic verse 6:145.

Some scholars, including the Al-Azhar Sharia Committee (Prof. Ahmad Ragab 2008[31]) and the Islamic Juridical Council, permit abortion for rape and severe congenital abnormality by utilizing the *fiqh* principles of *maslaha*[32] or *istisla*[33] and *istihsan*,[34] which makes abortion permissible. The Therapeutic Abortion Act of 2005 in Iran permits therapeutic abortion for familial or genetic disorders of the fetus that would lead to psychological affliction or an undesirable burden on the parents, or in the case of serious maternal disease (Zahedi and Larijani 2008). Others are more cautious in permitting abortion where the mother's life or health is not at risk. Sachedina (2009b) claims that the revelation-based principle of sanctity of life would appear to rule out termination of the conceptus's life even in the early stages. Results from this study revealed that most Sunni and Shia scholars interviewed did not permit abortion for rape or fetal abnormalities. Indeed, rape victims in Bosnia were denied abortions by such eminent figures as Shaykh Jad al-Haq and Shaykh Yusuf al-Qaradawi because the baby was innocent (Natour et al. 2005).

While contributions by medieval scholars from the Sunni *madhhabs*[35] form a vast repository of legal knowledge, contemporary juristic deliberations are hindered by having to incorporate four divergent views with each decree. It is pertinent that Sunnis do not choose their *madhhab* but are born into it. The current infrastructure results in a Sunni *mujtahid*, after painstakingly completing his or her juristic deliberations on abortion or embryo reduction, issuing a fatwa stating that, "For pregnancies not life threatening to the mother, the Hanafis permit abortion up to 120 days, the Shafi'is until 42 days, and the Malikis and Hanbalis not at all; if the ruling of your legal school [*madhhab*] is not conducive to you, you may change schools to one that may suit you better." Attempts to integrate and coalesce the doctrines of the four Sunni schools have not been successful (Professor Hameed 2007[36]). However, in the past two decades collective deliberations incorporating all Sunni and Shia *madhhabs* (Sachedina 2009c) by the *majma' al-fiqh* in Mecca have been a move towards the development of a more collaborative judicial process.

Another controversial area involves embryo research. Embryos can be obtained from supernumerary IVF embryos, those produced by somatic cell nuclear transfer (SCNT), and from induced pluripotent cells (iPS). Research on embryos needs to be assessed in the light of Islamic values of embryonic sanctity. Most scholars, both Sunni and Shia, maintain that embryos should not be created for research and that the embryo needs to be treated with dignity because of its "potential for life" status. However, some argue that posthumous, postdivorce, and surplus embryos that are destined to be disposed of could be put to more productive use in research. The manner of discarding embryos remains controversial; the opinion of most scholars in this study was that embryos <8 weeks (prior to completion of body form) do not need ritual burial but still need to be disposed with dignity.

Third-Party Reproductive Assistance

Sunni Islam prohibits all types of third-party assistance for conception, while a number of Shia scholars have endorsed the "official" position of Ayatollah Khamene'i, which permits third-party assistance in cases where infertility poses a threat to marriage. Third-party assistance for surrogacy or egg or embryo donation may be from a polygamous or *mut'a* wife, sibling, or outsider.

Polygamy and Mut'a Marriage

In Islam, all conceptions must be under the umbrella of a marriage contract, be it conventional, polygamous, or *mut'a* marriage.[37] Preservation of proper parental lineage (*nasab*) is essential and is part and parcel of a Muslim's identity, the goal, both in Islam and Muslim culture, being to safeguard the child's untainted identity through a legitimate conjugal relationship (see Griffel, this volume).

Polygamy, though still legal, is frowned upon and fast declining in the Muslim world, and is prohibited in Tunisia (Hallaq 1997a); however, both Sunnis and Shia approve of it, including its use to overcome infertility. Could the egg, embryo, or uterus from a co-wife in polygamy be employed in ART? The Sunnis declared a resounding "no" to the former two while their attempt to use the womb of a co-wife for surrogacy came to a premature end; after initially giving its approval in 1984 for the use of a polygamous co-wife as a surrogate, the *Fiqh* Council in Mecca (*Majma' al-Fiqh al-Islami*) rescinded it in 1986 (Yacoub 2001). Shia scholars, however, unanimously approve surrogacy and the cross-transfer of eggs and embryo in polygamy. In this special circumstance of a unique and close relationship of the husband with his two or more wives, they contend that in Islamic patriarchal society, the child's lineage is maintained and confusion in lineage and mixing of genealogy is minimal, being restricted to only the contribution by the co-wife, who, after all, is "family."

'Allamah Tabataba'i and Seyyed Hossein Nasr, both eminent contemporary Shia scholars, state that Shia Islam embraced the concept of pre-Islamic *mut'a* as a means of curbing promiscuity and channeling the inherent sexual desires within the *mut'a* arrangement (Tabataba'i 1971), thus providing a veil of legitimacy. The sharia validity of *mut'a* marriage practiced by the Shia is refuted by the Sunnis. The polemics of the debate regarding *mut'a* or its nonacceptance by the Sunnis do not concern us in the present context. What is important and controversial is that most, though not all, *marja'i* in Iran are congruent on extrapolating this *mut'a* arrangement for ARTs and all Shia scholars in this study showed unanimous support for it. However, there are cogent arguments against utilizing *mut'a* for ARTs. It is pertinent that currently *mut'a* arrangements for ARTs are devoid of all acts concordant with conventional marriage, and the parties need not even have any contact except to sign the agreement. To use this model of quasi-marriage for ARTs could allow it to come under "ruses" (*hiyal sharia*) and to be labeled as casuistry (Clarke, this volume). Not all Shia clerics or infertile couples subscribe to utilizing *mut'a* for ARTs in Iran, and in this study 60 percent of infertile couples in Iran vetoed this method, reflecting perhaps a natural reluctance on the part of the female partner to include another woman in her marital relationship.

The only equivalent to *mut'a* among the Sunni is *misyar* or unofficial temporary marriage, which is practiced in Egypt and some parts of the Middle East and where the woman voluntarily abandons any financial gain. According to Yusuf al-Qaradawi, an illustrious contemporary Sunni scholar, *misyar* should be viewed as a form of relationship between man and woman, though neither Islamically valid nor socially acceptable. Presently, *misyar* is not employed as an avenue for ARTs.

Sperm donation

> The depositing of semen in a place reserved by divine law
> for the husband is forbidden.
> –Imam Ja'afer Sadiq, the sixth Shia imam

Insemination with donor sperm is forbidden in Sunni Islam, and most Shia authorities concur with this in line with Imam Sadiq (quoted above); the exception to this is Ayatollah Khamene'i. The controversies lie in his fatwa permitting sperm donation and in the definition of *zina*. All scholars concur that the introduction of semen or sperm into another woman's vagina goes against Islamic sensitivity and propriety; Shia scholars make a distinction between seminal fluid and specially prepared sperm for ART, the latter understandably being more acceptable. The *ulama*'s abhorrence of the passage of semen or sperm via the vagina could be circumvented by the innovative yet pragmatic alternatives of gamete intrafallopian transfer (GIFT) and zygote intrafallopian transfer (ZIFT), where the sperm and egg or embryo respectively are injected into the fallopian tube via the abdomen, thereby avoiding passage through the vagina. However, these techniques make the procedure more complicated, invasive, and expensive.

The second controversy is on the definition of *zina*; Sunnis consider artificial insemination of donor sperm into the vagina as adultery or fornication (*zina*), while most Shia, including Ayatollah Khamene'i, argue that the word *zina* must be restricted to "penile penetration of the vagina" and therefore donor sperm insemination (DI) cannot be classified as *zina* (Al-Hakim 2008[38]). Though Ayatollah Khamene'i's fatwa on sperm donation was overruled by the Iranian *majlis* (parliament) in 2003 and hence prohibited in Iran, its jurisdiction does not extend to Lebanon where sperm donation is freely available (Clarke 2009). Despite this, sperm donation is used only as a "last resort" and no matter the religious sect, most Muslim men in Lebanon continue to resist both adoption and gamete donation, arguing that such a child "won't be my son," with 83 percent of Sunnis and 64 percent of Shia men opposing gamete donation (Inhorn 2006). A licit though convoluted and *hyal*istic[39] alternative pathway is for a woman to divorce her husband, marry someone else after the end of her *'iddah*,[40] artificially inseminate with the sperm of her new husband, then divorce him, wait until the delivery of the baby, and then remarry the first husband (Ayatollah Fadlallah cited by Garmaroudi Naef, this volume).

Egg and Embryo Donation

The Sunnis do not permit egg or embryo donation, but the Shia do under a *mut'a* arrangement. Also, after menopause, ovaries do not have eggs and though postmenopausal conception is not an option for Sunni Muslims, it is available for Shia. However, the use of one's own eggs or primordial follicles (precursors of eggs), cryo-preserved for use at a later date, does not create sharia problems for Sunni or Shia. Dr. Bahampour, the director of the Shia Centre for Advanced Studies in London, states that for Shia, age should not be a factor in denying this facility, provided both husband and wife are enthusiastic, mentally and physically fit, and make an informed choice; the eggs here would be obtained under a *mut'a* arrangement. Recently, the cytoplasm[41] from the egg of a younger woman has been injected into an older infertile female's egg (ooplasmic transfer) to correct mitochondrial deficiencies or enhance the reproductive potential in older women. Except for some messenger RNA[42] there is no transmission of nuclear DNA (genetic material), and therefore this should not raise any sharia objections.

While embryo donation is prohibited for Sunnis, the Shia are permitted to use an embryo formed by the union of husband's sperm with the egg of the *mut'a* wife. Though donor sperm outside the marriage contract is prohibited by almost all Shia jurists except Ayatollah Khamene'i, embryos with a donor sperm complement had a variable response; to help the desperate infertile couple, Shia clerics are prepared to overlook donor sperm when it is part of an embryo. Ayatollah Mo'men makes a distinction between the transfer of an egg fertilized by donor sperm for gestational surrogacy (permitted) and those that involve the injection of the sperm (traditional surrogacy), which he considers as *haram*. Ayatollah Khamene'i and some senior Shia *marja' al-taqlid* including Ayatollahs Sistani, Sadeqi, Mohammad Shiraz, Mosawi Ardebili, Qomi and Ayatollah Seyyed Mohammad Musavi Bojnurdi, have permitted the transfer of an embryo formed from donor sperm[43] as long as no *haram* act such as gaze or touch has taken place (see Garmaroudi Naef, this volume). The above notwithstanding, some Shia clerics are understandably concerned about embryos formed from donor sperm.

Embryos from relatives, though proscribed by all Sunni and some Shia, find their way into the wombs of the latter with approval by some clerics including Ayatollah Sadeqi and Ayatollah Yousef Sane'i, who permit embryo transfer among siblings (see Garmaroudi Naef, this volume). Even embryo donation with no *mut'a* arrangement is permitted by most Shia *marja'i* because it comes from a married couple (Clarke 2009).

Surrogacy

Where the womb (uterus) is absent or unable to carry a pregnancy, surrogacy provides a practical alternative. The surrogate may be a co-wife in a polygamous or *mut'a* relationship, a relative (mother or sister), or outsider. The embryo employed in surrogacy could be composed of sperm and egg from the commissioning couple, mother's egg and donor sperm, egg from a surrogate mother and sperm from a husband or donor (insemination or IVF), or both sperm and egg from a donor.

In surrogacy, there is no confusion of family lineage or mixing of genealogy. The Sunni prohibition of surrogacy, even where sperm and egg are from husband and wife, is based on Qur'anic verse[44] and hadith.[45] In addition, surrogacy involves the surrogate signing a contract to adopt the baby, but legal adoption is prohibited for Sunnis.[46] The Shia permit a polygamous or *mut'a* wife as surrogate, with Ayatollah Khamene'i permitting surrogacy even outside marriage.[47] Ayatollah Yousef Sane'i, a distinguished Shia scholar, upholds gestational surrogacy between siblings as permissible; a woman is allowed to deliver the child of her sister or carry the child of her brother in her womb and give birth to it.

The designation of motherhood, and how it is defined and articulated, is a critically important issue in any discussion of surrogacy.

Despite Islam placing a high value on genealogy, Sunni scholars accord motherhood to the gestational carrier and not to the owner of the egg; this has implications for assigning *nasab*. Frank Griffel (this volume) emphasizes the "clarity of one's *nasab* [which] is an important principle in Islamic law that the jurists cannot easily throw overboard."

Some scholars, including Ayatollah Mo'men, maintain that the Qur'anic verse, "Their mothers are only those who gave them birth" (58: 2) refers to men who pronounce *zīhār* and does not reveal the meaning of maternity (*me'yar-e madari*) and therefore assigns maternity to the originator of the egg (Garmaroudi Naef, this volume).[48] Also, according to Ra'fat Uthman, professor emeritus and past dean, Faculty of Sharia, Al-Azhar University, the hadith, "The child is for the bed, the adulterer the stone" (*al-walad li-l-firash wa li-l-ahir al-hajar*) was specifically referring to an adulterous illicit act of sexual intercourse (between two married illicit sex partners) with an intention of punishing the fornicator by not ascribing the child to him. Hence the Sunni analogy of the Qur'anic verse[49] and hadith[50] is controversial. Also, the denial of *nasab* means the child is punished for somebody else's illicit act, which some argue is not ethically justified (see Thomas Eich, this volume).

The majority of Shia authorities, including Ayatollahs Khamene'i, Fadlallah, the late Imam Khomeini, Yousef Sane'i, Mohammad Mo'men Qomi, Safi Golpayegani, Naser Makarem Shirazi[51] and Montazeri argue that maternity, similar to paternity, is established at conception[52] and therefore confer motherhood to the owner of the egg (Garmaroudi Naef, this volume) while Ayatollah Sistani adopts the Sunni line of designating the gestational carrier as the mother (Clark 2008). Some Shia scholars designate two mothers; the contributor of the egg (*saheb-e tokhmak*) and the carrying mother (Garmaroudi Naef, this volume).

Issues of kinship are also raised in debates on surrogacy. The Qur'an stipulates that breastfeeding five or more times confers kinship to the child. By analogy, Sunnis maintain that progeny resulting from surrogacy are considered "siblings" of the surrogate's children, because the surrogate provides nutrition, and hence are not marriageable. Ayatollah Khamene'i sweeps aside this Sunni sibling kinship of surrogacy, which he considers invalid since surrogacy entails a role only as an incubator and as a vehicle for the transmission of nourishment without any genetic contributions (Clarke 2009).

Experience has shown that surrogacy arrangements are a minefield in and out of the courtroom. The risks of pregnancy and con-

finement for the surrogate are usually underestimated, while monitoring the pregnancy of the surrogate is difficult to enforce. Other
ethical issues include "appropriate" compensation, nonacceptance
by both parties in case of an abnormal child, and psychological implications for the surrogate upon relinquishing the baby.

The current plurality of views on surrogacy among the *ulama* on
both sides of the Sunni-Shia divide poses a problem for professionals, both medical and religious, to provide guidance to the infertile
couple.

Marriage, Conception, and Donation

Islam prohibits conception outside marriage because the integrity of
the institution of marriage and family unit to provide a distinctive
family lineage is sacrosanct and is honored by both Sunni and Shia
as evident in the Qur'anic *ayat*.[53]

Although the Shia generally prohibit conception outside marriage,
the only and most influential *marja'i* in Lebanon, Ayatollah Fadlallah, supports Khamene'i in extramarital egg and embryo donation
(Clarke 2009) and in Lebanon, even Sunnis, are getting eggs from
young donors from the United States (Inhorn 2005), without even
resorting to *mut'a* arrangements and sometimes with close relatives
as donors (Tremayne 2009).

In Islam, the identity of the donor is important to identify and al-
locate paternity and motherhood, *nasab*, rights of maintenance, inheritance, and *mahram* issues relating to domestic privacy and veiling. Among the Shia, anonymity is often overlooked as is the rule in
Lebanon (Clarke 2009). The relationship between the participants
of a donor arrangement is complex and fraught with ethical, religious, and legal problems. Third-party donation confuses issues of
kinship, *nasab*, and inheritance, and holds the potential for incest in
anonymous donations (Inhorn 2003). Ayatollah Khamene'i's fatwa
permits both egg and sperm donation to overcome marital discord at
the expense of the mixing of genealogy. Despite his good intentions,
the impact on children who are conceived through gamete donation of egg or sperm on families and community differ (see Gürtin,
this volume) and the outcome for donor children, their parents, and
society not always has a happy ending (see Tremayne, this volume).
Moreover, the current Shia consanguineous practice of donation of
sperm, egg, and embryo among siblings leads to the propagation of
genetic diseases.

Sharia does not permit postdivorce or posthumous use of sperm,
egg, or embryo, even with written consent, because all conceptions

must occur under the marriage contract. Ayatollah Khamene'i's fatwa, which permits the posthumous use of sperm, is controversial and has not had support from his *marja'i* colleagues, the Guardian Council of Iran, or the Shia scholars interviewed in this study. However, this point merits further discussion. It must, however, be conceded that this is a special circumstance, wherein the husband's sperm was collected and cryo-preserved prior to his demise while the marriage contract was valid, with no confusion of family lineage or mixing of genealogy.

Preimplantation Genetic Diagnosis

Preimplantation genetic diagnosis (PGD) is a sophisticated technique to exclude chromosomal or genetic disorders by analysis of the genetic components of the cells in the very young embryo prior to implantation in the womb. It is employed in cases where the parents are known to be carriers of, or likely to be prone to, genetic or chromosomal defects. If a severe abnormality is detected, the affected embryo is not implanted, thus avoiding the need for a later abortion. This illustrates the Islamic principle of *sadd al-dhara'i'*, which in this case means blocking the means to abortion, which is a greater harm. Islamic scholars were slow to support the concept of prevention of severe congenital malformation by selection of disease-free embryos (Serour 2000); however, most Islamic jurists now approve of PGD.

Preimplantation genetic screening (PGS) employs an identical technique but is used to screen embryos for abnormalities that may manifest later in life. Using PGS for detecting Huntington's Disease[54] or genetic predisposition to breast cancer, and more recently to exclude aneuploidy in older women, received a guarded reception from Sunni scholars while Shia permitted PGS for all of the above. More contentious, however, is PGS for nonmedical indications, particularly for sex selection (Serour and Dickens 2001). Preconception gender identification is possible by sperm separation or PGS (which requires IVF) and postconception identification of y-fetal DNA by testing of placental tissue (chorionic villus sampling), or sampling of fluid around the fetus (amniocentesis). While Sunni scholars approved it in cases of sex-linked diseases, they unanimously rejected PGS for sex preference and sex balancing in accordance with the following Qur'anic *sura*: "He creates whatever He wills. He grants daughters to whom He wills, and sons to whom He wills; or He gives both sons and daughters to whom He wills and makes barren whom He wills" (42: 49–50).

However, unlike sex preference, sex balancing is where parents wish for a particular gender because they have many of the other. Some argue that sexing prior to implantation would lead to a happier outcome for both parents and baby. All Shia scholars approved PGS for sex selection and balancing; they have the added advantage of donating the unwanted embryos by *mut'a* arrangement to others or for research.

PGD for "savior siblings" is a special circumstance where the embryo is HLA-matched to provide stem cells or tissue for treating an existing sibling. The motive for conception and care of the child are matters for concern, but ethically PGD may be comforting to the couple morally and psychologically (Pennings and Liebaers 2002) in avoiding an abortion.

Gender of Attending Physician

Women place their faith and trust in their doctor and can feel vulnerable during gynecological examinations, particularly by male physicians. This sensitivity is not exclusive to Muslims, and it is the duty of male doctors to minimize their concerns by being gentle and professional and providing proper explanation, an adequate cover, and by not transgressing the boundaries of the doctor-patient relationship. "Prosperous are the believers who ... guard their private parts (by abstaining from sexual relations) except with their marriage partners" (Qur'an 23:5–6).

Mahram is an important Islamic concept designed to avoid opportunities of temptation that could lead to impropriety and fornication between the sexes. All scholars in this study, both Sunni and Shia, concurred on the need to observe *mahram* rules. Note for example Morgan Clarke's (2009) and Soraya Tremayne's (2009) excerpts of Ayatollah Khamene'i's fatwa of 1999, "He extended his approval to both egg and sperm donation, as long as there is no touch or gaze involved,"[55] which illustrates its importance. However, though Islam preaches modesty it also advocates the best possible medical care, therefore permitting examination, including of private parts, of the body by both male and female doctors with the proviso that if a female could serve equally well, it would be desirable for a female to attend. Further, if a female makes a request for a female physician, her wishes must be respected and adhered to (Hathout 1991).

In Islam, *mahram* issues are so sensitive that the Iranian government is planning to ban the training of male gynecologists. It is important to note that the Qur'anic verse 23:5–6 above refers to sexual impropriety and not to a professional examination by a physician. What is also relevant is that the doctor-patient gender relationship no longer appears to be contentious in Cairo or Iran, illustrated by the fact that in this study only 4 percent of those surveyed in Egypt and 15 percent in Iran requested a female physician. The large numbers of women not having any particular sex preference for their medical provider, though enlightening, is against the tide of current opinion among Islamic scholars.

Transgression of Prohibited ARTs

How important are religious rulings for Muslims? The desperation of the infertile drives some to transgress sharia boundaries to overcome statutory and religious obstacles in what is euphemistically termed "procreative tourism," which serves to gauge the barometer of religious zeal. Sharia in theory does not always relate to practice, and infertile couples do sometimes transgress sharia boundaries; the survey of infertile couples in this study indicated that 32 percent were would-be transgressors if they needed egg or embryo donation. Whether they would go through with this or whether more would transgress when actually faced with the problem is not clear. Currently, even in sharia-oriented countries, there are no statutory punitive measures for couples who transgress sharia in matters of ARTs, leaving transgression by Muslims to the tribunal of conscience and final arbitration to God. According to Gürtin (this volume), there is a serious discord between public discourse and private behavior regarding the demand for and acceptability of various ART procedures. She quotes Pennings (2002) in saying that "secret" pursuit of nationally banned ART treatments increasingly leads Turkish couples to demonstrate "moral pluralism in motion."

Lack of screening (for HIV,[56] hepatitis, and STDs[57]) exposes the recipients and child to genetic and medical defects. Moreover, the financial incentive for egg and embryo donors raises the question of exploitation. The extent of potential long-term psychological harm to recipient parents and their progeny has not been evaluated and may outweigh the benefits they are seeking through using the sperm or egg of a family member. There is no consensus among scholars on whether children should be given data about their genetic parents.

ART Funding

In this study, 70 percent of couples in Egypt and 40 percent in Iran expressed funding as the main deterrent to early attendance at ART clinics. Globally, subsidies for ARTs range from unlimited free treatment, as in many affluent countries in the Middle East and Israel (Kahn 2000), to little or no state support in low-resource nations. In Turkey, changing status from an "elective" to a "therapeutic" treatment and categorization of IVF as "compulsory health expenditure" carry great symbolic connotations, effectively medicalizing involuntary childlessness and normalizing IVF treatment (Gürtin, this volume). Schemes to alleviate funding problems include expediting state-funded nonurgent operations as a trade-off for donor eggs and egg-sharing schemes that involve trading surplus eggs from IVF patients to recompense the cost of IVF. Sharia proscription precludes egg sharing for Sunnis, but Shia can employ it by designating the egg donor as a *mut'a* wife.

Future ARTs

In my study, the willingness of different centers (and ART specialists) to consider future technologies was quite erratic and not obviously influenced by carefully considered religious implications. A few respondents indicated that the issues had not yet been adequately considered by their ethics committees while several centers responded with a blanket "no" to everything. Scholars of both Sunni and Shia persuasion show considerable disagreement even within their own ranks, with some recommending a "sunset clause" until more knowledge is available to make a final judgment. Of the future developments in ARTs, I discuss below transplantation, stem cell technology, the creation of germ cell lines, and cloning.

Uterine Transplantation

Where a woman has no womb or is incapable of permitting conception or gestation, transplantation of a donor uterus will enable her to carry her own pregnancy. Sunni scholars in this study rejected this procedure on the grounds of its prohibition by the *Fiqh* Academy in Mecca in 2006. There is no genetic transmission, and the oft-quoted analogy of kinship resulting from breastfeeding and the donor uterus supplying nutrition to the fetus does not apply here because the nutrition to the fetus, unlike with surrogacy, is supplied by the gestational carrier and not the donor. Also, there is no problem in the designation of motherhood, as the recipient provides the egg and also carries the pregnancy. It is therefore difficult to comprehend the reasons for the Sunni denial of this procedure. The Shia jurists do not have any objections to uterine transplantation.

Transplantation of Ovaries

Autologous[58] transplantation of ovaries has been successfully performed with seven pregnancies to date and is useful in cases of cancer where ovaries or ovarian tissue are frozen (cryo-preserved) and subsequently transplanted after chemo- or radiotherapy treatment has been completed. More recently, primordial follicles (immature eggs) obtained from ovarian tissue have been successfully matured in vitro (outside the body) and frozen for future use. This is permitted by both Sunni and Shia since no sharia principle is transgressed. Heterologous[59] transplants of genetic tissue, including ovaries, are not permitted by both Sunni and Shia scholars, due to mixing of genealogy and family lineage. However, ovarian tissue may be permitted for Shia by a donor under a *mut'a* arrangement. Donor testicular tissue transplantation, when it becomes technically feasible, would not be permitted except by Ayatollah Khamane'i.

Stem Cell Technology (SCT)

Advances in stem cell technology have opened up new horizons, paving the way for tissue replacement and revolutionizing the concept of regenerative medicine in addition to gene therapy and cloning. The technique involves programming early embryonic cells derived from natural or artificially created embryos and more recently from induced pluripotent cells (iPS)[60] to produce the desired cells for replacement in the treatment of diabetes, myocardial infarction, stroke, Alzheimer's and Parkinson's disease, spinal cord injury, extensive burns, and more. For research, it could provide a window for observing embryogenesis,[61] teratogenesis,[62] and embryo toxicity, in the process minimizing animal experimentation. Islam regards scientific research as discovering the laws of nature and works of God; scientific endeavor is considered God's grace (*baraka*) and not as an infringement in his work.

The enormous potential for treatment as replacement therapy was appreciated and approved by all scholars, both Sunni and Shia, with the proviso that embryos must be surplus and not created for the purpose of replacement therapy. Its use as a research tool, however, is contentious, with most approving it while a few disapproved of experimentation on living potential "humans." The latter stance by scholars is understandable except perhaps in the case of surplus embryos destined to be disposed of and also frozen embryos when the couple has no further desire to reproduce. "Are human embryos of such immense moral significance that we should never destroy them, even when research might contribute towards treatment and perhaps save the lives of human beings?" asks Mansooreh Sanei (this volume). Sachedina (2009c), however, argues that embryos, whether created for reproductive purposes or research, have no legal or moral basis to deny the dignity to the so-called spare embryos with total disregard of the inviolability of embryos or legal permission for the use of "spare" IVF embryos for research. He concedes, however, that stem cells derived from fetal tissue following abortion is analogically similar to cadaver donation for organ transplantation, and hence, the use of cells from that source is permissible.

Consequently, the moral significance of the early embryo, embryonic sanctity, and the respect to the preimplantation embryo remains at the center of the ethical controversy in stem cell research. The use of human embryos, which had raised ethical objections, may be overcome by somatic cell nuclear transfer[63] (SCNT) and induced pluripotent stem cells. Currently many of these are under clinical trials and should reach clinical practice in the near future.

Germ Cell Lines

The "flagship" of the ART specialist would be the creation of germ cell lines enabling the de novo production of sperm, egg, or embryo, obviating the need for donation of genetic material. However, according to Professor Austin Smith,[64] germ cell lines providing sperm and egg will not enter clinical practice for some time. Does artificial creation of sperm, eggs, and embryos have sharia approval? Though theoretically possible, all scholars surveyed in this study rejected it because not enough is known about it and were reticent on responding to a technology that is not yet available.

Cloning

Wilmut and colleagues at the Roslyn Institute in Edinburgh achieved a milestone in research into human embryology by successfully cloning Dolly the sheep in 1997 by somatic cell nuclear transfer (SCNT).[65] Its extension to reproductive cloning in humans is still in the experimental phase; however, therapeutic cloning has enormous potential for research and subsequent therapeutic applications. All Sunni and most Shia scholars rejected reproductive cloning, with Ayatollah Muhammad Hussayn Fadlallah of Lebanon and Shaykh Muhammad Sa'id Hakim of Najaf being exceptions (Natour et al. 2005). Some scholars expressed concern regarding the undermining of Muslim values and the status and social concerns of the cloned child (Sachedina (2009d). However, most scholars support therapeutic cloning because of its potential to treat many ailments, provided that embryos were derived from nonembryonic sources (SCNT or iPS)[66] or surplus embryos were used. In Iran, the National Ethical Guidelines for Biomedical Research were compiled in 2005 by experts in religion, law, ethics, medicine, and related fields of science; subsequently, state approval for stem cell research and cloning for therapeutic purposes has been achieved (Zahedi and Larijani 2008). A consensus statement by Sachedina (2009c) from Sunnis and Shia is that sharia has no problem with the concept of therapeutic cloning but that human reproductive cloning is regarded as suspicious or forbidden outright.

Conclusion

In Muslim society, fecundity is cherished, children highly valued, parenthood culturally mandatory, and childlessness socially unacceptable; hence, ARTs are generally warmly embraced by Muslims. Sharia evaluation of ARTs, which is mandatory for Muslims, is hindered by controversies due to differences in sharia interpretation between and within Sunni and Shia camps. While there is consonance for IVF, there exists significant dissonance on issues of third-party assistance (sperm, egg, and embryo donation and surrogacy), anonymity of donors, and conception outside the marriage contract, which all pose a sharia dilemma. Both Sunni and Shia scholars endeavor to alleviate the plight of the infertile couple, the Shia more so than the Sunnis because of their pragmatic utilization of *ijtihad* and *mut'a*. However, some innovative fatwas of the Shia and the use of *mut'a* for ARTs do not conform to conventional sharia norms. The desperation of some infertile couples can lead to transgression of sharia boundaries. Bioethics, a hitherto neglected discipline in ART evaluation, is gaining more recognition in the Muslim world.

While collective *ijtihad* practiced by the Sunnis is to be commended, their adherence to *madhhab*s that subscribe to a plurality of sharia rulings is not conducive to juristic deliberations. The Shia are reluctant to engage in formal collective *ijtihad* deliberations on vital issues of global importance, and they rely on the individual *ijtihad* of their *marja'i*, which lacks the expertise of a multidisciplinary team. Perhaps collective deliberations would have obviated unorthodox fatwas issued by the Shia *marja'i* pertaining to sperm donation and conception outside marriage.

The Sunni prohibition of uterine transplantation appears to lack clear sharia foundation. While their negative stance on sex preference is understandable both from an ethical and sharia viewpoint, sex balancing needs to be judged on the benefit to both the couple and the child. The oft-quoted Qur'anic verse[67] and hadith[68] that provide support for designating the woman who carries the pregnancy as the mother have recently been questioned by Islamic scholars and need to be clarified.

The Shia extrapolation of *mut'a* marriage for ARTs remains controversial, at least in the eyes of the Sunnis, and the Shias' tacit approval of donor sperm shielded by the veneer of an embryo label does not conform to conventional sharia norms. The legitimacy of anonymous egg and embryo donation without even a *mut'a* arrangement in Lebanon does not meet with the approval of most Shia scholars.

Scriptural hermeneutics and fatwas must give consideration to the plight of the infertile couple in line with the Islamic maxim, "Necessity overrides prohibition." The recent approval of abortion for rape, incest, or severe congenital abnormalities in Sunni Egypt and Shia Iran is in this sense commendable and hopefully will be followed by other countries. Sunnis appear not to share the Shia enthusiasm towards promoting sharia-compliant stem cell technologies, which may change with time. An increasing number of novel variations on genetic and molecular manipulation are in the research phase (with their clinical applications not too far away), which have the potential to create even more ethical, religious, and legal debate.

The current impasse across the Sunni-Shia divide appears difficult to reconcile, but at a minimum the dissonance within the Sunni and Shia camps needs to be addressed by encapsulating their differences within a pragmatic, workable framework to make interpretation easier for infertile couples, ART physicians, and Islamic scholars. The significance of religious dictates and the special nuances and controversies in the Islamic evaluation of ARTs that have been discussed in this chapter must continue to be placed on the agenda for meaningful intellectual debate.

Notes

1. "Wealth and children are the ornament of this life," Qur'an 18:46. "Children are God's *baraka*" (Qur'an 16:72).

2. "Marry those who can bear children. I will be pleased if you increase the numbers of the *Umma* [Muslim community]" Hadith—Ref Sonn Abu Dawood, 2/277–2050, Dar El-rayan Lltorath Publishing House, Cairo.

3. Sharia: Islamic law comprising Qur'an, hadith, *fiqh*, and contemporary fatwas.

4. *Maqasid al-sharia:* Imam Ghazzali, illustrious Islamic medieval theologian and jurist, condensed the essence of sharia to protection of life, religion, progeny, mind, and wealth, aimed at protecting humanity and providing the basis for most juristic deliberations.

5. *Istihsan:* juristic preference to provide a fairer solution where the conventional rule is detrimental or inappropriate for a particular case.

6. *Qawa'id al-fiqh (qawa'id kulliyah al-fiqhiyyah)* are epithetical abstracts of the vast edifice of *fiqh* and a valuable tool in "extracting the gems from the ocean of *fiqh.*" "Necessity overrides sharia prohibition," "No harm shall be inflicted or reciprocated," "No harm, no harrasment," are *qawa'ids* that command a general consensus of scholars, both Sunni and Shia, and are useful adjuncts in understanding the basis for evaluation of ARTs.

7. *Mujtahid:* an Islamic scholar learned in religion and sharia and capable of examining complicated legal issues and issuing appropriate fatwas.

8. *Ijtihad:* legal reasoning by Islamic jurists.

9. Fatwa: a legal response to a question by a *mujtahid.*

10. Shia *ijtihad* continued unabated, unlike that of the Sunnis who were denied this facility during the *taqlid* (blind imitation) era from the ninth to the nineteenth century.

11. *Marja'i:* the highest ranking Islamic jurist among Shia, well versed in both religion and sharia, who is selected or elected on his knowledge, competence, and piety.

12. Mufti: the highest ranking Islamic jurist among Sunnis, well versed in both religion and sharia, who is selected or elected on his knowledge, competence, and piety.

13. *Takhayyur:* borrowing doctrine from another *madhhab* (legal school).

14. *Siyasa sharia:* government in accordance with the goals and objectives of sharia.

15. Ayatholla Khamene'i's fatwa on extramarital conception and sperm donation.

16. Akham al khamsa: Fatwa ruling issued in a graded scale of five; permitted (halal).

17. "Do not take life, which Allah has made sacred except for just cause" (Qur'an 17:33).

18. "He has established the relationship of lineage and marriage" (Qur'an 25:54).

19. "Proclaim their real parentage. That will be more equitable in the sight of God" (Qur'an 33:4–5).

20. "Their mothers are those only who gave birth to them" (Qur'an 58:2).

21. Hadith, "The child is for the bed." In El-Bokari, in the book of El-Ahkam, 4/365–7182, Mansoura Publication House, Cairo.
22. Imam Ash'arī: Medieval Islamic scholar whose following constitutes 90 percent of the Muslim community.
23. Progressive scholars: elite largesse of erudite intellectuals, both Sunni and Shīa, educated in centers of higher learning and universities who challenge the restrictive dogma of the orthodox *ulama.*
24. *Tafsir:* interpretation of the Qur'an by adhering to accurate Arabic linguistics and lexicology, context of the revelation (*Asbab al-nuzul*) and abrogation (Rahman 2000).
25. *Ta'wil:* explanation of the Qur'an by understanding God's intentions (*maqasid*).
26. Ithna-Ash'ari Shia—mainstream Shi'a Islam who believe in the 12 Imams and form 80 percent of Shia mainly in Iran, Iraq, and Lebanon.
27. Hadith, "The creation of any one of you is … forty days as a drop (*nutfa*), then later a clot ('*alaqa*—forty days), then later a morsel of flesh (*mudgha*—forty days). The angel breathes the *ruh* into him." In El-Bokari, the book of El-Tawheed, 4/436–454, Mansoura Publication House, Cairo.
28. Complications of severe prematurity: neonatal deaths and prolonged neonatal intensive care with neurological handicaps, cerebral palsy, and retinal damage.
29 "But whoso is compelled by necessity, without wilful disobedience, not transgressing due limits, thy Lord is forgiving, most Merciful" (Qur'an 6:145).
30. *Rukhsa:* in special circumstances, concessionary alternative can replace strict sharia rule.
31. Prof. Ahmad Ragab, Al-Azhar University, personal communication, 2008.
32. *Maslaha:* public benefit; "God commands justice and good deeds" (Qur'an 27:90).

    Maslaha (public interest) for relieving hardship for the believers of Islam is an Islamic priority in all modern juristic deliberations. Law was dictated by divine wisdom for the promotion and protection of public good (Hallaq 1997b); "Wherever welfare is found, there exists the statute of God" (Hathout 1991).
33. *Istislah:* promoting and securing benefits and preventing and removing harm. Adaptability to meet the challenging needs of society. This is founded upon "circumventing hardship" as per Qur'anic verse, "God intends facility for you, and He does not want to put you in hardship" (2:185) and hadith, "The best of your law is that which brings ease to the people."
34. *Istihsan* is a breach of strict analogy for reasons of public interest (Schacht 1993b) to provide a fairer solution where the conventional rule is detrimental or inappropriate for a particular case. The basic intent of *istihsan* is to ensure that a literal application of the sharia must

not be allowed to defeat its higher objectives of justice and fair play (Kamali 2006a).

35. *Madhhabs:* —Hanafi, Maliki, Shafi'i, and Hanbali comprise the four Sunni legal schools.
36. Professor M. Hameed, Islamic College, Ealing, London, personal communication, 2007.
37. *Mut'a* marriage: a temporary marriage practiced exclusively by the Shia.
38. Al-Hakim, personal communication, 2008.
39. *Hiyal:* legal stratagem designed to circumvent a sharia obstacle.
40. *'Idda:* waiting period before remarriage after death or divorce.
41. Cytoplasm: intracellular medium surrounding the nucleus of the cell.
42. Messenger RNA serves as template for protein synthesis and carries information from DNA in the nucleus.
43. Embryo formed from egg of mother and sperm from donor.
44. "Their mothers are those only who gave birth to them" (Qur'an 58:2).
45. "The child is for the bed, the adulterer the stone," El-Bokari, in the book of El-Ahkam, 4/365–7182, Mansoura Publication House, Cairo.
46. Adoption: "Nor has He made your adopted sons, your sons ... Call them by (the names of) their fathers: that is more just in the sight of Allah" (Qur'an 33:5).
47. Ayatollah Khamene'i states that a surrogate is only providing a place to grow and need not even be a wife. It is not the same as *rida'* (milk kinship).
48. Mo'men (Ayatollah) 2006: 87, "*me'yār-e haqīqī-ye mādar būdan in ast ke nutfah-ye be wojūd āmadeh az tokhmak-e zan bāshad.*"
49. "Their mothers are those only who gave birth to them" (Qur'an 58:2).
50. "The child is for the bed, the adulterer the stone," El-Bokari, in the book of El-Ahkam, 4/365–7182, Mansoura Publication House, Cairo.
51. Correspondence by letter dated 11 October 2006, Qom.
52. Garmaroudi, this volume
53. "God has made for you (God's *baraka*) women (mates and companions) and out of them offspring" (Qur'an 16:72). "He has established the relationship of lineage and marriage" (Qur'an 25:54).
54. Huntington's Disease: genetic defect causing degeneration of brain cells.
55. Khamene'i' 1999: 281–83, question nos. 1271–72.
56. HIV: human immunodeficiency virus.
57. STDs: sexually transmitted diseases.
58. Autologous: ovaries from same individual.
59. Heterologous: ovaries from another woman.
60. Induced pluripotent cells: human cells reprogrammed to provide different cell types.
61. Embryogenesis: early embryo formation.
62. Teratogenesis: abnormalities of physiological development.
63. Somatic cell nuclear transfer is a process by which the nucleus from an egg is replaced by one from an ordinary body cell.

64. Professor Austin Smith, Stem Cell Institute, University of Edinburgh, personal communication, 2006.
65. Fertilization is initiated by injecting the nucleus of a cell (from the person to be cloned) into an egg.
66. SCNT: somatic cell nuclear transfer; iPS: induced pluripotent stem cells.
67. "Their mothers are only those who gave them birth" (Qur'an 58: 2).
68. "The child is for the bed, the adulterer the stone" (hadith).

References

Al-Hakim, A. H. 2005. "Flexible Marriage (Al-Mut'a)." In *Islam and Feminism.* London: Institute of Islamic Studies.

Asad, Muhammad. 1997. "A New Approach." In *This Law of Ours.* Gibraltar: Dar Al-Andalus.

Clarke, Morgan. 2009. *Islam and New Kinship: Reproductive Technology and the Shariah in Lebanon.* New York: Berghahn.

Coulson, Noel J. 1994. "Unity and Diversity in Conflicts and Tensions." In *Islamic Jurisprudence.* Chicago: University of Chicago Press.

Hallaq, Wael B. 1997a. "Crisis of Modernity." In *Islamic Legal Theories.* Cambridge: Cambridge University Press.

———.1997b. "The Legal Text, the World and History." In *Islamic Legal Theories.* Cambridge: Cambridge University Press.

Hathout, Hassan. 1991. "Islamic Derivation in Medical Bioethics." In *Proceedings of the First International Conference on Bioethics in Human Reproduction Research in the Muslim World.* Cairo.

Inhorn, Marcia. 2003. "Global Infertility and the Globalization of New Reproductive Technologies." *Social Science and Medicine* 56: 1837–51.

———. 2005. "Religion and Reproductive Technologies: IVF and Gamete Donation in the Muslim World." *Anthropology News:* 1–4.

———. 2006. "'He Won't Be My Son': Middle Eastern Muslim Men's Discourses of Adoption and Gamete Donation." *Medical Anthropology Quarterly* 20: 94–120.

Kahn, Susan M. 2000. *Reproducing Jews: A Cultural Account of Assisted Conception in Israel.* Durham: Duke University Press.

Kamali, M. Hashim. 2006a. "Characteristic Features of *Shariah.*" In *Shari'a.* Kuala Lumpur: Ilmiyah Publishers.

———. 2006b. "Goals and Purposes (Maqasid) of Shari'a." In *Shari'a.* Kuala Lumpur: Ilmiyah Publishers.

Mo'men (Ayatollah), 2006, p. 87: „ *me'yār-e haqīqī-ye mādar būdan in ast ke nutfah-ye be wojūd āmadeh az tokhmak-e zan bāshad".*

Nasr, S. Hossein. 1994. "Sunnism and Shi'ism." In *Ideals and Realities of Islam.* London: Aquarian Press.

Natour, Ahmed, Baha'eddin Bakri, and V. Rispler-Chaim. 2005. "An Islamic Perspective." In *The Embryo: Scientific Discovery and Medical Ethics,* ed. S. Blazer and E. Z. Zimmer. Basel: Karger.

Pennings, Guido, and Inge Liebaers,. 2002. "Parity for Donation—Conception with Subsequent Participation as a Donor." In *Ethical Dilemmas in Reproduction*, ed. F. Shenfield and C. Sureau. New York: Parthenon Publishing Group.

Rahman, Fazlur. 1979. "Origins and Development of the Tradition." In *Islam*. Chicago: University of Chicago Press.

———. 2000. "Later Medieval Reform." In *Revival and Reform in Islam*. Oxford: One World.

Sachedina, Abdulazeez. 2009a. "Introduction." In *Islamic Biomedical Ethics*. New York: Oxford University Press.

———. 2009b. "Terminating Early Life." In *Islamic Biomedical Ethics*. New York: Oxford University Press.

———. 2009c. "In Search of Principles of Healthcare Ethics in Islam." In *Islamic Biomedical Ethics*. New York: Oxford University Press.

———. 2009d. "Islamic Bioethics—Recent Developments." In *Islamic Biomedical Ethics*. New York: Oxford University Press.

Safi, Omid, ed. 2003. "Introduction." In *Progressive Muslims*. Oxford: One World.

Schacht. Joseph. 1993. "The Closing of the Gate of Independent Reasoning and the Further Development of Doctrine." In *An Introduction to Islamic Law*. Oxford: Clarendon Press.

Serour, Gamal I. 1993. "Bioethics in Artificial Reproduction in the Muslim World." *Bioethics* 23: 211.

———. 1995. "Bioethics in Medically Assisted Conception in the Muslim World." *Assisted Reproduction and Genetics* 12: 559–65.

———. 2000. "Pre-implantation Genetic Diagnosis." In *Ethical Implications of Human Embryo Research*. ISESCO.

Serour, Gamal I., and Bernard M. Dickens. 2001. "Assisted Reproduction Developments in the Islamic World." *International Journal of Gynecology & Obstetrics* 74: 189–90.

Serour, Gamal I., M. El-Ghar, and R. T. Mansour. 1991. "Infertility: A Health Problem in the Muslim World." *Popular Science* 10: 41–58.

Tabataba'i, Allamah MH. 1971. "Mut'a or Temporary Marriage—Appendix 11." In *Shi'a*. Qum, Iran: Ansaryan Publications.

Tremayne, Soraya. 2009. "Law, Ethics, and Donor Technologies in Shia Iran." In *Assisting Reproduction, Testing Genes: Global Encounters with New Biotechnologies*, eds. Daphna Birenbaum-Carmeli and Marcia C. Inhorn. Oxford: Berghahn Books.

Yacoub, Ahmed. 2001. "Reproduction and Cloning: Surrogate Wives and Polygamy." In *The Fiqh of Medicine*. London: Taha Publishers.

Zahedi, Farzaneh, and Bagher Larijani. 2008. "National Bioethical Legislation and Guidelines for Biomedical Research in the Islamic Republic of Iran." *Bulletin of the World Health Organization* 86(8): 577–656.

Part II

FROM SPERM DONATION TO STEM CELLS
THE IRANIAN ART REVOLUTION

PART II INTRODUCTION

Narges Erami

This next section includes chapters that simultaneously set challenges and elaborate on Muslim views on ARTs. Concentrating on Islamic bioethics, state law, theological verdicts and edicts, Shia Iran becomes the arena where people affected by the inability to have children must mediate between state legal latitude and theological moral longitude. Collectively the chapters offer a myriad of explanations and explicate the manifestations that permeate discussions in Iran about ARTs and the feasibility of third-party donations as overseen by the *ulama* and the nearly seventy clinics that have sprung up throughout Iran. Key issues that guide and motivate the questions that arise throughout the following section are how Shia Iran is different from other Muslim nations and how the various parties involved absorb those differences. It is a combination of Persian culture and Shia law, be it personal or state law, which guarantees the debates to take on new meanings in the Islamic Republic of Iran.

Robert Tappan's chapter lays out the challenges faced by families, clinicians and the *ulama* in regard to ARTs. The author elaborates upon the dynamic processes of Islamic bioethics in response to ARTs and how Shia law is practiced through specific cases at fertility clinics. The importance laid upon fatwas and the *marja' al-taqlid*, the one living religious leader whose work must serve as guidance for his followers, is often not enough in determining the answers to third-party donations. Tappan demonstrates how fatwas, casuistic clinic decision making, and theocratic state laws mitigate various factors. Maneuvering what appears to be complicated laws actually mirrors everyday life in Iran where decisions are made based on moral, societal, and legal barriers that appear often fluid and dynamic. Tappan draws on Islamic academician Abdulaziz Sachedina's scholarly intervention in developing a more "conservative" view upon reaching consensus on the ethical telos of ARTs.

Soraya Tremayne's clear and in-depth analysis echoes Tappan's argument on questioning the speed with which ARTs have been embraced in Iranian society. Tremayne massages the complexities that families must face when embracing third-party donations. What does it mean for the Islamic Republic of Iran to open up to third-party donations? By accounting detailed personal stories, Tremayne provides heart-wrenching life decisions faced by families and children who were products of third-party donations. The author elaborates on how such choices are gendered and alter realities of life for those seeking these technologies, explaining that "the use of third-party donation provides ample scope for a reinforcement of the patriarchal values in relation to reproduction."

Such patriarchal values take on new meanings with the practice of gestational surrogacy. Shirin Garmaroudi Naef's chapter is groundbreaking in detailing this practice in Muslim nations in general and Iran specifically. The author begins her analysis by first analyzing various Shia *ulamas'* conclusions on ARTs, and what takes precedence in establishing paternal rights, especially in the case of third-party donations. It is the case of establishing maternity with a surrogate's uterus where opinions differ. Ultimately by interviewing jurists and families involved in surrogacy, Garmaroudi Naef reveals the complex world of legality and illegality of illicit sex when it comes to bearing children. The ethico-moral dilemma of kinship and incest at times takes an inferior position to the birth of a child.

Mansooreh Saniei's chapter in many ways captures the essence of Iran's national vision of being at the forefront of technological advances and science in the twenty-first century. Human embryonic stem cell (ESC) research has been hotly debated globally, and theocratic Iran has embraced this technology in spite of the moral and ethical implications that surround new technologies. Saniei's research follows the inspirational message of Ayatollah Khamene'i, the supreme leader of the Islamic Republic, publicly applauding stem cell research with residual embryos from IVF procedures. ARTs and the resultant ESCs reveal cleavages in Iranian society that have left various clerics, clinicians, and families grasping for answers. The chapters in this section depict a discursive tradition that is burgeoning in Iranian society, but which has left more questions than clear directions for those afflicted by infertility and other forms of suffering.

Chapter 4

More Than Fatwas

Ethical Decision Making in Iranian Fertility Clinics

Robert Tappan

Introduction

The study of the bioethical decision making regarding the use of assisted reproductive technology (ART) in Iranian fertility clinics provides a lens with which to simultaneously examine the wider conception of Islamic bioethics. While the notion that Islamic bioethics is simply Islamic law, as expressed in the Muslim jurist's fatwa, is widespread among both Western academics and many Muslims themselves, clinical practices provide a glimpse of a more complex and involved process. Though Islamic law plays an important, even foundational, role in bioethical decision making in the clinics, Islamic bioethics cannot be reduced to and equated with the fatwas of the jurists.

Instead, clinicians and bioethics consultation groups[1] consider a range of justificatory sources, including civil laws, fatwas, reason, and bioethical cases from the West. But even as the clinical decision-making process in some clinics goes beyond mere reference to the fatwas, it does not seem to encompass the full scope and range of moral concern in bioethics, nor of bioethical reflection on the use of ART specifically.

Thus we do not find the clinics considering larger questions, such as the morality of certain techniques and technologies, or the ethical elaboration of their long-term effects on patients, society, and, especially, on the resulting children. So while clinicians deploy legal and rational resources beyond the fatwas, they are doing it largely in an instrumentalist manner, in order to bridge the gap between the fatwas, which simply say a procedure is permissible or impermissible, and the complex nature of the cases faced in clinical practice. But like the jurists, they are not addressing questions about the ethical rightness or wrongness of an action—why an act is morally justifiable or not, prior to its being ruled permissible or impermissible by the jurist, or before a clinical policy is adopted or a procedure is undertaken in a specific patient's case. Neither group has been able to articulate an Islamic bioethics that accounts for the deontological (duty-based ethics, judging an act as right or wrong because of its own nature, and not its effects) and teleological (an act is judged right or wrong based on its consequences) norms regarding the status of any particular act, as informed by the religious and cultural tradition in Islamic Iran.

However, a recent work by Abdulaziz Sachedina sets out to provide such an accounting of Islamic bioethics, and includes a discussion of ART. In the first section of this chapter I will present a descriptive overview of the state of infertility in Iran, as well as the clinical decision-making process as it stands currently. In the remainder of the chapter I will present Sachedina's approach to Islamic bioethics in a point-by-point manner, contrast it with the previous presentations, and examine how its principles and methods might impact ART in Iran, specifically.

Infertility in Iran

With rates of infertility averaging 14 percent worldwide (Bentley and Nicholas Mascie-Taylor 2000: 18), it should be no surprise that many Iranian couples are among those facing difficulty conceiving. Infertility in Iran probably ranges somewhere between a bare minimum of 5 percent and a high of 20 percent,[2] and upwards of fifty fertility clinics have sprung up throughout Iran in order to address the problem (Abbasi-Shavazi et al. 2008). These facilities are quite advanced in their technology and methods, with success rates comparable to the West.

Much as in the Western world, the rapidly developing biotechnologies that enable ART also raise complex moral and religious questions in Iran, particularly when a third party is involved, as in gamete or embryo donation or surrogacy. While Western academics have explored some of these issues in the Muslim world, until very recently most have been restricted largely to Sunni and Arab Muslims. Iran is different in key ways since it is a religiously Shia-majority country and its culture is predominantly Persian, not Arab. In addition, the Iranian state is an Islamic republic, which means religious-legal considerations are at play not only in the conscience of the individual believer but also in the state law, which is controlled by the religious establishment. Furthermore, there is a religious duty incumbent upon each Shia believer to follow the rulings of one high-ranking *marja' al-taqlid*. This leads to a plurality of equally authoritative religious rulings, which might differ greatly from one another, and may vary from the state law as well.

Iranian Fertility Clinics: General Points

Iranian fertility clinics are the loci where state law, culture, society, and religion intersect on ART. It is in the clinics that we can see some of the ways in which the Islamic juridical tradition is being articulated with reference to the fatwas, though with only limited reference to their underlying moral reasoning. But before looking at the clinical setting, we should first consider the general attitude toward ART among the religious scholars. This is crucial for several reasons. First, as mentioned above, every believer is supposed to refer to one of the high-ranking scholars for rulings on controversial issues in the interpersonal realm, including on matters such as ART. This applies not only to patients seeking guidance on these technologies but also to the medical staff who provide them. Second, the opinions of the jurists, represented by their fatwas on ART, serve as the primary grounds upon which clinical decisions are made. In the absence of the articulation of the moral foundations of the fatwas, or of another source of moral guidance altogether, the fatwas hold the de facto role as the major source of guidance for clinical decisions. This view is pervasive. As one of my informants in the clinics explained to me, even Iranians who do not care about religion in any other aspect of their lives attempt to make sure they follow the fatwas when it comes to birth, death, marriage, and divorce.[3] Finally, the fatwas require our consideration because they play a major part in shaping Iran's civil law.

In contrast to Catholicism, for example, Muslim scholars of both major schools—Sunni and Shia—agree on the permissibility of using any sort of ART methods as long as the techniques involve a married couple and their own gametes. When it comes to the issue of third-party donation of gametes or the use of a surrogate, Sunni scholars oppose all such procedures, while most Shia jurists permit many of them (see Mahmoud, this volume). The Shia jurists differ among themselves on the permissibility of the different procedures, though on certain issues, such as sperm donation, there is near unanimous opposition. The majority of the jurists' discussions regarding these procedures are focused on external considerations, such as the permissibility of using opposite-sex providers, masturbation to obtain semen, looking at and touching the patient's private parts, or the possible need for temporary marriage when an egg donor or surrogate mother is used. Despite these discussions, the jurists have failed to explore the very issue of the morality of ART (and its outcomes) itself.

Fatwas play an important role in the discussion of ART with regard to the individual believer's choices, as well as in each clinic's decision about which services it chooses to provide. Because the practice of referring to the *marja' al-taqlid*'s ruling is considered an obligation on the believer, and is so ingrained in Shia culture, we find constant reference to their rulings. Patients often bring in rulings approving or forbidding certain procedures (and insist on presenting them to clinicians, even when clinicians say the fatwas are not necessary for them to carry out the procedure), and clinics keep the scholars' legal guidebooks on hand to use with patients during pretreatment consultation (alongside civil legal and psychological counseling). Often patients will change their chosen scholar in order to use a procedure he forbids but another permits. Typically, the individual is expected to select and stick with one scholar, so making such a switch is not taken lightly and is one indication of the enormous pressures felt by infertile patients. As for the clinics, some choose to limit their procedures and services strictly in accord with the major religious-legal rulings. Individual physicians may elect not to perform particular procedures if forbidden by their chosen scholar, even if the clinic itself offers the treatment.

The fatwas are also of particular importance with regard to the Iranian legal system. In postrevolutionary Iran, an effort has been made to bring the state's civil law into conformity with Islamic law.

Indeed, the ultimate arbiter for what can be done in Iranian fertility clinics is the law of the state, despite the ruling of any individual scholar's fatwa for or against any particular technique. It must be remembered that in Iran, any civil law passed by the parliament must be approved by the Council of Guardians, a body of Islamic and civil jurists who can send legislation back to the parliament if they feel it violates Islamic law.

Certain procedures relevant to ART, such as embryo donation, have been legislated by the state. Where a civil law exists, the clinic cannot perform any procedure forbidden by that law, even if such an act is permitted by a religious scholar. However, there are some gray areas in the civil law where a procedure has been neither forbidden nor authorized by the civil law. In these instances where the law is silent, such as on gamete donation, the clinician and the patient can refer to the fatwas of the jurists and proceed according to those rulings.[4]

This means that the fatwas play two roles in relation to the state law. In the first instance, when the civil law permits or is silent on an issue, patients and clinicians can refer to the religious-legal rulings to decide which procedures to use or to avoid. In the second case, there is an effort by clinicians and institutes to seek fatwas from the highest ranking scholars on contentious points of ART. The medical experts attempt to educate the authoritative religious scholars through meetings and presentations, in an attempt to communicate the complex scientific aspects of a new technique, in order to facilitate a fatwa permitting its use. These rulings are then presented to the government's legislative organs in order to pass a law, like the Embryo Donation Act mentioned above.

The Clinical Decision-Making Process

As we saw, both civil law and religious-legal rulings affect the pursuit of ART methods in Iranian clinics. But the decision-making procedure involves more than that. Similar in some ways to their Western counterparts, Iranian fertility clinics have ethics consultation groups or oversight committees that decide which procedures the clinic will offer. The typical composition of a committee includes a religious scholar in addition to the standard mix of physicians, lawyers, and psychologists. This religious scholar will provide a sense of the religious-legal issues at stake regarding a certain procedure, as well as the rulings of a range of Islamic scholars on the topic under consideration. Again, this is primarily limited to presentation of the permissibility or impermissibility of certain procedures, and the concerns related to touching, the need or not of temporary marriage for donors, from whom the child will inherit, and so on. According to one of my contacts, if the clinic or committee is "secular," they might well approve of and offer any legally permissible technique, as well as any technique on which the law is silent. If the clinic or committee is "religious" or "ethical," in his terms, they will try to follow the well-known fatwas on any particular procedure.

In some clinics the committees simply stop at the level of religious rulings. Their religious discourse about any particular procedure ends by reference to the rulings of the religious scholars, without arguing, reasoning, or asking further about them. However, the discussion in some clinics goes beyond reference to state law and religious-legal opinions. After considering both of these elements, the committee then holds open-ended debate using any rational sources, including reference to philosophical or bioethical arguments articulated in other countries, or analyses of similar cases from foreign countries.

At the two major ART clinics I visited, committee members were said to be familiar with European and American bioethical approaches and issues, for example, but they did not simply adopt these elements wholesale. Rather, they incorporate them into the larger religious and cultural system as seems relevant in the Iranian context. However, it appeared that this usage was largely limited to functional outcomes. In other words, there did not seem to be a thorough engagement with Western bioethical systems in a cross-cultural manner to evaluate their theoretical and foundational approaches. Instead, the encounters seem to be confined to consideration of particular cases seen in the Western bioethics literature. Thus, a clinic might decide to only use anonymous donors, because of declines in donor participation seen in Western countries when donor anonymity was removed.

The Limitations of Fatwas as Seen in the Clinics

We have seen so far that certain religious sensibilities symbolized by the fatwas play a central role for the oversight committees in the Iranian clinics. Those rulings serve as the starting point and overarching guide for their discussions, even among those committees that consider themselves flexible in utilizing a number of sources.

However, even when the religious rulings serve this foundational role, there is still a sense that the scholars' rulings that a particular procedure (such as embryo donation) is either permitted or forbidden "in itself" (in the language of the jurists) are insufficient to address all of the ethical concerns that will result from its use. Usually these rulings are given in a discrete form, without a sense of a systematic overview—just if permitted in the general case at hand or not. Often a jurist may extrapolate on some of the immediate effects of an issue. In the case of embryo donation, for example, they often discuss religious-legal points that historically have been prominent considerations in Islamic law, such as from whom the child should inherit or whom the child can touch or marry.

But these rulings fail to consider a host of other issues. Fatwas alone seem incapable of encompassing the full range and scope of complex bioethical concerns. In the case of embryo donation, little, if any, attention has been paid to questions such as whether children should be given data about their genetic parents later in life, or if donors should remain anonymous, or how to prevent accidental incest among the children of anonymous donors, and similar problems that are addressed in the Western bioethical literature. This confirms Sachedina's point that while Islamic law includes rulings classified as "medical jurisprudence," this is not equivalent to the contemporary notion of bioethics as a field (2008: 244).

The efforts of the clinics to address the concerns of the fatwas when faced with the clinical realities of specific cases represent one aspect of the attempt to articulate a more comprehensive system of Islamic bioethics. One element of this is the attempt to work with jurists in order to avoid arbitrary or inconsistent fatwas. Several clinicians complained that the way a question is put to the jurist might affect the response, even leading the same jurist, given the same question, to provide a contrary answer in two different instances, simply due to the phrasing of the question (Clarke 2005). It seems the clinicians want more reliable and thought-out religious-legal guidelines with which to work. Mahmoud's chapter in this volume further highlights the difficulties faced by clinicians as they attempt to navigate between a range of often widely varying fatwas and the needs of their patients.

This is also the reason that clinicians make detailed presentations of ART issues to the religious scholars. Employing the findings of international conferences involving Islamic religious scholars, psychologists, lawyers, physicians, sociologists, anthropologists, and many other types of specialists, along with videos, case studies, and other media, clinicians and institutes attempt to provide the scholars with a thorough overview of the issues, as they see them, involved with ART. As mentioned earlier, they then seek to use those rulings to promote state law.

Thus we find the clinicians are faced with addressing a number of bioethical issues that have fallen outside the purview of the rulings of the religious scholars. Using rational methods and with reference to international bioethical cases and solutions mentioned earlier, the clinicians and oversight committees attempt to flesh out these points. A cluster of issues jumps out from the subject of egg donation, for example. While a number of high-ranking Islamic scholars have approved the process, for the most part, those religious-legal rulings have simply said that the act is "permissible in itself," meaning it is religiously acceptable to give or receive a donor egg. While some scholars may have provided a few subsidiary rulings, such as who is considered the mother from the religious perspective (donor mother, gestational mother, or both), or from whom the resulting child should inherit (the owner of the genetic material or the gestational mother), they cannot, or at least have not, addressed other points normally considered under the rubric of bioethical concern with regard to ART.

This includes discussion over whether egg donation should be anonymous or if it can be done with known donors. If it is done anonymously, how can one protect against accidental incest between the child of a donor egg and the birth child of the donor? If a known donor is used, should the resulting children be told? Do the possible psychological harms to the recipient parents outweigh the psychological benefits they are seeking through using the eggs of a family member? Should egg donors be paid, and if so, does that expose them to exploitation? The fatwas are unable to weigh and balance these competing interests, which lie at the heart of bioethics.

In the absence of guidance from the fatwas, the oversight committees look to other sources for direction and craft their own responses. Thus one clinic sets a limit of five eggs from any one donor to ensure a statistically insignificant chance of accidental incest. Another clinic allows known donation so that they can provide the service to couples who will only use an egg from a trusted relative, while another clinic only allows anonymous donation in order to avoid the problems that can arise from such a close transaction. These are reasonable steps to take, and reflect various clinical bioethical policies and decisions found in other countries.

Problems and Shortcomings on the Clinical Side

These are the sorts of issues that illustrate how Islamic bioethics encompasses more than reference to the fatwas, including the active role of the clinicians and their contributions to Islamic bioethics. But here too we find some notable shortcomings. In much the same way that the religious jurists' fatwas are general and focused mainly on ruling whether a procedure is religiously permissible, in order to attempt to alleviate the very real suffering of their followers, the clinicians are highly motivated to aid their patients as much as possible. As Tremayne wrote regarding the clinicians, their main concerns are the health of their patients and their success rates (2009: 159–60).

However, in their sincere desire to provide ART services to infertile couples, the clinicians might be overlooking other key bioethical points. One major issue in particular stuck in my mind—the absence of discussion about the children who will be born from these procedures. The clinicians, like the religious scholars, are focused on providing whichever legally permissible services they can so that the suffering patients can try to have a child. Thus, they might prefer to use unknown donors in order to protect the donors from the claims of these children for inheritance later in life, or to protect the parents who receive embryos or gametes from the owners of those materials staking a claim to the child at a later date. Anonymous donation also makes the supply of gametes larger, since donors do not have to worry about later repercussions and so are more inclined to participate. The emphasis on anonymity might also include a sense of trying to keep the child from the psychological trauma of learning that his "real" parents are not raising him.

Yet, at the very least, it neglects the child's right to information about his genetic health. If clinics fear to keep donor records in the event a child subpoenas them for inheritance claims, this lack of information can have deleterious effects on the lives of the children. We have already seen tragic cases in the Western bioethical literature of children who develop severe genetic illnesses from gamete donors.[5] Less dramatic, but perhaps more important, are genetic gauges of health—histories of heart disease, diabetes, cancer, or psychological problems that offspring ought to be aware of for their own medical treatment. Yet neither of the major clinics I researched had a system in place to maintain this genetic information.

The efforts of both religious scholars and clinicians in addressing ART in Iran provide a case study for a different approach to Islamic bioethics. Perhaps the most detailed example of a different perspective can be found in Abdulaziz Sachedina's recent work on Islamic bioethics, which culminated in his book *Islamic Biomedical Ethics: Principles and Application* (2009). Sachedina is one of the leading contemporary Muslim public intellectuals, alongside scholars such as Khaled Abou El Fadl and Abdulkarim Soroush. His undergraduate training occurred partly in Iran, where he studied with the renowned Iranian intellectual Ali Shariati. Sachedina received his PhD from the University of Toronto, is a professor in the Department of Religious Studies at the University of Virginia, and spent much of the first part of his academic career working on Shi'ism. More recently he has written a series of books presenting his approach to Islam and democracy, religious pluralism, Islam and human rights, and Islamic biomedical ethics. His opinion is often sought in the public sphere, such as when he provided testimony on Islam and human cloning to the United States Senate.

Sachedina's approach is important in that it is one of the very few that gives a detailed picture of the complexity of Islamic religious concerns in light of biomedical advances. The approach is already gaining traction among some Muslim thinkers, and despite the anticipated defensiveness of the Muslim seminaries (Sachedina 2009), it is likely that Sachedina's arguments will occupy a place of primacy in the discussion of Islamic bioethics for some time to come. Both his theoretical approach to Islamic bioethics generally, as well as his specific arguments about ART and related topics, will be applied here to the case of ART in Iran.

Which Islam?

The first point of value for the discussion of Islamic bioethics generally, and our specific case of ART in Iran, is found in Sachedina's discussion of Islam and Muslims. One of the shortcomings of the study of ART and Islamic bioethics thus far has been a rather simplistic classification of Muslims (in this case, Iranian Muslims) as either "religious" or "nonreligious," with attendant effects on the decisions they make about their health care. While there are certainly those who were born as Muslims and have left religion and religious concerns completely, this number is quite small, and is in any case not merely the opposite of being "religious," which is typically portrayed in the social scientific literature as scrupulous adherence to the religious-legal rulings of the Muslim jurisprudent. Instead, it is more appropriate and useful to perceive and acknowledge various types of Islam and Muslims.

Sachedina offers three broad, but not exhaustive, categories, and it is the third that seems to have been identified as "religious Muslims" by social scientists. This classification includes the perception of Islam as the unique and exclusive experience of the truth, with morality and religious fulfillment essentially limited to adherence to traditional interpretations and methods of religious law. This type is identified with the seminaries and traditional religious scholars, and with the majority of the members of any particular Muslim society (Sachedina 2009). This shares many similarities with Soroush's tripartite division of the "types of religiosity." In Soroush's classification, this type of Islam would be called "utilitarian" or "pragmatic" and is characterized by being legalistic, hereditary, and identity based. Like Sachedina, Soroush holds that this approach is favored by the clergy and the masses, and largely ignores morality in favor of amassing religious merit through sheer volume of religious ritual performance and obedience to religious law (Soroush 2000).

This also makes clearer the position of those Iranian patients mentioned earlier whose only religious concern involves securing a guiding fatwa at certain critical life stages, or who change out their former religious scholar for one with a more permissive fatwa on an ART technique that the person hopes to use. These are not people and actions that can be regarded as simply either "religious" or "nonreligious," but of a particular approach to religion. The presentation in this volume on ART in Turkey by Gürtin provides another opportunity to go beyond simple contrasts of "religious" and "nonreligious," or "religious" and "secular."

Whether these authors' remaining categories overlap, and to what degree, is beyond the scope of this chapter. However, the arguments of both highlight the fact that we do not find a simple split between "religious" and "nonreligious" Muslim patients, but that, except for a limited number of cases where the person has totally forsaken religion, we are instead talking about varieties of religious orientation. Furthermore, to identify religion as solely the fatwa or ritual runs the risk of reductionism. So while the fatwa-focused description of many Iranian Muslims is correct to a degree, consideration of the religious lives of Muslims ought to encompass more than the body of fatwa literature and ritual practices. This is especially important if we are to identify an Islamic bioethics that can provide deep and systematic ethical justifications for medical practices in light of Islamic beliefs, as well as provide common points of moral understanding and dialogue with medical ethicists from non-Muslim countries and cultures.

What Ethics?

Another element missing from the discussion of Islamic bioethics, including the literature about ART in Islam, is a thorough presentation of Islamic ethics itself. We saw earlier that as a practical matter, the fatwa literature cannot encompass the full range of bioethical concerns that confront clinicians and that stand to impact the wider society. While the clinicians have attempted to use the fatwas as a basis from which to elaborate an Islamic bioethics, we saw that they too ran into significant problems. The issues faced by the clinicians, as reflective of bioethics on a wider scale, do not seem resolvable by either more fatwas or more oversight committee debates on issues not covered by the fatwas. In both cases it seems that these methods, while they should be a part of the process of Islamic bioethics, are insufficient on their own to impart confidence in a full reflection of the moral and religious consequences of ART.

Sachedina has initiated a critique and analysis of the relationship between juristic rulings and ethics, and their respective roles in Islamic bioethics, which departs from the fatwa-centered presentations of other authors, and to which we now turn. Ultimately, limiting Islamic bioethics to collecting and reporting the fatwas, as has been done by both Western and Muslim scholars and physicians, has failed to address the underlying and essential question of "what is ethical conduct in Islam?" (Sachedina 2009: 27).

Throughout his work, Sachedina makes the case that, despite the ultimate grounding of juridical rulings in theology and theological ethics (which we will examine below), jurists have largely ignored the ethical issues at stake in any particular bioethical case when they issue their fatwa (Sachedina 2009). Thus, even though the jurists are basing their fatwas on legal principles with grounds in theological-ethical principles, they are not engaging in any reflection on those ethical roots, but are instead simply working from within the well-established legal principles that are familiar to them (Sachedina 2009). So we find that despite rulings forbidding or permitting the use of various new biotechnological procedures, the scholars have not engaged with the moral teachings in the foundational Islamic sources (Sachedina 2009).[6]

This criticism is a more refined take on the approach to law and ethics presented by the late Fazlur Rahman. Rahman claimed that jurists had favored the easily identifiable legal principles from the revelatory sources over the broader but more significant and more frequently mentioned ethical teachings found there. Rahman's suggestion was that the theological-ethical principles of the revelation ought to first be elaborated, and only then should legal principles and rules be derived from them (Rahman 1983).

Both views are vindicated in the actions of the clinicians we saw earlier. The clinicians, desperate for more detailed guidance for their clinical practices, host conferences where religious scholars participate and make detailed presentations of new ART procedures to scholars in the hopes of receiving fatwas based on the scientific realities of the technologies in order to guide their clinical practices in a religiously ethical manner. But perhaps they are asking the wrong questions.

We can see also how limiting the ethics of ART in Islam to the fatwas can be misleading to Western researchers. If it is assumed that the fatwa literature represents the full depth of Islamic bioethical thought on a matter, then when an Islamic scholar issues a ruling stating, for example, that egg donation is permissible, this seems like a major shift in the religious culture. Claims of changing notions of kinship among Muslims or similar conclusions might be reached that, while perhaps reflective of the use by desperate patients to treat their infertility through recourse to a fatwa stating a given procedure is permissible, are not ultimately indicative of any sort of coherent thinking about the range of ethical quandaries related to the act of egg donation or to well-conceived notions of new forms of kinship and relatedness. In fact, the desperate use of such techniques might actually indicate the lack of serious reflection on kinship. Serious issues involving relatedness might only rear their heads much later after the use of the technology.

Likewise, this spills over to claims of bold *ijtihad* in some of the Western literature on ART in Iran. On the one hand, yes, Iranian jurists (and Shia jurists generally) are issuing rulings that are often quite at odds with Muslim jurists elsewhere, particularly with regard to the permissive use of third-party donation and surrogacy. One might argue that *ijtihad* in the specific legal definition of the act of providing a new ruling based on reasoned jurisprudence does occur with these fatwas. But the changes identified as vibrant *ijtihad* are not representative of the far-reaching and innovative thinking about new biomedical ethical cases and technologies that these scholars might have expected to find. *Ijtihad* of that scale and substance would need to come through the engagement of Islamic scholars with the theological-ethical underpinnings of the legal principles and methodology. This grander movement has yet to materialize among the scholarly classes in Iran and other Muslim societies, although it parallels what Sachedina argues for below.

Culture and Religion

The continuum of culture and religion provides another ground for examining the inadequacy of the assumption that fatwas are indicative of Islamic bioethics. If we understand ethics in its traditional sense, then we must acknowledge that it is the evaluation of the rightness or wrongness of human actions. Islamic ethics is no different. It too is the search for ways of making decisions regarding the goodness or badness of any particular act (Sachedina 2009). One of the key factors in evaluating an act is the role of context—the act's location in time and space. While there may be certain a priori valuations applied to acts, principles, or rules irrespective of context, those must be reevaluated on a case-by-case basis depending upon relevant contextual circumstances. Thus, Islamic bioethics, like Islamic ethics itself, is going to be a mix of these timeless and time-bound norms (Sachedina 2009).

Yet the typical fatwa, in its evaluation of an act as either permissible or forbidden, does not lend itself to this understanding of Islamic ethics. The categorical nature of the fatwa brings an end to the exploration of the rightness or wrongness of an action. In bioethics, it limits the contextual considerations of the factors unique to each clinical case, which must be part of the moral calculus (Sachedina 2009). In doing so, it fails to resolve convincingly the conflicting claims presented in the case (Sachedina 2009).

This gives us further insight into the actual problems we saw clinicians wrestling with earlier. Even armed with the fatwas, the clinicians still find themselves without an adequate sense of the religious-ethical parameters when implementing certain techniques or when considering the unique factors of a particular patient's case. We witnessed the clinicians being forced to do much of the heavy lifting as they tried to elaborate moral guidelines without much religious input beyond an act's being permissible or forbidden, and perhaps some subsidiary rulings on inheritance or veiling, which led them towards some potentially serious ethical shortcomings.

This also accounts for the efforts the clinicians undertake in order to inform the jurists about the specifics of certain types of ART in order that the fatwas they give might better reflect these considerations, and hence be more useful to the clinicians. Yet even if specific rulings are given on specific techniques, and even if those are enshrined in law in the hopes of making their use ethically clear and to protect the clinicians from any legal judgment, they have failed so far to address the moral dilemmas of ART in a wholly satisfactory manner.

Clarke's dissertation on ART in Lebanon touches on some of these points as well. His work led him to question the wisdom of focusing solely on the fatwas. In the course of his research, he found that the fatwa was just one of the ways that religious scholars gave advice and responded to the dilemmas faced by their followers. Very often their guidance was based on considerations of the local sociocultural norms rather than on explicit reference to the revelatory texts, legal principles, or theological points (Clarke 2005). He later concludes that despite any officially stated ruling on a topic, the jurists will always have to give situation-specific guidance for individual cases (Clarke 2005). While this analysis is somewhat different from what Sachedina is suggesting, it does indicate the importance of the sociocultural context to the resolution of a moral dilemma, and further illustrates the pitfalls of limiting the investigation of Islamic bioethics only to the fatwas. So while we must avoid inadvertently equating culturally based beliefs and practices with religion on the one hand, we must also recognize that the contextual setting of an ethical question plays a central, often determining, role in its resolution, and that this context is provided by the culture.

An Alternative Approach to ART and Islamic Bioethics

Having seen the problems and snags of most previous approaches to Islamic bioethics, we can now take up Sachedina's arguments for what Islamic bioethics should include. Most essential is his presentation of the relationship of Islamic ethics to Islamic law. Rather than reading ethics as the outcome of the legal rulings, he makes the case that ethics, grounded in theology, precedes (and ideally is reflected in) the fatwa. However, this ideal has been largely unrealized due to the widespread disinterest of the jurists in pursuing these foundations of jurisprudence (Sachedina 2009).

Beyond that, he argues that bioethics in Islam is properly explored under the rubric of social ethics, rather than merely through
the fatwas, as most have done so far (Sachedina 2009). This is important not only for the methodology that he will elaborate but
also because it is the only way to make Islamic bioethics commu-
nicable across cultures, which then permits Muslims and others to
find rational common ground from which to address global biotechnological issues (Sachedina 2009). At its core, the fatwa cannot do
this. Although a fatwa ultimately does (or should) embody rational
moral principles, elaborated in a reasoned way (particularly in the
Shia tradition), at the practical level of cross-cultural discussion, the
fatwa literature alone is mainly a conversation stopper. Thus to really give Islam a place at the table of global ethics, we must look at
the steps and grounds that precede the ruling.

The source of Islamic ethics that ought to inform the fatwas is not
simply an amalgam of Islamic-themed analogues of the dominant
Western bioethical paradigm of the four principles.[7] In Sachedina's
estimation, these Muslim scholars (who are frequently physicians)
have not paid proper attention to the theological-moral discourse
that then manifests in the legal-ethical system of Islamic law (2009).
Just as with the jurists and those who only locate Islamic bioethics
in the fatwas, the scholars who have tried to import the four principles methodology directly into Islamic biomedical ethics have also
missed the mark.

Part of the problem with the approach above revolves around the
historical development of biomedical ethics as a field of inquiry in
the West, particularly in the United States. Historically, all cultures
have had expectations of virtuous behavior and professionalism of
their healers, which were called "medical ethics." In 1960s America,
a confluence of social issues, technological advances, and research
scandals led to the creation of the field of biomedical ethics. No longer were issues of medical import regarded as limited to a physician's
virtuous behavior and professional duties. Instead, matters related
to biomedicine in its broadest form came to the fore, as technology
enabled the use of respirators and ventilators—raising the new issues of brain death and organ transplantation—contraception and
abortion became more widely available, and dialysis machines could
prolong life, but were scarce resources that needed to be fairly allo-
cated. Research scandals at the Jewish Chronic Disease Hospital and
the Willowbrook State Hospital, and in Tuskegee, Alabama, raised
questions first seen at the Nuremberg Trials following World War II.
The general social atmosphere of civil rights, feminism, and antiwar

sentiment led to increased scrutiny of medical and related scientific matters, thus going beyond medical ethics into biomedical ethics (Kuhse and Singer 2001).

This context was not replicated throughout the world, and hence we can see the problem in elevating autonomy, for example, as a key bioethical principle in societies with a strong communal ethic. However, there was also a shift in Muslim countries from medical ethics towards biomedical ethics in the contemporary period (Rahman 1998). In this case, the importation of these new technologies required engagement at the sociocultural and religious levels, and necessitated public policy discussions about their use and distribution. Hence we find a growing discussion of a field of Islamic biomedical ethics—rather than simply the medical ethics of physicians—among Muslim thinkers, with those like Sachedina attempting to formulate an approach that is based in the normative religious sources and sociocultural concerns of Muslims.

While a full presentation and analysis of Sachedina's proposed approach to Islamic bioethics is more than can be explored in this chapter, we should be familiar with the key points so that we can understand how they might shape the future course of discussion on ART in Iran. Despite his earlier criticism of jurists, and especially of their fatwas that simply identify various aspects of ART as permissible or impermissible, Sachedina is not calling for jurisprudence to be left out of the equation of bioethics; in fact, quite the opposite. While there is a certain strain of thought among some Iranian intellectuals that calls for the limitation of the scope of jurisprudence to the *'ibadat,* or religious observances that occur between the believer and God (such as prayer and fasting), and the removal from their purview of the *mu'amalat,* or realm of social transactions (and also the location of social ethics in Islam), Sachedina holds that this sphere is indeed within the influence of the jurists (Sachedina 2009).

What he is attempting to do is to get Muslim jurists to take the moral discourse seriously. He ties ethical reflection to the field of jurisprudence and its process of searching the normative sources in order to find support for new legal-moral decisions (Sachedina 2009). This is not to say that jurisprudence is solely an exercise in taking a clear textual proof on a matter and then relating that to a new case. Rather, particularly in the Shia and Mu'tazila Sunni theological schools, reason is given a substantive role in the process (unlike in the Ash'ari Sunni school where reason simply serves a formal purpose to understand the scriptural directives). This creates a linkage between human moral judgment and divine commandments (Sachedina 2009). As such, this means that human reason very often can discover and know the moral status of an act, assessing it to be good or evil, right or wrong, even without reference to revelation, or that reason can identify underlying principles in revelation, such as justice, as entities in their own right, rather than defining justice solely by a literal mention in the religious texts (Hourani 1971).

This foundation allows Sachedina to move towards a presentation of several key legal principles, which are bounded and informed by theological reflection, and which can facilitate Islamic bioethical decision making. The most important of these is *maslaha*, a general principle that gives rise to several other principles and rules key to Islamic bioethics (see Houot, this volume). This principle can be employed to find solutions to the majority of bioethical conundrums and contains the rational obligation to weigh and balance any particular act's possible harms and benefits (Sachedina 2009).

While *maslaha* is a legal principle, its parameters and nature are defined through theology. As touched on above, there is a difference in approach between the divine command ethics (i.e., "good" is what God says is "good" in the revelation) of the Ash'ari Sunnis and the objectivist rationalist ethics (i.e., God-given human reason and intuition can identify what is "good," even without revelation) of the Mu'tazila Sunnis and Shia. Relevant for our case, this means that, theoretically, the Shia school prominent in Iran would be able to employ the principle of public interest inductively to make legal-ethical judgments about technologies not discussed in the revelatory sources, and which are located in changing contexts. It also implies that the competing interests that naturally arise in the consideration of the public good need to be thoroughly examined before any ruling is given (Sachedina 2009).

Though Sachedina is advocating for the status of public good as a key principle in legal-ethical thought, traditionally Shia scholars did not consider it as such. However, and apropos to our considerations here, public good came to the forefront in Shia jurisprudence with the Iranian Revolution and the need to provide legal-ethical rulings in the administration of the state (Sachedina 2009). A related notion, that of *'urf* or custom, plays a similar role in Sachedina's thinking, and was likewise influenced in the Shia world by the post-revolutionary circumstances in Iran. Custom is related to the public good in that rationally determining the common interest at any point in time necessarily must factor into consideration the unique contextual setting of that time. While custom is also controversial in its status as a jurisprudential principle, again, the Iranian Revolution led Ayatollah Khomeini to recognize the prime role of custom and time and place in jurisprudence. In fact, Khomeini declared that time and place are the two most important elements for the jurist to consider in formulating a ruling (Sachedina 2009). Thus, these elements of Sachedina's approach to Islamic bioethics may well find relatively easy acceptance among Iranian scholars.

A final, though essential, principle Sachedina identifies for Islamic bioethics is "no harm, no harassment in Islam." The principle of "no harm, no harassment" is widely accepted by all schools of Muslim thought and is key to rulings of Islamic social ethics, including bioethical dilemmas (Sachedina 2009: 66–67). It also gives birth to ethically important subsidiary rules such as "Hardship necessitates relief," "Preventing harm has a priority over promoting good," and "Protection from distress and impairment" (Sachedina 2009: 71, 74). Custom also plays a role with regard to "No harm, no harassment" by serving to define "harm" and "harassment." Having indicated the key jurisprudential principles in Islamic bioethics, we can now move to consider them in relation to ART, and to ART in Iran in particular.

ART in Light of Islamic Bioethics

With the framework of this new approach to Islam bioethics established, we will first examine Sachedina's general comments about ART, and then view our earlier points about ART in Iran in this new light. It is worthwhile to start with a brief examination of why infertile Muslim couples are willing to undergo ART procedures that are often invasive, expensive, embarrassing, and ineffective. The question of reproduction illustrates the need for Islamic scholars to investigate the nature and purposes of marriage further, particularly in the current day. This chapter cannot go deeply into this question, but we can touch on some of the points of tension.

On one side of the equation we have some evidence from the religious sources indicating the desirability, perhaps even the obligation, for a married couple to have children. While the Qur'an itself does not explicitly define the goal of marriage and sexuality as reproduction, the connection is made implicitly.[8] Two important Islamic prophets, Abraham and Zechariah, have the burden of their infertility displayed in several Qur'anic passages. In both cases, the men and their wives overcome their infertility with God's aid. Beyond this, many commentators of the Qur'an as well as Muslim scholars writing on family, whether in the classical period or even today, insist that producing offspring is a major purpose of marriage, if not the main purpose altogether. Cultural attitudes reflect this, seeing reproduction as a sort of "divinely ordained obligation" (Sachedina 2009: 127).

Yet the Qur'an is quite explicit that procreation is not the sole purpose, nor perhaps even the highest purpose, of marriage. Rather than being portrayed as reproductive partners, the husband and wife are presented in the Qur'an as loving supports for one another:

> And of His signs is this: He created for you spouses from yourselves that you might find rest in them, and He ordained between you love and mercy. In this indeed are signs for people who reflect. (Q 30:21).

> They [your wives] are garments for you and you are garments for them. (Q 2:187)

> He it is who did create you from a single soul, and from it made his mate that he might take rest in her. (Q 7:189)

Here the Qur'an has presented us with a deep sense of the essential relationship between spouses. The wife and husband, according to these verses, have a role to play that goes beyond anything else that might arise from the marriage bond and that supersedes any other role. That role is to serve as a source of comfort, rest, love, and mercy to the other. Sachedina agrees with this view (2009).

In fact, the pressures felt by infertile couples to reproduce stem from Muslim cultures, not from Islam. We can find ample evidence of this in the case of Iran. Tremayne has discussed the relationship of reproductive capacity with the notion of "face" or social standing in Iranian society. The inability to have children is a major blow to one's social position in Iran, with many negative consequences for the infertile (Tremayne 2006: 29). There is also a lingering pronatalist tendency in Iran that is conditioned by the country's unique recent history. Iran undertook a formal family planning program in 1967 at the behest of Shah Reza Pahlavi. Many Iranian clerics saw population control programs as Western imperialistic efforts to limit the number and strength of Muslims. Hence, with the Iranian Revolution of 1979, this program fell out of favor (though contraceptives remained available and religiously permissible), and the Islamic government began to promote policies such as early marriage (and the religiously permissible temporary marriage) that aimed to prevent religiously illicit sexual relations and to strengthen the family, and thus the society, through population growth (Hoodfar and Assadpour 2000). An additional factor was the nearly decade-long Iran-Iraq war. Iran suffered heavy casualties, and thus Iranian women were strongly encouraged to marry early and to have children (Obermeyer 1994). Though the Iranian government has reversed its pronatalist policy in the wake of a population boom, it would not be unreasonable to assume that the effect of the previous policy on the cultural and religious sensibility of Iranians continues to inform their desire for children. Thus, Sachedina is correct in his assessment that infertility in Muslim societies needs to be treated for social and psychological reasons (Sachedina 2009).

But Sachedina's bioethical analysis leads to a dramatically different stance on the use of ARTs, particularly those involving third-party donation of gametes or embryos, than that of many Iranian clinicians and jurists. He ultimately bases his position around the right of any child born to have an "unblemished lineage." He identifies this issue of the protection and clarity of lineage to be so strong in Islam that it is considered one of the main purposes of the religious law and to be an "inalienable right" of the child (2009: 103).

This is not so different from what many of the traditional jurists who are opposed to third-party donations have stated. But Sachedina has gone further than their responses, which are typically limited to superficial statements about the child's lineage and inheritance. He provides a theological-ethical basis for this, based on prophetic guidance to parents to raise children to become "virtuous and healthy member[s] of the family and society." Because of the Muslim cultural stigma against children without proper lineage, those children will face a lifetime of discrimination, psychological suffering, and other violations of their human rights, in addition to the financial instability posed by being cut of from their father's property (Sachedina 2009: 107).

He raises related points that have not been treated in previous discussions of ART in Islam as well. Much like my own observation regarding anonymous gamete donation in Iran, Sachedina argues that such donations deprive the resulting child of important genetic information about his biological parent(s), leaving the child susceptible to a range of medical and psychological problems (Sachedina 2009). Again, this is not a mere violation of an obscure point of Islamic law, but a violation of the child's essential human rights. Tremayne's chapter in this volume further illustrates the very real harms suffered by these children (as well as the parents) in her detailed case studies.

The discussion of third-party donation allows us to see how some of Sachedina's Islamic principles of bioethics play out in the realm of ART. The ultimate outcome of his analysis of the use of donor gametes and embryos is that such practices ought to be forbidden, for the reason of protecting the resulting child's lineage and rights. Despite the permissive rulings of many Shia scholars, there are those who advocate a similarly cautious approach to third-party donation. Sachedina's stance also appears to converge with the position of the Sunni authorities (Inhorn 2003). What makes his approach different from others who have taken a conservative stance on the matter is that he provides discussion about the weighing and balancing of the relevant Islamic bioethical principles involved.

Regarding the rule of "Necessity overrides prohibition," he claims that it cannot be invoked by jurists to justify gamete or embryo donation because it does not outweigh the harms visited upon the child (Sachedina 2009: 114–16). Elsewhere he invokes the ethical rule of "Protection from distress and impairment," which, like "Necessity overrides prohibition," comes from the principle of "No harm, no harassment." In this case he applies the rule to the question of the effect of the use of ART on the relationship of the family. If the technology causes "distress and impairment" to the family relationship—not only of the child, but of the husband and wife—then Muslims ought to be very cautious in employing it (Sachedina 2009: 118–19).

These sorts of ethical critiques lay the foundation for further evaluation of the conflicts inherent in, but so far overlooked in, the discussion of ART in Iran. As we saw earlier, both clinicians and jurists are trying their best to alleviate the mental and physical suffering of those facing infertility. The jurists provide rulings that allow ART procedures, sometimes even permitting third-party donation of gametes and embryos. Clinicians aim to provide any available ART treatments that have even a sliver of justification (or silence) through the fatwas and/or civil law.

In both cases they are weighting the treatment of the suffering of the patients above and beyond the other stakeholders, namely, the possible children and the society at large. But it seems now that, even if the jurists were justifying their rulings based to some degree on the principles Sachedina has elaborated, such as public good or "No harm, no harassment" and its derivative rules, an equal or stronger case can be made against questionable ARTs on the same grounds. A more thorough ethical analysis might well show weightier harms arising from these techniques rather than the alleviation of the harms associated with infertility. Is the prevention of harm applicable only to the would-be parents, or to the child, or to the society? Those possible harms include the genetic pitfalls of anonymous gamete donation, such as unintentional incest among donor offspring, genetic disease or general lack of genetic information in the children of anonymous donors, or the psychological and social harms that might result to both child and nongenetic parents as a result of using these procedures, even if all attempts are made to preserve anonymity. Clearly these points need to be factored into any discussion of ART, but such a discussion is not served in the mere issuance of a fatwa.

Sachedina takes the jurists to task for their failure to initiate this discussion. In assessing their rulings and supporting evidence, he claims that most simply gave nonethical textual interpretations to support their views of the varieties of ARTs. In doing this they justified their ultimate position on the ART in question simply by reference to procreation or sexual modesty. So even though they provided the permissive or prohibitive fatwa, they failed to give adequate consideration to the social and individual factors that are also in play (Sachedina 2009). It is the reconciliation of such competing claims that is the hallmark of bioethics, and such dilemmas cannot be handled simply through fatwas.

Conclusion

Sachedina's new presentation of Islamic bioethics, the most comprehensive to date, raises many important points with regard to ART in Iran. Its elaboration of the theological, ethical, and legal principles comprising Islamic bioethics serves to take the discussion of ART beyond the limited range of the fatwa literature, and serves to frame the discussion in a way that addresses the shortcomings of previous analyses of ART in Iran, as well as providing guidance to clinicians and jurists grappling with the ethical implications of this technology.

Unlike the sensational rulings permitting the use of a range of third-party donations in ART in Iran, and in contrast to the eagerness of clinicians to use these rulings to treat their patients, Sachedina has taken a considerably more cautious stance, based on his understanding of the relevant principles. He justifies this position in general by reference to the religious law's own precautionary approach to scientific advancement (Sachedina 2009). While he has supported this approach well, and we have seen its important critique of certain segments of ART, it would have been helpful to see this conservative stance in dialogue with another well-known Islamic approach to science and medicine that is reflected in the prophetic tradition that "there is no disease that God has created, except that he has also created its treatment." He has touched upon this concept (Sachedina 2009: 167), but its implications in Islamic bioethics generally, and especially for ART, are well worth investigating further. In any case, his evaluation of third-party donation, as carried out in Iran, sets a high bar for those in favor of such practices to overcome. So far they have not met this ethical challenge in a satisfactory way.

In fact, we might ask if there are not better solutions to the problem of infertility in Iran than religiously and socially questionable third-party donations. With the stakes so high for the status of the children born of these procedures, we must really question if even the most vigorous attempts at anonymity, even if religiously sanctioned, are morally justifiable. Genetic problems aside, the social consequences will remain and would be devastating if at any point the child's secret is not maintained.

Though there are efforts, largely from the major fertility clinics and research institutes, to educate Iranian society on these practices and thus remove the stigma from these children and their parents, this will be a difficult road. Until the cultural attitudes are changed, it would seem morally and religious-legally wrong to permit children to be exposed to such stigma. Perhaps those resources ought to be put towards changing Iranian sociocultural views on the practice of guardianship of orphans. Such children already face innumerable social stigmas and are most in need of kind protection and support.

The Islamic practice of fostering or guardianship is not equivalent to adoption, as commonly understood. This means that while Muslims are exhorted by the Qur'an and other normative sources to care for orphans, they are not to create a fictive relationship with the child (Q 33:4–5), wherein the adoptive parents give the child their own name, or otherwise imply that the child is their biological offspring. These foster parents are responsible for the majority of duties incumbent on the child's biological parents, though neither party inherits from the other in the standard Islamic manner.

While secret or informal adoption has been practiced in Muslim societies (Sonbol 1995),[9] most Muslim nations maintain a ban on adoption. However, Iran has a civil adoption law that has been on the books since 1975. This law goes so far as to grant the adoptive parents the child's birth certificate, in the parents' name, and institutes inheritance rights between them and the child (Abbasi-Shavazi et al. 2008). Thus, while adoption in this sense might appear to be one solution available to infertile Iranians, it still raises the same problematic ethical concerns, according to this presentation of Islamic bioethics, as does involvement of third-party donation. Thus, even though promoting increased guardianship will not fully assuage the suffering of those who wish to have "their own" child, it seems a morally preferable and religiously laudatory option, and avoids the expense, complications, and limited success of ART while providing an outcome not dissimilar in the end from the child born from donor gametes, or especially from a donor embryo.[10]

Sachedina's approach to bioethics has already been noted in Iran. To the extent that it is engaged with by the ART clinics and among the religious scholars, it may have a dramatic impact on the practice of these technologies. It should certainly provide clinicians and religious scholars with much of the understanding and direction they have been missing. Future discussion of ART in Iran will have to take note of this perspective and will require discussion and analysis considerably different from what has been found in other examinations so far.

Notes

1. Though often referred to as "ethics committees" by themselves and in academic literature, the status of these committees in Iran is open to some debate. Staff from both of the clinics I examined, the Avicenna Research Institute and the Royan Institute, described themselves as having ethics committees. Likewise, a recent study described a "Medical Ethics Committee" structure at the Avicenna Research Institute, which functions like an Institutional Review Board in the West (Abbasi-Shavazi 2008: 11). However, it is likely that these groups are actually more akin to bioethics consultation groups, meeting in an ad hoc manner to address specific cases arising in the clinic, as compared to an ethics committee, where the larger ethical questions of the rightness or wrongness of an act are addressed. The validity of this distinction will become more apparent in the course of this chapter.
2. Mohammad Rasekh (PhD faculty member at Shahid Beheshti University and on staff at the Avicenna Research Institute), in discussion with the author, May 2006.
3. Ibid.
4. Ibid.

5. For details on several of the most notorious cases, see Kotler 2007.
6. See also his similar criticism of the Sunnī-Shīʿī Islamic Juridical Council of the World Muslim League, 221–22.
7. Justice, beneficence, nonmaleficence, and autonomy. See Beauchamp and Childress 2001.
8. *Encyclopaedia of the Qurʾān*, s.v. "Parents."
9. See also the *Encyclopedia of Women in Islamic Cultures*, s.v. "Adoption and Fostering."
10. An analysis of Sachedina's chapter on suffering in light of ART might be an especially interesting study. This would be complemented by reference to the recent interviews with infertile Iranian women in Abbasi-Shavazi et al. 2008.

References

Abbasi-Shavazi, Mohammad Jalal, Marcia C. Inhorn, Hajiieh Bibi Razeghi-Nasrabad, and Ghasem Toloo. 2008. "The 'Iranian ART Revolution': Infertility, Assisted Reproductive Technology, and Third-Party Donation in the Islamic Republic of Iran." *Journal of Middle East Women's Studies* 4(2): 1–28.

Beauchamp, Tom L., and James F. Childress, eds. 2001. *Principles of Biomedical Ethics.* Oxford: Oxford University Press.

Bentley, Gillian R., and C. G. Nicholas Mascie-Taylor, eds. 2000. *Infertility in the Modern World: Present and Future Prospects.* Cambridge: Cambridge University Press.

Clarke, Morgan. 2005. "Islam and 'New Kinship': An Anthropological Study of New Reproductive Technologies in Lebanon." PhD diss., University of Oxford.

Hoodfar, Homa, and Samad Assadpour. 2000. "The Politics of Population Policy in the Islamic Republic of Iran." *Studies in Family Planning* 31(1).

Hourani, George. 1971. *Islamic Rationalism: The Ethics of ʿAbd al-Jabbār.* Oxford: Clarendon Press.

Inhorn, Marcia C. 2003. *Local Babies, Global Science: Gender, Religion, and In Vitro Fertilization in Egypt.* New York: Routledge.

Kotler, Steven. 2007. "The God of Sperm." *LA Weekly* (26 September).

Kuhse, Helga, and Peter Singer. 2001. "What Is Bioethics? A Historical Introduction." In *A Companion to Bioethics,* ed. Helga Kuhse and Peter Singer. Oxford: Blackwell Publishers.

Obermeyer, Carla Makhlouf. 1994. "Reproductive Choice in Islam: Gender and State in Iran and Tunisia." *Studies in Family Planning* 25(1).

Rahman, Fazlur. 1983. "Law and Ethics in Islam." In *Ethics in Islam,* ed. Richard G. Hovannisian. Malibu, CA: Undena Publications.

———. 1998. *Health and Medicine in the Islamic Tradition.* Chicago: Kazi Publications.

Sachedina, Abdulaziz. 2008. "Defining the Pedagogical Parameters of Is-
    lamic Bioethics." In *Muslim Medical Ethics: From Theory to Practice*, ed.
    Jonathan Brockopp and Thomas Eich. Columbia: University of South
    Carolina Press.

———. 2009. *Islamic Biomedical Ethics: Principles and Applications*. Oxford: Ox-
    ford University Press.

Sonbol, Amira al-Azhary. 1995. "Adoption in Islamic Society: A Historical
    Survey." In *Children in the Muslim Middle East*, ed. Elizabeth W. Fernea.
    Austin: University of Texas Press.

Soroush, Abdulkarim. 2000. "Types of Religiosity." *Kiyan*, no. 50 (March).
    http://www.drsoroush.com/English/By_DrSoroush/E-CMB-20000300-
    Types_of_Religiosity.html.

Tremayne, Soraya. 2006. "Change and 'Face' in Modern Iran." *Anthropology
    of the Middle East* 1(1).

———. 2009. "Law, Ethics, and Donor Technologies in Shia Iran." In *Assist-
    ing Reproduction, Testing Genes: Global Encounters with New Biotechnologies*,
    eds. Daphna Birenbaum-Carmeli and Marcia C. Inhorn. New York and
    Oxford: Berghahn Books.

Chapter 5

THE "DOWN SIDE" OF GAMETE DONATION
CHALLENGING "HAPPY FAMILY" RHETORIC IN IRAN

Soraya Tremayne

Introduction

The use of assisted reproductive technologies (ARTs) for infertility treatment has been made possible in the Muslim countries of the Middle East by the endorsement and strong support of the religious leaders, as observed by Inhorn (2003) who also notes that "the global spread of these technologies is nowhere more evident than in the 22 nations of the Muslim Middle East." These technologies, however, have remained limited in their application in most Muslim countries to IVF treatment for married couples only, and no third-party donation is allowed among Sunni Muslims (Inhorn 2005; Clarke 2006a). Iran, which is a Shia theocracy, on the other hand, has adopted these technologies with open arms and has legitimized almost all forms of third-party donation including that of sperm and egg donation, embryo donation, and surrogacy, and more recently stem cell research and sex selection. ARTs have been practiced in Iran for over twenty years, and demand for them continues to grow. As Inhorn notes, "Iran is definitely in the lead among the Muslim countries in the Middle East in the application of these technologies."[1] The reasons for and the process of legitimizing ARTs in the Muslim Middle East have been documented extensively elsewhere (Inhorn 2003, 2005, 2006a, 2006b; Clarke 2006a, 2006b, 2009; Serour 1993; Tremayne 2005, 2006a, 2006b, 2009 among others). A brief explanation of the difference between Shia Iran and the rest of the Muslim world is that the majority of Sunni Muslims, in considering such practices, have concluded that the practice of third-party gamete donation would lead to confusion in the lineage (*nasab*), which forms the foundation of the Muslim family, and would be equal to incest or adultery and, therefore, a threat to the stability of social relations (Inhorn 2005; Clarke 2009; Tremayne 2009).

The Shia religious leaders in Iran, on the other hand, have been able to find solutions to legitimize third-party donation without breaking any of the Islamic rules concerning adultery and incest. In doing so, they have focused on an in-depth examination of what constitutes *nasab*,[2] and whether the practice of ARTs with all its ramifications would confuse the line of lineage. To do so, the senior Shia clerics resorted to *ijtihad*, and concluded that certain forms of third-party donation could be allowed without breaching any divine rules (Tremayne 2009). ARTs are therefore currently practiced in Iran with the full approval of the ruling religious leaders, although the use of donor sperm remains a more contentious issue, as will be discussed further down, and its practice is limited. However, not all religious leaders in Iran are in agreement with the interpretations that have led to legitimizing third-party donation. Similar to the Sunni religious leaders, the opponents of such practices in Iran remain uncompromising in their interpretations of the Qur'an and forbid the use of third-party donation. Iran being a theocracy, a distinction has to be made between the views of those leading clerics who are also the political rulers and law makers and represent the "official" position on religious and juristic matters, and those who are equally, if not more, qualified in *fiqh* and are sources of emulation with a large following, but are not in a position to enforce their views.[3] It is therefore the ruling of the religio-political rulers, with support from some of the more progressive apolitical clerics, that has opened the door for the use of ARTs.

The official endorsement of third-party donation of gametes, issued by the supreme religious leader Ayatollah Khamene'i in the late 1990s, is generally taken as the starting point for third-party donation (Inhorn 2006a; Clarke 2009; Tremayne 2009). However, prior to this fatwa, several Shia scholars had debated at length the legitimacy of third-party donation and had issued their views on it.

One example, which proved an important landmark in influencing the decision-making process, was a conference organized by Dr.
Mohammad Mehdi Akhondi, the Director of the Avicenna Research
Institute and head of one of the leading fertility treatment centers,
which resulted in the publication of its proceedings in *Modern Human Reproductive Techniques from the View of Jurisprudence and Law*
(2001).[4] The book, the first in this field, includes several chapters
by senior clerics and jurists in which they examine closely the legitimacy of third-party donation. Some of the chapters had been
published a few years earlier and preceded the above conference.
Indeed, those deliberations in the book which favored third-party
donation themselves may have been the inspiration behind the late
1990s fatwa. Likewise, in addition to the views of the religious leaders of both convictions (for and against such practices), and long before the official decisions were announced in favor of such practices,
experts from a variety of other disciplines in the legal, medical and
social sciences had also engaged in exploring the consequences of
third-party donation and whether these breach any legal, religious,
and social rules. The initial condition set for third-party donation
was that it should take place between the married couple. A solution was found within the Shia practice of temporary marriage so
that the gamete donor and recipient could get married temporarily
to legitimize the donation.[5]

While debates on most aspects, hypothetical and real, of the implications of ARTs continued, and long before the supreme leader's fatwa, many clinics took their cue from those clerics who had
endorsed them and started the practice of third-party gamete donation.[6] The 1990s fatwa proved very "liberal," to use Clarke's expression (2009), and allowed the donation of both sperm and egg
based on the religious edict[7] that "as long as no gaze or touch takes
place between the donor and recipient, donation is allowed." Essentially, such endorsement served as the basis for all future forms
of donation, such as embryo donation and surrogacy, and removed
any suggestion of incest or adultery as long as no bodily contact
took place between the two parties (Tremayne 2009: 148; see also
Garmaroudi Naef on surrogacy, this volume). While third-party egg
donation did not provoke any fierce reaction, the approval of sperm
donation met with such uproar among the majority of the *ulama*
(Muslim legal scholars), as well as the general public, that its practice
did not become widespread and only a few private clinics discreetly
continue with sperm donation. Currently the majority of clinics
practice egg donation only, though sperm donation does continue

in some private clinics. Also, with the passage of time, temporary marriage is used to a lesser degree at the clinics.

The rationale behind the approval of ARTs was the stability and happiness they bring into the family by treating infertility. In legitimizing the use of ARTs, the initial deliberations by experts predominantly focused on issues concerning biological and social belonging and inheritance and their implications for donor children. But, they did not address the long-term impact of the donor child on the dynamics of family relations, between the child and the parents, between the spouses and genders, and on the larger social group. Such a gap stemmed from the fact that the donor children had not yet reached the age to make a study of this kind possible, but, more importantly, the assumption behind the approval of third-party donation was that once lineage and other legal and practical matters are resolved and the child is born, a happy and stable family will be formed, which will function as any "normal" family (Tremayne 2009, 2008; Abbasi-Shavazi et al. 2008).

The hitherto limited research on donor families in Iran suggests that ARTs have saved thousands of marriages by helping couples conceive. However, no known in-depth research has been carried out to follow the life trajectories of the donor children and their families, to assess the actual outcome of their presence on their families and social group. This chapter will follow the life trajectories of a few selected cases who present the other side of the coin to the happy families. The cases presented here are extreme ones, and while the findings do not suggest that all donor cases are similar, they will try to demonstrate that focusing on the cases of happy families alone would be only a half-veiled truth about the full impact of ARTs. The findings and conclusion in this chapter are substantiated by tens of similar cases from a larger study carried out from 2004 to 2009.

ARTs in a State of Flux

The research that serves as the basis for this chapter started in 2004 in Iran. Third-party donation was still relatively new at that time, and donor children were few and far between and too novel to assess their impact. It was clear that the wider implications of third-party donations would be known only when the donor children come of age (Tremayne 2005). The follow-up research between 2004 and 2008 revealed that reproductive technologies have had so many unexpected and unintended outcomes that they seemed to remain in a constant state of flux (Tremayne 2009). The findings of one phase of research seemed to be overruled within six months, and new situations emerged frequently. For example, in 2004, according to the official figures, only twelve cases of surrogacy were known publicly, and the practitioners complained that due to cultural taboos it was difficult to find surrogate mothers. A year later, this number had gone up several fold. In 2004 many cases of same-sex sibling donation existed where sisters donated eggs to each other, but I did not come across siblings of the opposite sex who donated gametes to each other. Two years later, evidence came to the fore that many brothers and sisters had started donating gametes to each other and making embryos together following the fatwas that gave legitimacy to such donations, namely, that "as long as there is no touch or gaze third-party donation is allowed" (Tremayne 2009; personal interviews 2006–2008; Garmaroudi 2008).

In 2003 the law for embryo donation was approved and specified that embryo donation should come from a married couple and be donated as a gift. Three years later, in 2006, at a conference held in Tehran on gamete and embryo donation, one of the leading practitioners expressed his dismay publicly that some agencies had started selling embryos that were the result of prostitutes' eggs and unknown men's sperm, and that these agencies had tried to sell these embryos to his clinic. So, the changes are continuing in such unpredictable ways and at such speed that they leave the researcher in doubt as to the validity of his/her original findings. As Nancy Scheper-Hughes, in an editorial on a different topic, wrote: "One major obstacle to public anthropology is our [anthropologists'] reticence to describe events before we have gained a deep understanding of their context. By the time we finally feel we have something to say, the moment has passed into history. In a sense all ethnography is historical—a history of the present—always trailing well behind the moment" (2009: 4).

However, in spite of the apparently rapid changes mentioned earlier, the present study shows that ARTs, which on first sight seem to have affected the landscape of kinship, have served to confirm and in some areas reinforce cultural values and practices. While the constant changes in the use of ARTs may be interpreted as confusing and paradoxical for their users, in reality these are mirroring a complex set of relations, which have their roots in cultural values but which, when faced with modern technologies, embrace them readily and gain strength from them. As Becker puts it, "Because new reproductive technologies reflect cultural meanings and become a conduit for changing cultural practices, they signify both a challenge to and a reinforcement of the moral order" (2000: 236).

Third-party donation of sperm and egg has been practiced for several years in Iran, and the donor children are now old enough to make it possible to assess their impact on their parents and the wider social group. In doing so, this chapter focuses on two different but related areas, and asks, first, whether conceiving through such modern technologies, and having received information on the scientific realities of procreation from the clinics, has really transformed the cultural values, beliefs, perceptions, and behavior of the users in a significant way. Second, whether it is correct to assume that proving their fertility and reproductive abilities to themselves and to their social group has resulted in the infertile users forming a "happy family," which, as mentioned earlier, has been the main driving force behind legitimizing third-party donation (Abbasi-Shavazi et al. 2008: 2; Tremayne 2009). Finally, I suggest that the wish for having a child, per se, is not limited to making a family happy or otherwise. It is seen as the duty of the individual to undergo the ritual of reproducing (see also Abbasi-Shavazi et al. 2008: 3), to contribute to the social reproduction of the group, before an adult is accepted as one of its members. To this end, I surmise that children become pawns in such cultural practices to be used for different purposes at different times, by different members of the social group.

Methodology

This chapter is based on two sets of data. The first were collected in Tehran and Yazd (central Iran), between 2004 and 2008 in the course of several field trips. Information from these data is used as the background to support the analysis and conclusion in this chapter. The second were data collected between 2007 and 2009 in the United Kingdom, and were based on case studies of Iranian women refugees whom I had come across in my role as an expert witness to courts during their claims for asylum. These women had undergone third-party donation, and their donor children were old enough to allow an assessment of the long-term effect of their conceptions on their families and their wider social group. I have chosen two particular cases, from among several others, because they are representative of the large number of families whom I have come across who are users of third-party donation and whose stories remain untold. Although these two cases can be considered as "extreme," they epitomize the hidden lives of numerous families with similar social and cultural backgrounds, and can be considered the tip of the iceberg. They are exceptional in that these women have been able to leave Iran and tell their stories, and not because they are unique. One of the cases is that of third-party egg donation, and the other, sperm donation. The choice was made to examine whether and how the children who are conceived through gamete donation of egg or sperm differ in their impact on the families and community. Although these stories are written with the explicit permission of both women, I have tried to disguise their identity as much as possible.

Finally, as is clear from the above, the data presented in the case studies in this chapter have not been collected using the usual anthropological methods of fieldwork. For those of us who carry out research in fertility treatment clinics, we are less likely to encounter stories such as the ones told here. But, even when as anthropologists we live with our informants on a daily basis, as opposed to interviewing them at clinics, we are not always likely to be a party to the kind of stories the women in this chapter have recounted. I would have never been privy to these stories in such detail had it not been for the fact that, unknown to these women, I had read their stories and commented on them as an expert witness to the courts. The stories seemed to be so extreme that, to begin with, I doubted their veracity, but on cross-examination I was convinced of their being genuine and not fabricated to obtain asylum. The point is that, these kinds of cases do not come to the fore frequently because those who are affected by them, especially women, are often willing parties to perpetuating and protecting the cultural values to which they belong by conforming to what is expected of them by their social group.[8] While such motivations do not reduce the emotional desire for having a child, it is above all the sense of belonging and identity that is the driving force for such submission and silent cooperation. Women in this study appear to have submitted of their own so-called volition[9] to the hardship of undergoing IVF treatment to contribute their shares to the social reproduction of the family and social group, and in doing so they have been greatly assisted by modern reproductive technologies. Unnithan-Kumar's study of female-selected abortion in India shows that "[reproductive] technologies in themselves do not bring about social transformation but it is in how they are made socially meaningful that their power lies" (2009: 13). Likewise, Thompson, in her analysis of feminists' theorization of infertility, illustrates the dilemma created by the modern infertility treatment technologies:

> On the one hand, the burden of involuntary childlessness is considered especially heavy for women, and prominent feminists call for it to be taken seriously as a feminist issue. On the other hand, feminists are also interested in disrupting the gendered role expectations and the essentialist connection between motherhood and women's identity that greatly intensify infertile women's suffering. Contemporary infertility and its treatment are conceptualized and structured on a strongly coupled, ultra-heterosexual, consumer-oriented, normative nuclear family scenario. When successful, treatment enables women to reinscribe themselves into that logic. The paradox of infertility for feminism, then, is this: feminists are well placed to understand the special burden of involuntary childlessness, but they are ambivalent about supporting women who seek infertility treatment because it seems to lend implicit support to conventional gender roles and gendered stratification (2002: 52).

As is clear from the above, ARTs can become a new form of coercion to which women submit willingly.

Creating a Culture (*Farhang Sazi*)

The health care system and the fertility clinics in Iran have taken a proactive role to educate infertile users of ARTs about the facts of procreation (Abbasi-Shavazi et al. 2008). In their view, this is the first step towards normalizing the use of ARTs by familiarizing infertile couples with the biological facts, as opposed to the common understanding and general beliefs about infertility and its causes. This education is generally referred to as "creating a culture" or "building a culture" (*farhang sazi*). The first time I came across such an educational program was in May 2004 when I walked into a private fertility clinic in Tehran. Around fifty men and women were sitting silently in the waiting hall, staring impassively at a giant TV screen. At first, I did not pay any attention to what they were watching, assuming that it was the usual TV program advocating the correct Islamic values. I was looking for the midwife, who was supposed to show me around. She was late, and while waiting for her, I turned my attention to the TV screen. To my disbelief, I saw a live transmission of the fertilization of a woman's egg from the operating theater of the clinic, with the patient's name written on the screen and the doctor's voice explaining how Mrs. X's egg was being fertilized. I looked around anxiously, expecting a reaction from the crowd of men and women watching this. Iran is a country where sex segregation is supposed to be in force in theory. Here, at the fertility clinic, I see men and women watching the reproductive organs of a woman, who is being named, without any reaction. This was even more surprising because most of the couples seemed to come from conservative and, most likely, religious backgrounds.

The fertilization of the egg went on, and when the midwife finally arrived, I expressed my astonishment at such a demonstration. She did not seem particularly worried and just said, "Yes, we show these operations live for the patients to teach them what to expect." I then persisted, asking, "But what do the patients think of this?" She said, "We think it is good for them." I realized that my point was missed and did not continue. I then raised the question of why the clinic was called the center for the cure of *na-zai*, meaning the inability to give birth, which is the term used for female infertility. I wanted to know whether it implied that infertility is a uniquely female affliction, which seemed to be in direct contrast with the aims of the educational programs trying to explain that infertility could affect both men and women. The doctors looked blankly at me and then said, "This is a strange question, we have never thought about it in this way." But, they added, "Perhaps we should change this as we do try to tell men that they could be infertile, too."

Two years later, in 2006, I met with the director of a leading private fertility clinic. On my way to his office, I noticed the same giant TV screen in the waiting hall with a similar large crowd of people sitting watching similar scenes of the fertilization of an egg. I raised the same question on the prohibition of women's bodies being displayed in such a public way. The director looked uncomfortable at first, then said, "Islam has said that the outside of women's bodies should not be seen, but it has never said that the inside cannot be displayed." Faced with the look of disbelief on my face, and realizing that taking refuge behind an implicit religious explanation was not going to prove convincing, he laughed and said: "To tell you the truth, we have never thought about this aspect of the display. Our intention is to create/build a new culture (*farhang sazi*), so that people understand how babies are conceived and how infertility can be treated. We need to make these new techniques fit into the culture (*ja andakhtan*)." He went on, "Our intention is to teach these people scientifically that infertility should not be a stigma and to make them come forward without any shame about their infertility."

In 2008, during an interview with one of the practitioners, whom I had interviewed previously and who had proudly claimed that "we are building a new culture," I found him disillusioned and subdued and having second thoughts about "making a culture" and "creating babies." He mentioned that in starting his fertility clinic, he wanted to make happy families, allow people to have children, and save as many couples from their miseries of being infertile as possible. "What have I achieved?" he says in a low voice. "I have just come across brothers and sisters who have started making embryos together, some to help their siblings, but many for the purpose of making money. Is this what I have worked for so long and so hard? What have I managed to teach these people?" He mentions several cases whereby, in his judgment, norms have been breached and rules broken by both the donors and users of gametes. He repeats the story of the growing number of agencies that make embryos illegitimately (meaning from unmarried couples) and sell them.

Consequently, I heard similar stories from other practitioners. Such breaches seem to have led the clinics to try to take control of the process of donation, wherever possible, by minimizing contact between donors and recipients to prevent the "misuse" of gamete donation. As practitioners, the doctors are more concerned with the biological and genetic outcome of these breaches than the social and cultural rules, which they consider to fall outside their responsibilities. There are other instances whereby the education of users has produced opposite results too. For example, a counselor psychologist from a different private clinic mentioned: "We can familiarize our own users to these technologies, but the practice of ARTs is widespread now and we have no control over who learns in the right way about them. Doctors with minimum training are practicing IVF and third-party donation without any respect for the rules" (personal interviews 2006).

From the limited research carried out among the successful recipients of gametes on the long-term effect of the education they have received, there are indications that the education has served the immediate interest of all parties involved to justify their resorting to ARTs. Beyond that, as soon as the baby is taken home, the "cultural education" fades into the background, and the new parents fall back into their "normal" lifestyle and behavior. However, this area remains underresearched and is in need of further monitoring and verification.

Case Studies

The use of third-party donation among Iranian couples goes back many years before the technology reached Iran. Infertile Iranian couples used to come to the United Kingdom to seek IVF treatment, partly because these technologies did not exist in Iran, but mainly because they did not want anybody back home to find out that they could not conceive. In one case, I acted as interpreter for a couple and when, after long trials, the doctors told the husband that the problem was with him and not his wife, he started subjecting his wife to intolerable violence. When I asked the wife why she did not divorce him, she said that she had been married and divorced before, and a second divorce was simply not an option, "because even if my father and brothers don't kill me, they will not let me back into their house, and how am I going to live with my parents, neighbors and friends, all of whom will blame me? Divorce will be an added stigma to being infertile and one that I cannot live with." Research in Tehran's infertility clinics also highlights the stigma of infertility, especially male infertility (Abbasi-Shavazi et al. 2008: 14). Divorcing a violent husband who shifts the blame for infertility to his wife, as described by Inhorn (2003), would be "to thrust them [divorced women] into an extremely vulnerable position."

Batoul's Story

The following case studies of two women form the second part of this chapter. Batoul is a forty-five-year-old woman who comes from a highly religious and conservative family. She was seventeen when her father forced her to marry a man several years older than herself. She had no say in the decision. Her husband was an engineer and went to work in the United Arab Emirates. In 1988, by the time she was twenty-two years old and had not conceived, her husband decided to take her to the United Kingdom for treatment. The couple received gamete intrafallopian transfer (GIFT) assisted reproduction. Batoul did not speak any English and did not understand anything about the procedures she underwent, so her husband took charge of the entire negotiations. The treatment proved successful, and she became pregnant. They returned to the United Arab Emirates, where she gave birth to nonidentical triplet girls in 1989. The triplets had blonde hair, two with brown eyes and the third with green eyes. It was obvious that the husband was not the biological father of the children. At such a finding, he accused Batoul of having slept with the doctor in the clinic, and became violent and started beating her.

They returned to Iran, where he told the members of his and her families that she had slept with the doctor and the children were bastards. Batoul's father and brothers sided with the husband, and became abusive and threatened to kill her and the children because "they were not Muslims" and because "she had brought shame upon the family." Batoul was summoned by the security forces to account for what had happened at the clinic in the United Kingdom. During this time, she was subjected to extreme violence by her husband, who beat and injured her regularly. Over the years, in addition to the routine beatings, she suffered various fractures and burns, including: two broken legs; a sewing machine thrown at her head, which knocked her unconscious; burns with hot oil; and being frozen by having buckets of ice poured over her. The children were also beaten regularly and called bastards. Mina, the daughter with green eyes, developed a heart problem when she was eighteen months old and underwent an operation. After three years Batoul managed to get a divorce, but the court did not instruct the father to pay any maintenance for the "bastards." Legally, he could have claimed custody of the children, but did not do so and was happy for her to keep the children, but did not see it as his duty to contribute financially towards their upkeep.

Over the following five years, Mina had three heart operations. Every time Batoul had great difficulty in getting Mina admitted to the hospital, because no hospital would admit her without the father's permission and confirmation that she was his daughter. None of the members of the father's family were prepared to help with the "illegitimate" children. Batoul had to make a living by sewing and doing various jobs. As the children grew up, they were subjected to constant abuse at school because the father turned up and told the school that these girls were bastards and were Christians. The children were bullied, and once thrown out and told to go to a school for Christian children. The appearance of blonde hair and green eyes in Mina's case made it credible that they were not "Muslim" or from an Iranian father. Batoul kept changing location and moving from one school to another, only to find that her husband had turned up again and asked the school to throw them out. Eventually they moved to Batoul's native village, and Batoul managed to convince the head teacher that her children were Muslims. But, the bullying continued by other children. Mina, who I met recently in the United

Kingdom, added that, in order to be allowed to stay at school, she even joined the Basij[10] at her school to prove that she was a Muslim. Finally, Batoul's husband told her that if she wanted his help with getting the children to schools or hospitals, she should remarry him. Batoul seemed to have little choice but to accept this. But, although she was now married to him, he refused to support the family financially. Throughout this time the only person who supported Batoul both financially and morally was her mother, despite the disapproval of her husband, Batoul's father.

After the renewal of the marriage, the husband did not live at home but came home occasionally and without warning. Batoul was lonely and miserable, and met another man with whom she fell in love and started an affair. One day, when he was visiting her, the husband came back home accompanied by three men from the security forces and caught Batoul and her lover in bed. The men were to be witnesses to adultery, and duly took photographs and took Batoul and her lover to their headquarters. She was held for two days in a dark cell, and while in custody was raped by the officers. Both she and her lover were sentenced to be stoned to death. By now, Batoul's father was dead and her mother sold her house to pay a heavy bail for her temporary release while waiting to be stoned. Batoul hid two of her children and fled from Iran and came to the United Kingdom with Mina to allow her to have a fourth urgent operation for her heart. On arrival, she applied for asylum. At first she and Mina were kept in a notorious detention center, where she attempted suicide twice and has suffered mental ill health since.

Soon after she left Iran, Batoul's husband started harassing her mother to discover Batoul's whereabouts. Mina is now twenty years old and is at the university, while her two sisters are in Iran and still on the run from their social father. I heard recently that Batoul has gone back to Iran, clandestinely, to save her children from her husband, who was trying to sell them to some dealers in the United Arab Emirates. One of them was held at gunpoint recently by a man, who was employed by the husband to abduct them and take them to the United Arab Emirates. According to Batoul and Mina, the husband is still calling the girls "bastards" and wants to "wash this stain of shame from the family" by either forcing them into marriage or actually trafficking them as sex workers. Batoul said that she had no choice but to rescue her daughters, whose lives are in danger. She is still wanted by the courts in Iran, and if her husband finds her, he will make sure that she is arrested and the death sentence is carried out. Her own brothers maintain their threat that they too will kill her. So, twenty-one years after Batoul underwent IVF treatment, her life, and that of her daughters in Iran, has gone from bad to worse, with no end in sight as yet. The two girls in Iran have now completed their secondary education, against all odds and with help from their grandmother. They wish to go to university, but do not have the financial means. The grandmother is old and frail and has run out of money, and the girls are still hiding from the father.

I met with Mina, to hear her side of the story. She is still under medical surveillance for her heart problems, but is determined to make her life a success. She said that her maternal uncles are still telling the two sisters that if they ever catch Mina, they will kill her "because of her green eyes, because she, Mina, is the perfect testimony for our sister's shameful adultery." Mina told me: "I do not consider 'that man' to be my father. Apart from the fact that he is not my biological father, he never gave me any love or affection." To date, Batoul's brothers attack their own mother and abuse her verbally and throw stones at her house, where Batoul's two remaining daughters live. They are angry with their mother for helping Batoul. Batoul's relatives also reject the girls. On one occasion, when the two sisters ran away from their father's violence and took a bus to a town where their paternal aunt lived, they were cross-questioned by the police on the bus, asking what two young women were doing traveling by themselves and where were they going. The sisters gave their aunt's address and on arrival were delivered by the police to the aunt's house. She attacked them and beat them up and threw them out. One last remark from Mina was about her paternal uncle's youngest brother, who has married recently, and has realized that *he* is the infertile party. Since this discovery, his behavior has changed drastically towards Mina's sisters, saying that he now realizes that perhaps infertility runs in the family and, after all, it must have been his brother who was the infertile party.

In Batoul's case, the fact that her husband had been shown not to have been the biological father of the children dealt such a devastating blow to him, and made him lose face so seriously, that for the following twenty years he made Batoul and her three daughters' lives a misery and has kept them under constant threat. The recent investigations at the clinic that carried out the donation twenty years previously in the United Kingdom indicate that the clinic had explained fully to Batoul's husband about the procedure of third-party donation. The conclusion, therefore, must be that the husband was aware that Batoul's egg would be fertilized with another man's sperm, but that he had hoped to pretend that the child was his own as the result of the IVF treatment. Furthermore, what seems to matter more to him is to show his ability to reproduce, at all costs, even by secretly agreeing to use another man's sperm. Several other examples among the cases in this study show remarkable similarities. In one case the couple had gone abroad and on return claimed that the wife was pregnant. When the baby was born he was black, and it became clear that they had undergone third-party donation. Or, in another case, the infertile man had made a deal with the doctor and his brother to receive the brother's sperm, without his wife's knowledge. In the latter case, I have previously argued that, whenever possible, infertile men and women resort to their families for gamete donation to keep the lineage intact (Tremayne 2009). At the same time, consistent with the stigma of infertility, if an infertile man can possibly hide his infertility even from his kin group, he will do so. Batoul's husband did not seek his brother's help for donation because the technologies did not exist in Iran then, but possibly also because he did not imagine that his "secret" will be revealed in such an unexpected way, or he might have resorted to his brothers for help. Data from previous research also testifies that even when men have willingly chosen to receive sperm from other men, after the children are born men find it hard to accept them, and in the case of those who do not resort to violence against their wives, some have been known to have developed serious psychological problems themselves and have had to resort to treatment and counseling. One such man told his psychologist, "I cannot help looking at him and thinking that he is not my child. I cannot stand having him around." Inhorn also provides substantial evidence of such deeply ingrained adversity elsewhere (2006c; see also Tremayne 2009).

Sahar's Story

Sahar's story is a contrast to that of Batoul in some respects. She is fifty-three years old and comes from a wealthy and moderately religious and conservative family. When she was thirteen, she was given in marriage to a man who raped her before the marriage ceremony had taken place. As a result she became pregnant, and gave birth to a disabled child; her family made her divorce the man and give the child to the husband's family. Sahar never saw her son again. A few years later, she married a wealthy man who told her that he was impotent and could not satisfy her sexual needs. "But, he was a fair man and told me that I could have lovers if I wanted to, but I was so traumatized by my past experience that I was content living with him." Sahar lived in "real style," as she puts it, traveling everywhere with her husband, owning several homes, and employing an army of helpers. The marriage lasted a few years, but he was posted to other countries and she did not want to leave Iran. So, they separated. She started a property management business that became very successful, and she purchased several homes for herself, including some in the United Kingdom. She then married her third husband, who came from a highly conservative background, and had a senior position as the mayor of a district in a major city in Iran. Soon after they were married the husband became violent and started beating her severely. As a result, she had a miscarriage, two broken legs, and is lame in one leg and deaf in one ear.

By the time Sahar was forty-one years old, in 1997, she thought that having a child might help improve the marriage and reduce her husband's violent behavior. Due to her age, she resorted to third-party egg donation. To do so, a temporary marriage[11] arrangement was used between the donor and Sahar's husband at the fertility clinic. The egg donor was married to Sahar's husband for three days, until the doctor was satisfied that the egg was fertilized. Sahar became pregnant with twins, but during one of the severe regular beatings from her husband, she had a miscarriage and lost one child and only just managed to keep the second one. She gave birth to a son in 1998. But, giving her husband a son did not improve his behavior, and after five years she was forced to separate from him and live on her own with her son. Her husband then came to the United Kingdom to seek asylum, claiming that he had converted to Christianity. Their son was desperate to see his father, and Sahar brought him to the United Kingdom. While visiting her husband, he asked her to give false evidence to the courts about his conversion to Christianity, which she refused to do. He beat her up so badly that she needed hospital treatment. Her injuries were so severe that the authorities in the United Kingdom, realizing that she was the victim of domestic violence, offered her asylum. But, she refused this offer and returned to Iran.

The husband, having had his asylum turned down, returned to Iran too. Once in Iran, he banned Sahar and their son from leaving the country, since women need their husband's or father's permission to leave the country. He then took the son away to live with him in a town 1,200 kilometers away. Since legally the child belongs to the father, she could not protest and was given visitation rights of thirty-six hours every three months. He started using the son to blackmail Sahar financially and managed to obtain some of her properties, but refused to return the child. In effect, the child had become a bargaining chip in the relationship between Sahar and her husband.

The husband then complained to the courts that she had falsified papers to implicate him as having sought asylum in the United Kingdom on the grounds that he had converted to Christianity. This is a very serious accusation since conversion from Islam in Iran carries a death sentence. The husband and his father also made an attempt to kill her by driving a car towards her and trying to run her off the road. At this point, Sahar, who had succeeded in getting a divorce but whose court case on her husband's accusations was still pending, left the country for the United Kingdom and sought asylum. In the meantime the husband had taken the son away to an unknown location. In spite of appealing to international agencies to track the child down, she has not been able to find him and is thinking of returning to Iran even at the risk of having to face the Revolutionary Courts. She says that "life without my son is meaningless." Unlike Batoul, Sahar's parents and relatives are supportive of her, but her in-laws, especially her mother-in-law, have gone to great lengths to make life difficult for her.

Discussion

In this chapter I have examined the implications of the use of third-party donation of sperm and eggs on the life of some families who have gone home with a child. I have considered whether the use of the state-of-the-art reproductive technologies has altered the values that are the driving force behind the reproductive decisions infertile couples make. The effect of the donor child on the parents and the wider social group was also considered. To this end, two cases were selected on the basis that they reflected the "other side of the coin" to the successful cases and happy families. These cases are extreme ones, but by no means unique or even rare. The findings presented in this chapter are supported by a larger study of donor technologies, which include tens of other cases and which serve as the main source for the analysis in this chapter. Other studies also support some of the findings in this chapter (see for example Abbasi-Shavazi et al. 2008).

Several points emerge from the combination of the studies mentioned above. In general, men's and women's approaches to ARTs have been shown to differ, and the way donor children are treated depends upon whose biological child they are in the family. Women seem to have invariably welcomed egg donation, and have submitted to the treatment and cherished the child afterwards. In some of the cases of egg donation the couple returned with the same donor to have another child. Such reactions, viewed in their cultural context, support the suggestion that the way the ARTs have been used reflect the users' understanding of what constitutes kinship, families, lineage, and relationships (Inhorn 1996, 2006a, 2006b; Inhorn and Van Balen 2002; Becker 2000; and others). In the case of Iranian donor parents and children, although in Shia Islam a child takes its lineage from both parents, it belongs to the father whose lineage takes precedence over that of the mother (Mir Hosseini 1993; Ebadi 2003). It is therefore understandable why the clerics and jurists went to such trouble to establish the lineage of donor children before allowing third-party donation. However, the prevailing cultural values have proved more powerful and have undermined the legal and religious endorsements.

The use of third-party donation provides ample scope for a reinforcement of the patriarchal values in relation to reproduction. This mirrors the experience of infertile Iranian women, and is highlighted in the practice of third-party donation, more specifically that of sperm donation, which has been shown to result in further widening of an existing gender gap depending on who the infertile party is. In the case of egg donation, society's reaction has proved, by and large, to be consistent with patriarchal values. No hostile reaction is known to have been provoked in such instances towards the mother and child on the grounds that the child is a donor child. But, third-party sperm donation does not follow a symmetrical pattern. In spite of the initial legitimization of sperm donation, this remains frowned upon, the approval or disapproval of religious leaders notwithstanding. Having a donor child who is the result of sperm donation often leads to the child's rejection by the social father and often other male members of the social group, or, at its best, does not lead to the "happiness" and "stability" of the family, which are considered as the two cornerstones for a "perfect" family.

It follows, therefore, that the donor children's future depends on whether they are the result of egg or sperm donation. In both of the cases studied, not only had the donor children not brought happiness to the couple, or reduced the violence inflicted on the women who bore them, they had increased the violence to an intolerable level. To use Inhorn's argument, (cited in Abbasi-Shavazi et al. 2008: 21) in the case of infertile Egyptian women, "infertility experience is a form of 'lived patriarchy.'" Finally, the use of third-party gamete donation, which aims at improving the quality of life of the couple and ensuring the stability of the family, has so far also resulted in reinforcing the patriarchal family where gender inequality remains a social reality. In reproducing in a patriarchal culture, men and women are expected to fulfill different duties, which Inhorn (2003: 221), citing from others, calls "infertility: his and hers" (Greil et al. 1988).

The intervention of reproductive technologies has been shown in various studies to increase the collective social control over women's bodies (Unnithan-Kumar 2009; Martin 1987; Petchesky 1995; Thompson 2002; Inhorn 2006c; among others). In general, in Middle Eastern countries, pressure on married couples to have children starts from the first day of marriage. Iran is no exception to this, and while a woman's personal desire to have a child is not disputed, studies at clinics in Iran show time and again that women undergo third-party donation under immense pressure from the kin group, predominantly that of their in-laws. To find out at what stage of marriage women are forced to seek infertility treatment, during one of my visits to a fertility clinic in Tehran I asked whether any of the infertile women were under the age of fifteen.[12] The clinic's record showed that it had received several females below the age of fifteen. These girls must have been at least thirteen years old, if not younger, at marriage, and when they had failed to produce children, their husbands and in-laws had brought them to the clinic to seek treatment.[13] Abbasi-Shavazi et al.'s study (2008: 14) of Tehran's fertility clinics also confirms the extent of coercion by in-laws on women to seek fertility treatment. Finally, as Unnithan-Kumar's study (2009) of the case of lack of choices for female selective abortions (FSA) in India explains: "This is not an autonomous choice at all. But, by focusing on the freedom of choice alone, we are foreclosing the ability to understand the more complex aspects of how women's agency works in collectively oriented patriarchal contexts."[14] Unnithan-Kumar continues, "In the conjugal context where notions of self and control over one's body are both collectively constituted as they are individually desired, crafted and experienced, the willingness of women to take part in the use of biotechnologies is often a reflection of wider social processes in which women continually participate, which serves their own interest as well as those of the wider social group to which they belong" (2009: 12).

This kind of participation is what Lock and Kaufert (1998), cited in Unnithan-Kumar (2009), refer to as "pragmatic agency," whereby individuals do not necessarily either comply with or resist the "disciplining" that accompanies technological interventions but often act in accordance with pragmatic considerations. Accordingly, the donor children, in turn, become a tool to exercise control over women by the male members of the larger family. Batoul's example shows how all the male members of her own family took sides with her husband. The support for the husband was so strong that as long as her father was alive, her mother helped her secretly, and it was not until he died that she openly supported her. The case of Sahar epitomizes the life of several other women among the cases studied and shows a different kind of control exercised by men, by using the donor children as a pawn to retain control over the family and women in particular.

Previous studies on the causes of rejection of donor sperm by infertile men have convincingly argued that in the Middle East, with predominantly patriarchal values in relation to reproduction and fertility, men have a strong desire to maintain their *nasab* and reject the idea of sperm donation (Inhorn 2006c; Tremayne 2009; Clarke 2009). However, the combination of research from the larger study of third-party sperm donation carried out between 2004 and 2009 and from the present study provide unexpected insights into the behavior of infertile men who resort to donor sperm. They raise the question of whether in reality it is the biological infertility that matters more to infertile men, or the fact that they are seen to be infertile and not fulfilling their social role and losing their identity and status in society. Key to such use, however, remains anonymity. As long as the "secret" is not revealed, men with strong conservative values in this study seem to have been willing to compromise the "purity" of their biological lineage when faced with having to choose between remaining childless or using a stranger's sperm.

ARTs in cases of sperm donation have generated two kinds of responses by infertile men. There are those who have chosen openly to opt for donor sperm. Most of these men come from the more-educated and less-conservative layers of society. Even some of these men have rejected the donor child later as they "could not bear to see another man's child roam around their home." This rejection has taken various forms, from violence towards the mother and child to falling into depression by the social father, who could not blame anybody else but himself (Tremayne 2009). Often conceiving through sperm donation transcends the boundaries of fertility and reproduction and becomes a form of symbolic sexual transgression in the mind of these infertile men. Such reactions, however, are predictable and do not come as a real surprise. It is the unanticipated responses of the second group of infertile men, who come from highly conservative layers of society and who have decided to use donor sperm, which challenges the previous findings that mention that "men refuse to compromise their lineage by resorting to donor sperm." Infertile men in this study, who have used donor sperm, seem to have overcome their dilemma of keeping their purity of lineage intact or having to live the life of a barren man with all its ramifications, and have opted for donor sperm to prove their fertility, fulfill their duty to their social group, and maintain their social status, masculinity, and identity. While such solutions have existed historically, and examples are known of infertile men who have resorted to their brothers to impregnate their wives, the emergence of new possibilities in the form of ARTs has made it possible for infertile men to hide their infertility more easily and pass off another man's sperm as their own.

What is emerging strongly from this analysis is the interface between reproduction as a means of personal achievement and love of one's own biological child, against one's sense of social identity as a member of the social group. Clearly, the importance of reproducing socially is paramount for individuals, who are prepared to go to any length to demonstrate that they have fulfilled their reproductive duties and to secure their rightful place in society. For those who do not wish to reveal their infertility, even to the close members of the kin group, ARTs have provided the perfect way out, and it is not until something goes wrong that the true extent and implications of such practices become evident.

Conclusion

The data in this chapter have shown that the use of ARTs has led to a reinforcement of cultural values among infertile couples rather than altering them. Further, ARTs have been a contributory factor in the broadening of the gender gap among infertile couples of a certain social group. The findings of the earlier data clearly indicated that the efforts of the practitioners to break some of the cultural molds and alter attitudes towards infertility have had limited effects on the recipients, especially in the case of men. The deeply rooted values on fertility/infertility, acting as cultural barriers to further penetration and acceptance of ARTs, were shown not to have been dislodged beyond their immediate use. To date, infertile men seeking treatment seem to be so imbued with their cultural understanding of what constitutes masculinity that the clinic's education has little significant effect on them. The use of reproductive technologies, and the information that goes with them, become a medium that may help these men achieve "their" ideas of masculinity, rather than transform them.

In addition to highlighting the role of ARTs in deepening the gender gap among certain layers of society, some unanticipated facts in cases of third-party gamete donation have also emerged. One such finding shows that the ground is beginning to shift for many infertile men to move towards a compromise on the "purity" of their lineage in favor of being "seen" to be fertile, by resorting to reproductive technologies to make them be, or appear to be, fertile. ARTs provide the perfect "secrecy" they need to disguise their infertility, something that the traditional method of resorting to one's brother could not. Infertile men's reluctance and hostile reaction to publicizing their infertility (by being seen to receive another man's sperm) stems not just from a feeling of humiliation or inadequacy, but also from deeper cosmological and metaphysical beliefs in relation to procreation. Furthermore, while the resistance of infertile men towards sperm donation has been understood all along to derive from a lineage, gender, and "face" issue, in reality it also lies, in great part, in the fact that in resorting to other men's donated sperm to gain progeny, men become passive spectators, watching their wives being impregnated by what they may view as a "symbolic act of sexual transgression" without playing any role in such a process themselves. The consequent feeling of alienation is what often drives the infertile men to violence towards women or self-deprecation. For women, on the other hand, the IVF treatment takes a totally different meaning since they take an active part throughout the process of procreation. Third-party donation for women, to use Hadolt's (2009) expression, "is a process which is an ensemble of body parts, machines, techniques to which women unavoidably make a corporeal contribution,"[15] and in which they fully participate. In this sense, women's relationships with their donor children differ too from that of men, and make them cherish and treat the children as their own even though such children may be the result of donor eggs.

The future of men and women users of third-party gamete donation and that of their children will therefore continue to be shaped by the fragile balance between disempowered infertile men and their wives who are at the receiving end of their husband's shortcomings. It must be expected that as these technologies continue to reach a higher number of users and the range of class, education, and generation of their users continues to broaden, further research will be needed to assess their impact on kinship, gender relations, donor children, and family, and on the ongoing dialogue between these technologies and their users.

Notes

1. Opening Speech given at Reproductive Disruptions Conference, Ann Arbor, MI, 2005.
2. For a clarification of the meaning of *nasab* see Clarke 2009: 40. As he explains, *nasab* refers to agnatic and uterine relations of filiation in legal discourse. It is also commonly used as "genealogy", i.e., purely agnatic descent, projected backwards in time. In Shia Islam, a child can take his *nasab* from both his parents, but belongs to the father and his lineage. For details of this see Mir Hossieni 1998, and Ebadi interview with *Yas e No* daily paper (in Persian), 10 October 200.
3. Also see Abbasi-Shavazi et al. 2008.
4. The conference was organized by one of the two major leading clinics, the Avicenna Research Centre, (the other being the Royan Institute), and has paved the way for the legitimization of several ARTs by engaging some of the more "progressive" clerics to openly debate and endorse ARTs.
5. The practice of temporary marriage is a form of marriage whereby a man and a woman agree to get married for a fixed length of time between one hour to ninety-nine years (Haeri 1989; Tremayne 2009: 148–49). In the case of the wife's infertility, the husband would marry the egg donor without any sexual contact, to receive her egg to be fertilized with his sperm. Polygyny being allowed in Islam, this would not necessarily cause any complications. But, in the case of the husband's infertility, the wife, not being able to be married to two men at the same time, would divorce her own husband, marry the sperm donor without any sexual contact taking place, receive his sperm, and remarry the first husband. In both cases the embryo is fertilized outside the womb and planted in the uterus.
6. When I first started my field research on third-party donation in 2004, I came across couples who had used temporary marriage before the supreme leader's fatwa and had children who were three or four years old.
7. This procedure has been explained fully in a previous chapter; see Tremayne 2009.
8. Cases of women in Tehran clinics who help cover up their husbands' infertility are documented in Abbasi-Shavazi et al. 2008: 14. According to the study, some of the women interviewed mentioned that they

were infertile, but "they soon disclosed that their husbands were the infertile ones; both had been threatened with divorce if they disclosed the male infertility or refused to shoulder the blame."

9. What may appear to be a voluntary act to undergo treatment often turns out to have been coerced, on close examination.

10. Basij is the paramilitary volunteer militia working under orders from the Revolutionary Guards. Basij have local organizations in every town, government offices, and schools.

11. Temporary marriage is used by Shia only and is an arrangement for marriage between a man and a woman with a time limit on it (see note 5). Temporary marriage has been used as a solution to legitimize third-party donation of sperm and eggs in Iran. For more details on temporary marriage see Haeri 1989.

12. The minimum age of marriage in Iran is 13 for girls and 15 for boys. Following the Islamic Law (sharia) the minimum age of marriage used to be 9 for girls, but, in 2003, under pressure from female members of the Iranian Parliament, the age was increased to 13 for girls. This remains conditional to date. If the girl's father or her guardian or a medical doctor judges her ready to be married earlier, this can be done.

13. For more details on links between age, marriage, sexuality, family, and Islam see Moghadam 1994 and Tremayne 2004. As Moghadam argues, traditionally marriage and the formation of the marital union in patriarchal Muslim societies were viewed as a transaction, with female sexuality as a commodity traded by men. She argues that the legal commoditization of female sexuality should be incorporated in the analysis of gender economics in Muslim societies.

14. Although the Iranian family is moving towards the nuclear family form, the essence of family and kin relations has not changed accordingly. The assumption that an educated, secular couple seeking to have a child is an independent unit and free from the influence of its social group is untrue. The collective involvement of the larger social group prevails, regardless of the lifestyle or physical distance of the couple from its larger social group. The influence of the kin group remains so strong that, the educated and secular as well as the less-educated and conservative layers of society, alike, conform to its will. Young Iranian men, who have grown up in the West, come back to Iran often "because I want to marry a virgin and have children by an innocent [presumably meaning sexually inexperienced] girl." To do so, their families in Iran find the right girl in advance and arrange for him to return, marry her, and take her back with him. The influence of the family, however, continues from across the oceans, and firm control is exercised over most of the couple's decisions through daily contact by telephone, for both sides of the families. In this sense having a child for a couple goes beyond the mere fact of biological reproduction between them and remains a matter for the social group. Having a child becomes an obligation and a necessity towards the social reproduction of

the group and the continuity of the lineage. It is clear that unless the way donor children are conceived fits into the cultural understanding of what constitutes parenthood, their presence creates hostilities and proves disruptive for the family and the wider social group.

15. Seminar on "Age and Reproduction," Fertility and Reproduction Seminars, Institute of Social and Cultural Anthropology, University of Oxford, 30 November 2009.

References

Abbasi-Shavazi, Moḥammad Jalal, Marcia C. Inhorn, Hajiieh Bibi Razeghi-Nasrabad, and Ghasem Toloo. 2008. "The 'Iranian ART Revolution': Infertility, Assisted Reproductive Technology, and Third-Party Donation in the Islamic Republic of Iran." *Journal of Middle East Women's Studies* 4(2): 1–28.

Becker, Gay. 2000. *The Elusive Embryo: How Women and Men Approach the New Reproductive Technologies*. Berkeley: University of California Press.

Clarke, Morgan. 2006a. "Islam, Kinship and New Reproductive Technology." *Anthropology Today* 22(5): 17–20.

———. 2006b. "Shiite Perspectives on Kinship and New Reproductive Technologies." *ISIM Review* 17: 26–27.

———. 2009. *Islam and New Kinship: Reproductive Technologies and the Shariah in Lebanon*. New York and Oxford: Berghahn Books.

Ebadi, Shirin. 2003. *Women's Rights in the Laws of the Islamic Republic of Iran* (in Persian). Tehran: Ganje Danesh Publishers.

Garmaroudi, Shirin. 2008. "Sibling Intimacy in the Age of Assisted Reproduction: An Ethnography of New Reproductive Technologies in Iran." Master's thesis, University of Berne.

Greil, Arthur L., Thomas A. Leitko, and Karen L. Porter. 1998. "Infertility: His and Hers." *Gender & Society* 2(2): 172–99.

Haeri, Shahla. 1989. *Law of Desire: Temporary Marriage in Shi'i Islam*. Syracuse, NY: Syracuse University Press.

Hadolt, Bernard. 2009. Seminar delivered at Fertility and Reproduction Seminar Series, Institute of Social and Cultural Anthropology, Oxford University.

Inhorn, Marcia C. 1996. *Infertility and Patriarchy: The Cultural Politics of Gender and Family Life in Egypt*. Philadelphia: University of Pennsylvania Press

———. 2003. *Local Babies, Global Science: Gender, Religion, and In Vitro Fertilization in Egypt*. New York: Routledge.

———. 2004. "Middle Eastern Masculinities in the Age of New Reproductive Technologies: Male Infertility and Stigma in Egypt and Lebanon." *Medical Anthropology Quarterly* 18(2): 162–82.

———. 2005. "Religion and Reproductive Technologies: IVF and Gamete Donation in the Muslim World." *Anthropology News* 46(2): 14–18.

————. 2005. "Reproductive Disruptions." Paper presented at the International Conference on Reproductive Disruptions: Childlessness, Adoption, and Other Reproductive Complexities, 19 May, University of Michigan, Ann Arbor.

————. 2006a. "Making Muslim Babies: IVF and Gamete Donation in Sunni versus Shia Islam." *Culture, Medicine and Psychiatry* 30(4): 427–50.

————. 2006b. "A More Open Mind toward Iran." *Chronicle of Higher Education* B12.

————. 2006c. "He Won't Be My Son." *Medical Anthropology Quarterly* 20(1): 94–120.

Inhorn, Marcia C., and Frank van Balen, eds. 2002. *Infertility around the Globe: New Thinking on Childlessness, Gender, and Reproductive Technologies.* Berkeley: University of California Press.

Lock, Margaret, and Patricia Kaufert. 1998. *Pragmatic Women and Body Politics.* Cambridge: Cambridge University Press.

Martin, Emily. 1987. *The Woman in the Body: A Cultural Analysis of Reproduction.* Milton Keynes: Open University.

Mir-Hosseini, Ziba. 1993. *Marriage on Trial: A Study of Islamic Family Law.* London: I.B. Tauris.

Modern Human Reproductive Techniques from the View of Jurisprudence and Law (in Persian). 2001. Book based on papers presented in a symposium of the same title. Tehran: Published by the Avisena Research Institute and in association with the Academic Publishing House for the Social Science.

Moghadam, Fatemeh. 1994. "Commoditisation of Sexuality and Female Labour Participation in Islam: Implications for Iran 1960–90." In *In the Eye of the Storm*, ed. M. Afkhami and E. Friedl. London: I. B. Tauris.

Petchesky, Rosalind. 1995. "The Body as Property: A Revision." In *Conceiving the New World Order: The Global Politics of Reproduction*, ed. Faye D. Ginsburg and Rayna Rapp. Berkeley: University of California Press.

Scheper-Hughes, Nancy. 2009. "Editorial." *Anthropology Today* 25 (August): 4.

Serour, Gamal I. 1993. "Bioethics in Reproductive Health: A Muslim Perspective." *Middle East Fertility Society Journal* 1: 30–35.

Thompson, Charis M. 2002. "Fertile Ground: Feminists Theorize Infertility." In *Infertility Around the Globe: New Thinking on Childlessness, Gender, and Reproductive Technologies*, ed. Marcia C. Inhorn and Frank van Balen. Berkeley: University of Californian Press.

Tremayne, Soraya. 2004. "And Never the Twain Shall Meet." In *Reproductive Agency, Medicine and the State: Cultural Transformations in Childbearing*, ed. Maya Unnithan-Kumar. New York and Oxford: Berghahn Books.

————. 2005. "The Moral, Ethical and Legal Implications of Egg, Sperm and Embryo Donation in Iran." Paper presented at the International Conference on Reproductive Disruptions: Childlessness, Adoption, and Other Reproductive Complexities, 19 May, University of Michigan, Ann Arbor.

————. 2006a. "Whither Kinship? New Procreative Practices, Authoritative Knowledge, and Relatedness: Case Studies from Iran." Paper presented at the Conference on Gamete and Embryo Donation for Infertility Treatment, 2 March, University of Tehran, Iran.

———. 2006b. "Not All Muslims are Luddites." *Anthropology Today* 22(93): 1–2.

———. 2009. "Law, Ethics and Donor Technologies in Shia Iran." In *Assisting Reproduction, Testing Genes: Global Encounters with New Biotechnologies*, ed. Daphna Birenbaum-Carmeli and Marcia C. Inhorn. New York and Oxford: Berghahn Books.

Unnithan-Kumar, Maya. 2009. "Female Selective Abortion—Beyond Culture: Family Making and Gender Inequality in a Globalising India." *Culture, Health and Sexuality* 12(2): 153–66.

———. 2010. "Learning from Infertility: Gender, Health Inequities and Faith Healers in Women's Experiences of Disrupted Reproduction in Rajasthan." *South Asian History and Culture* 1(2): 315–27.

Chapter 6

GESTATIONAL SURROGACY IN IRAN
UTERINE KINSHIP IN SHIA THOUGHT AND PRACTICE

Shirin Garmaroudi Naef

Anthropologist: "When you carry the baby inside you for nine months, don't you think that the baby is yours?"

Surrogate: "No, it is not mine. The egg is someone else's. The baby is just nurturing from me. Neither the sperm is from my husband. It is from another man. The baby is like a deposit [*amanat*] to me. I safeguard it in my womb for 9 months. It is a good deed [*savab dareh*]."

(Excerpt from an interview with a gestational surrogate)

Gestational surrogacy, in which the surrogate is not the provider of the female gamete and only gestates another couple's embryo, as a solution to infertility is being practiced in Iran and has become an ongoing issue in the public debate. The practice demands the involvement of another woman in the process of childbearing and delivery—a woman who is able to carry the baby of another married couple in her womb for nine months and ultimately gives birth to it. In this respect, it is of utmost importance that the majority of Shia *fuqaha* (legal experts in *fiqh*) allow this form of assisted reproduction as legitimate from the viewpoint of Islamic law, albeit only for infertile married couples.[1]

In Sunni Islam, as shown by Marcia Inhorn (e.g., 2003, 2006) and also as demonstrated in several chapters of this volume, the use of donor gametes and surrogacy is unacceptable and is regarded as analogous to *zina* or "adultery."[2] The resulting child would be considered illegitimate with no paternal relations, although she/he is still related to the mother. In Shia thought, the issue is more complex and diverse. Most Shia authorities disagree with this position and do not regard assisted reproduction involving a third party—whether legitimate or not—as analogous to adultery or *zina*, since it does not involve the physical act of sexual intercourse, as addressed extensively by scholars who have worked on third-party donation in Muslim societies (Tremayne 2006, 2007, 2009; Abbasi-Shavazi et al. 2008; Inhorn 2006; Clarke 2007, 2009; among others).

On the basis of my analysis of Shia legal positions on the appropriateness of gamete donation and surrogacy, which will be the major concern of this chapter, I explore the fact that central to this divergence is the question of *nasab*[3]: whereas Sunni notions of *nasab* take a more agnatic form—which passes through the male—Shia notions take a more gender-balanced structure and recognize a bilateral filiation, under which maternal (*nasab-e madari*) and paternal filiation (*nasab-e pedari*) are clearly distinguished and in many regards symmetrical. According to the majority of Shia authorities, both male and female reproductive substances play a symmetrical role in the procreation of a child as well as in producing the line of descent, ties of agnatic and uterine kinship. So, as I wish to show in this chapter, the juridical meaning ascribed to the physiological facts and bodily substances, either male or female in this account, leaves room for the legal permissibility of third-party donation and surrogacy.

However, the opinions are not monolithic and centralized, and Shia scholars' responses to the questions posed by assisted reproduction are controversial, although one should also note that certain principles remain the same. In this chapter, I argue that the Shia notion of *zina* does not depend on the biological act that occurs through the contact and transfer of bodily substances. It depends on the illegitimate physical act that occurs through illicit sexual intercourse between a man and a woman and not on the act of conception itself.[4] In this manner, a considerable number of Shia scholars have authenticated the application of third-party donation and surrogacy arrangements (even among sibling sets) under specific conditions.

Certainly, the rapidly growing number of research centers in Iran and new supporting medical approaches addressing infertility, as well as the increasing number of infertile couples seeking proper treatment, created a ground for debates on jurisprudential (*fiqhi*) and legal (*hoquqi*) aspects of the social uses of new reproductive technologies in order to pave the way for constituting a proper law.[5] In 1999, the Avicenna Research Institute in cooperation with the Faculty of Law and Political Sciences of Tehran University presented the jurisprudential and legal aspects of embryo donation for the first time in a symposium called "Jurisprudential and Legal Issues Concerning Embryo Donation." According to Dr. Mohammad Mehdi Akhondi, director of the Avicenna Research Institute, the religious deliberations by Islamic legal scholars at this symposium played an important role in presenting a provision on embryo donation to the parliament and in the parliament's decision to approve the bill for embryo donation (personal communication, Tehran, November 2006). Finally, in 2000, a provision was presented to the Iranian Parliament (*majles*) titled "Embryo Donation to Infertile Spouses" in five clauses, which consequently resulted in the ratification of the bill on 20 July 2003. As for all regulations approved by the parliament in Iran, this was sent to the Guardian Council (*shora-ye negahban*)[6] to decide whether such laws were based on Islamic principles (*mavazin-e islami*).[7] However, shortly after its approval by the parliament on 30 July 2003, the Guardian Council endorsed a legislative act governing embryo donation, and the law became fully operative in 2005.

Along the same line, the following symposiums on various fields of reproduction and infertility have been organized by the Avicenna Research Institute in association with several universities in Tehran: Gamete and Embryo Donation in Infertility Treatment, March 2006; the National Congress on AIDS, November 2006; the Interdisciplinary Seminar on Surrogacy, October 2007; and Fertility Preservation, January 2010.[8] I attended the National Congress on AIDS in the course of my field research in Tehran. One of the most interesting subjects discussed in this symposium was in regard to patients with HIV/AIDS who wanted to have a healthy child through IVF and other assisted reproductive technologies (ARTs). I attended the Interdisciplinary Seminar on Surrogacy as well, which was also held in Tehran. The two-day conference was also organized by the Avicenna Research Institute in association with the Faculty of Law and Political Sciences (Allameh Tabataba'i University, Tehran) and the School of Theology and Philosophy (Islamic Azad University, Science and Research Branch, Tehran). The conference focused on issues related to surrogacy from a multidisciplinary perspective. Like the above-mentioned conference on embryo donation, it played a key role in

presenting a legitimate solution for the practice of gestational surrogacy in infertility treatments in Iran. Subjects related to surrogacy contracts, rights of infertile couples, rights of the child, rights
of gestational surrogates, surrogacy and abortion, surrogacy in the
law of Iran, issuing birth certificates to newborns from surrogacy,
and kinship relations resulting from the act of surrogacy were discussed and further studies and actions were proposed.[9] In discussing
the legal framework for gestational surrogacy, participating jurists in
the conference offered a bill to issue a birth certificate for a child's
legal parents and not for the woman who delivers the child (see
also Milanifar et al. 2008).[10] An edited volume titled *Essays on Medical, Legal, Islamic Jurisprudential, Ethical-Philosophical, Sociological, and
Psychological Aspects of Surrogacy*, which included twenty-nine articles,
was published as the result of this conference. One can thus assume
that the relationship between Islamic legal scholars and physicians,
indeed between religion and biomedical science, contributes to the
enhancement of the social patterns of relatedness in Iran by abolish-
ing infertility as a source of disorder in the constitution of kinship
relations.[11]

The first part of this chapter is an analysis of some leading Shia
scholars on the appropriateness of gamete donation and surrogacy.
Clearly, a full examination of this complexity is beyond the scope
of this chapter. Through close reading of Islamic legal texts, as well
as extensive ethnographic field research, I attempt to show how
the juridical meaning ascribed to physiological facts and bodily substances, either male or female, leaves room for the legal permissibility of gestational surrogacy. The second part of this chapter further
explores the way in which gestational surrogates attempt to transform surrogacy from a controversial issue into a normative concept
in infertility treatments in Iran.

Methodology

I began to study infertility and ARTs in 2005. I started with participant observation in infertility and IVF clinics in Tehran, which
took place during several research trips to Iran. Furthermore, I began to carry out conversations with men and women who were directly or indirectly faced with the problems of infertility, both those
who already had experience with ARTs and those who were seeking
to have children through assisted reproductive methods. In Qom
(the center of Shia scholarship in Iran) I was able to meet and in-

terview Shia religious scholars who had differing views on assisted reproduction.

Moreover, through the kind cooperation of the medical staff in Tehran's infertility clinics, I was able to undertake many in-depth interviews with persons undergoing ART procedures, and I kept in contact with most of them. I also spent long hours of participant observation in different infertility clinics, which gave me additional insight into the topic. I conducted over one hundred in-depth, open-format interviews with both infertile couples undergoing ART procedures using donor eggs, donor embryos, donor sperm, and surrogacy, as well as people such as gamete donors and surrogates. Furthermore, I discussed assisted reproduction many times with more than twenty people (directors, doctors, social workers, nurses, lab workers, and consultants) working at five well-known infertility clinics and one hospital where I conducted my research. I also presented a paper based on the collected data and some of the arguments discussed in this chapter at the two-day Interdisciplinary Seminar on Surrogacy in Tehran in October 2007 (see Garmaroudi 2008b).

Bodily Substances

In recent years, the anthropological analysis of the notions of contact and transfer of bodily substances has become an approach for studying kinship and assisted reproduction in Muslim societies (e.g., Conte 2000, 2003; Clarke 2009, 2007; Fortier 2007; Parkes 2005), associated in particular with the works of the French anthropologist Françoise Héritier (1999). In a general retheorization of incest in her monograph, "Two Sisters and Their Mother: The Anthropology of Incest," Héritier argues that the prohibition of marriage and sexual contact between kin and affines in fact derives from the taboo on identical bodily substances being mixed, an incestuous element in these type of relationships: "The fundamental criterion of incest is the contact between identical bodily fluids" (Héritier 1999: 11). Thus, the worst part of Oedipus's crime, as Héritier seems to demonstrate, is not that he married his mother, Jocasta (incest of the first type), but that he had sexual relations with a woman with whom his father has already had sexual relations (contact of identical substance, incest of the second type). Hamlet, too, according to Héritier, is a story of incest of the second type that ended in blood. Thus, the vital part of Hamlet's tragedy is not a question of the father's murder by his brother, but the contact of the two brothers' identical fluids in the same womb through the intermediary of the same woman, Queen Gertrude.

Héritier analyzes ancient Near East, Greek, Roman, and Judeo-Christian-Islamic texts, on the one hand, and ethnographies of African societies, on the other. Inspired by Soraya Altorki's (1980) pioneering article on milk kinship created through suckling breast milk (*rida'*) in urban Saudi Arabia, Héritier expands upon her thesis to elucidate the logic underlying marriage prohibitions resulting from suckling, as stated in Islamic jurisprudence. In Islamic legal tradition, the act of breastfeeding constitutes a basis for kinship relations other than relationships created through ties of marriage and descent. Islamic rules forbid marriage not only between the child and the milk mother but further, between all the other members of the milk mother's kin, including the milk mother's husband and his kin (see e.g., Clarke 2007 for full references). According to Héritier such alliance prohibitions can only be understood by means of "incest of the second type," which implies contact of identical bodily substances. From a folk and juridical saying that "the milk is from the man," which implies that the milk of the woman takes its source from a pregnancy, Héritier argues that in the Islamic rules of milk kinship, the male substance transmitted by lactation ultimately appears to be decisive in establishing kinship ties: "The breast-feeding relationship reinforces the agnatic relationship and extends it" (Héritier 1999: 276).

Héritier's work on the Middle East has been endorsed by several like-minded French anthropologists (e.g., Conte 2000 and Fortier 2007), but also has attracted some criticism (e.g., Parkes 2005 and Clarke 2009). Most recently, Corinne Fortier (2007) has published an article on the subject of milk kinship, descent, and medically assisted procreation; her review is again another reaffirmation of Héritier's thesis and the importance of bodily substance in the definition of incest. Inspired by Héritier's idea of substantial identity, Fortier repeatedly appeals to agnatic forms of Arab kinship as biologically based, arguing that in Sunni Islam, "sperm appears as an essential biological determinant of patrilineal descent" (2007: 16). She argues that in all stages of conception, gestation, and lactation in the physical creation of the child is the male agnatic substance, which plays a primary role. Thus, "In these representations, woman plays no substantial role in either conception or pregnancy" (2007: 26). Furthermore, "they are dispossessed of the substance visibly flowing from their breast" (2007: 26). Based on Marcia Inhorn's IVF and infertility studies in Egypt (2003), Fortier adopts this approach to demonstrate and clarify why Sunni Islam forbids sperm donation but allows artificial insemination for married couples and why Sunni Islam forbids sperm banks but allows blood banks. Her conclusion is:

> Any form of procreation involving a third person is related to adultery and any child who is born from it is regarded as illegitimate. This explains why oocyte or embryo donation, or surrogate motherhood, are also forbidden in Sunni Islam. Furthermore, the absence of a female biological substance in procreation and the importance of gestation in the definition of maternity as shown in the analysis of descent in Sunni Islam explain how it is that, in the theoretical case of disjunction between conception and gestation, in the case of oocyte donation or surrogacy, jurists ascribe full maternity to the woman who bears and delivers (*wilādah*) the child (Fortier 2007: 29).

Again, the analysis of ties of kinship in this approach is restricted to the study of the definition of bodily substances, as Fortier further argues that "these contemporary questions can be clarified by an analysis of the meaning of sperm, blood and milk in Sunni Islam" (2007: 15). In this chapter I problematize Héritier's thesis of contact and transfer of bodily substances for the study of incest and its implications for kinship thinking and practice. By doing so, I wish to show that rhetoric of incest does not follow a "universal grammar." I argue that the definition of incest in Shia thought and practice does not depend on the transfer or contact of bodily substances. Rather, it depends on the illegitimate physical act of illicit sexual intercourse, and not on the act of conception itself.

Assisted Reproduction in Contemporary Shia *Fiqh*

The Shia scholars justify assisted reproduction on the basis of the need to define kinship relations (*nasab*, both agnatic and uterine) resulting from the use of ARTs. The issue of assisted reproduction has raised many questions, and the religious scholars have controversial opinions regarding it. However, the following questions are primarily addressed in the arguments of Shia scholars regarding assisted reproduction: Is artificial insemination (*leqah-e masnu'i*) religiously allowed? Are the procedures such as the use of donor sperm, eggs, or embryos and surrogacy arrangement permitted? Does artificial insemination with donor sperm constitute *zina*? Is it allowed to fertilize the woman's egg with the sperm of a man other than her husband? And if so, what is the legal status of the child conceived with donor gametes? Should a child conceived this way be considered a *walad al-zina,* a bastard? Who would be the father and mother of the child: the owner of gametes and uterus or the recipients of the gametes? How should the rules of inheritance (*ahkam-e erth*) and marriage (*ahkam-e ezdewaj*) be applied? However, the most important question is the issue of the *nasab* of the child, both agnatic and uterine (*pedari* and *madari*), and how paternity and maternity would be constituted.

Artificial Insemination and Traditional Surrogacy

Artificial insemination could be either by the husband's sperm or by a donor's sperm—in Islamic legal texts, a "stranger" (*biganeh* or *ajnabi*). The majority of Islamic scholars, both Sunni and Shia, argue that fertilizing the ovum of a woman with the sperm of her husband outside her body, and implanting it in the wife's womb, is not forbidden in Islam, and the resulting child is the legal offspring of the married couple (Inhorn 2003). Artificial insemination by donor, which involves the insertion of sperm from a man other than the husband into the woman's uterus, is forbidden in Sunni Islam (Inhorn 2006), but is argued differently in Shia legal thought. Most Shia scholars, however, argue that the act of fertilization of the woman's egg with the sperm of a man other than her husband's is not allowed (*ja'ez nist*),[12] but this process is not regarded as analogous to *zina* and the resulting child would not be considered illegitimate (e.g., Rezaniya Mo'allem 2005). For many Shia authorities, but not all, the originator of the sperm, however, would be considered as the father of the child.

Yet, some Shia authorities have adopted a different stance on the issue of artificial insemination. They authorize the insemination of the woman's egg with the donor's sperm in a lab dish, and then implantation of the fertilized egg (zygote) into the wife's uterus. For example, according to the fatwas of Ayatollah Khamene'i, the supreme religious leader of Iran (Samadi Ahari 2004: 33) and some senior Shia clerics like Ayatollahs Mohammad Shirazi (Samadi Ahari 2004: 39), Mosawi Ardebili (Samadi Ahari 2004: 46), Qomi (Rezaniya Mo'allem 2005: 196), and Ayatollah Seyyed Mohammad Musavi Bojnurdi (Rezaniya Mo'allem 2005: 197), in the case that the husband's infertility leads to difficulties in marriage, fertilization of the woman's egg with the sperm of a man other than her husband outside of the woman's body and then the implantation of the fertilized egg (*janin*) in the woman's uterus is allowed as long as no forbidden act (*fe'el-e haram*), such as gaze or touch, has taken place. So, in response to the question concerning the artificial insemination by a man's sperm other than the husband's, some above-mentioned scholars give the following explanations:

> **Question:** "Is it allowed to fertilize the wife with the sperm of a stranger [*biganeh*, here 'a man other than the husband'], by placing the sperm in her womb?"
>
> **Ayatollah Khamene'i:** "There is no problem as long as no forbidden act [*fe'el-e haram*] such as touch and gaze has taken place." (Samadi Ahari 2004: 33)
>
> **Ayatollah Mohammad Shirazi:** "It is permissible with the consent of the husband and as long as no forbidden act [*fe'el-e haram*] has taken place." (Samadi Ahari 2004: 39)
>
> **Ayatollah Mosawi Ardebili:** "There is a problem to the placing of a stranger's sperm (*biganeh*, 'donor's sperm') directly into a woman's uterus, but there is no problem to the fertilization of an egg outside of the womb and then implanting the embryo (*janin*) into the woman's uterus." (Samadi Ahari 2004: 46)

Again, the distinction made here between physical contact (such as a gaze, a touch, or illicit sexual intercourse) and the transfer and contact of bodily substance in definition of adultery makes the fertilization of the woman's egg with the sperm of a man other than her husband and then the implantation of the embryo in the woman's womb religiously permissible. As a result of this permissibility, sperm donation is practiced in some clinics in Iran (Garmaroudi 2008c).

Traditional surrogacy, which also involves the insertion of sperm from a man other than the husband into the woman's uterus, is not allowed according to the majority of scholars. In contrast, the practice of gestational surrogacy, in which the surrogate woman is not the contributor of the egg and just carries the embryo of a married couple, is, among the majority of Shia authorities, an accepted form of assisted reproduction.[13] Again, a clear Shia distinction can be made here between the act of placing sperm directly into the female's uterus, which according to the majority of religious scholars is not allowed, and the act of implanting an embryo into the womb of a woman, a new technological procedure in which the sperm and egg of a married couple are combined outside the woman's body and the resulting embryo is placed in a surrogate woman's womb, for which there is clearly religious permissibility. In other words, the prohibition is against putting the seed in a womb, which is forbidden to a man, and not against putting an embryo into her uterus. Thus, the use of gestational surrogacy and embryo transfer for married couples unable to produce a child is, according to the majority of scholars (see e.g., Musavi Bojnurdi 2007: 102–24), permissible.

Ovum, Uterus (*Rahem*), and Maternal Relatedness

In the cases of egg donation and gestational surrogacy, which involve one woman's egg and another woman's uterus, the question arises: Who will be considered the mother? The woman who carries the child in her uterus, the producer of the egg, or both? This is an important question in the kinship system that determines the maternal filiation of the child. In this regard, Shia jurisprudence recognizes a bilateral filiation in which maternal filiation acquires the same importance as paternal. Here, I examine the construction of maternity in the context of assisted reproduction in Shia thought. As we will see below, the juridical meaning ascribed to egg and womb shows the important role that the female portion plays in the creation of a child and in producing the line of descent, the ties of uterine kinship.

In an interpretive and juridical framework, a group of Shia scholars argue that the maternity of the child should be assigned to the woman who carries the pregnancy and gives birth to the child. This is the opinion of late Grand Ayatollah Khu'i, late Ayatollahs Ma'refat (correspondence by letter, 20 October 2006, Qom), Tabrizi (correspondence by letter, 9 October 2006, Qom), Araki, and the majority of Sunni authorities (Rezaniya Mo'allem 2003: 317–62). Those who hold this opinion argue that the Qur'anic verse "Their mothers are only those who gave them birth"[14] relates directly to the point that the gestational carrier and deliverer of a child should be considered as the mother. Therefore, these scholars hold that only the woman who carries the child in her uterus and subsequently gives birth to it is the mother, whether she is the producer of the egg or not. Following this interpretation, maternity should be established only at parturition (in Persian *zayeman:* the act of giving birth to a child).

Another opinion held by the majority of Shia scholars (Rezaniya Mo'allem 2003: 355) is that the producer of the ovum should be considered the mother. They argue that maternity, similar to paternity, is established at conception. This is the opinion of many leading

Shia Ayatollahs like the late Khomeini, Yousef Sane'i, Mohammad Mo'men Qomi,[15] Musavi Bojnurdi (Musavi Bojnurdi 2007: 113), Safi Golpayegani (correspondence by letter, 9 October 2006, Qom), Naser Makarem Shirazi (correspondence by letter, 11 October 2006, Qom), Montazeri, Sistani, and Khamene'i. They give equal emphasis to both the maternal and paternal seed in the procreation of a child; so, ovum and sperm play an equivalent role in the conception. Following their interpretations, the definition of maternity is identical to the legal father-child relationship, considering the fact that the father is the owner of the sperm; thus, the owner of the egg should be considered the mother (Rezaniya Mo'allem 2003: 317–62). They support this view by the Qur'anic verses, which indicate the constitution of *nasab* (both agnatic and uterine) and the origin of the human being:

And it is He who created of water [*al-ma'*] a mortal, and made him kindred [by *nasab*], and marriage [*sihr*] ...[16]

We created man of a [*nutfah*], a mingling.[17]

In their discussion of these verses, they refer to the definition of *khalaga men ma'* (created from water) and *men nutfah emshaj* (from mixed semen) to explain the Qur'anic description of the creation of human life by God from mixing male and female fluids, the sperm and the ovum respectively. In their interpretation, the term *ma'* (water in Arabic) refers to the male and female fluids (*ma' al-rajol* and *ma' al-mar'at*) and it is from their mixing that the fetus is formed. In this interpretation, the male's sperm and the female's ovum have a symmetrical role in the formation of the fetus and the creation of the child and subsequently the constitution of *nasab*. Furthermore, in reference to *emshaj*—literarily, "mixed" in Arabic—they argue that the phrase "*men nutfah emshaj*" means "from mixed *nutfah*" and indicates the fertilized ovum (zygote), resulting from the ovum of the woman and the sperm of the man.

According to these Shia scholars (Rezaniya Mo'allem 2003: 327), the Qur'an does indeed make it clear that the construction of the human being starts with a single cell called *nutfah emshaj* (zygote), which is a mix of an ovum from a female and a sperm from a male (two *ma'*). Thus, in the case of egg donation or gestational surrogacy, the majority of Shia opinion ascribes the maternity to the originator of the egg (*saheb-e tokhmak*). Among scholars, Ayatollah Yousef Sane'i, a Shia *marja'* widely renowned as a theologian, Islamic philosopher, and reformist scholar, is one of the most distinguished holders of this opinion. I collected his views regarding assisted reproduction published in different sources (e.g., Rezaniya Mo'allem 2005: 449–55; *Essays on Modern Human Reproductive Techniques from the View of Jurisprudence and Law* 2003: 396; and Sane'i 2006), which can be summarized as follows:

1. Ayatolla Yousef Sane'i argues that the implantation of the fertilized egg (zygote, *nutfah-e emshaj shodeh*) of a married couple into another woman's uterus to grow in it is allowed. According to him, in this case, the father and mother of the child are the originators of the zygote (*saheban nutfah emshaj*). This permissibility would facilitate gestational surrogacy arrangements. In this situation, the resulting child would be assigned to the couple providing the embryo (the intended parents for whom pregnancy is impossible) and not to the woman who carries it and gives birth to the child (gestational surrogate).

2. According to Ayatollah Sane'i, the child conceived through gestational surrogacy is not *mahram* (unmarriageable member of kin)[18] to the woman who carries the child in her uterus as well as the woman's husband (*farzand be zan-e saheb-e rahem wa shoharash mahram nemi-bashad*), since the surrogate woman only carries the child in her uterus and is not the contributor of the egg and her husband is not the contributor of the sperm. In fact, in the case of gestational surrogacy, the child should be considered to be related to the married couple who emitted sperm and egg for his or her conception, and not to the woman who carries and delivers the child.

3. According to Sane'i, a gestational surrogate can be either a married or unmarried woman (*farqi bein-e zan-e shohar-dar wa bi-shohar wa mahram wa gheyr-e mahram nemi-bashad*); she can be either *mahram* (unmarriageable) or *namahram* (marriageable); even the wife's sister (*khahar-e zan*) and the husband's sister (*khahar-e shohar*) could act as a gestational surrogate. In other words, gestational surrogacy between siblings is permissible: a woman is allowed to deliver the child of her sister or carry the child of her brother in her womb and give birth to it.

Finally, another opinion held by Shia legal scholars is that maternity is established by two principles: one through bringing into existence (*ertebat-e takwini*) and one through gestation and birth (*ertebat-e hamli wa weladati*). Some Shia scholars suggest that the child born as a result of gamete donation and gestational surrogacy should be considered to have two real mothers: one is the "contributor of the egg" (*saheb-e tokhmak*) and the other one is the "gestational carrier" (*saheb-e rahem*). This is the opinion of Ayatollah Mosavi Ardebili

(Rezaniya Mo'allem 2003: 355) and Ayatollah Sadeqi Tehrani (Interview with Ayatollah Sadeqi Tehrani, 19 December 2006, Qom). I interviewed Ayatollah Sadeqi Tehrani, a distinguished scholar of the Qom Seminary and a Shia *marja'*, at his residence. He argues that maternity is established by two principles, a biological and a gestational one, and that the Qur'anic revelations have taken both principles into consideration (*Sura* 86:7 and *Sura* 2:233). Therefore, the child born through assisted reproduction using one woman's egg and another woman's uterus has two mothers and inherits from both of them.

Furthermore, Ayatollah Sadeqi Tehrani differentiates between the act of gamete donation on the one hand and the legal status of the child originating from gamete donation on the other. In the course of the interview, he explained to me that a third-party donation in the form of sperm and egg donation is not allowed. In these forms of third-party donation, another "man's sperm" or another "woman's egg" enters a place to which it does not belong. Such procedures are against the Qur'anic text (*Sura* 23:5–7), which, according to Ayatollah Sadeqi Tehrani, gives strong clarification about the immorality of such actions. However, the child conceived this way would be the legal offspring of the provider of the sperm and egg and should inherit from the sperm donor, egg donor, and the woman who carries the child in her uterus and gives birth to it.

Ayatollah Sadeqi's opinion opposing sperm and egg donation, however, supports embryo donation that involves both sperm and egg from another married couple and gestational surrogacy, which involves the uterus of another woman. In other words, he separates the status of egg and sperm from the status of the embryo and identifies embryo donation as a fully legal religious act. He does this by considering the embryo as a result of a legal marriage between a man and a woman. Following his arguments, both embryo donation and gestational surrogacy are allowed in order to overcome both male and female infertility of another married couple. According to him, it is even necessary (*wajib*) for an infertile married couple, who would like to have a child and do not have another opportunity to attain true parenthood, to take gestational help into account and to be ready for the implantation of an embryo into the uterus of another woman.

The Law on Embryo Donation to Infertile Spouses approved in 2003 in Iran has restricted embryo donation and reception to married Iranian couples, without linking this to a prohibition of embryo donation among kin groups, for instance among siblings. In

the course of the interview, I told Ayatollah Sadeqi about my ethnographic fieldwork in Tehran's infertility clinics that enabled me
to observe embryo transfer among siblings (same or opposite sex),
especially when male infertility was present. I was interested, therefore, in his view on the practice of embryo donation between siblings
and whether it was allowed. According to Ayatollah Sadeqi, embryo
donation between siblings is permissible, in the case that it does not
involve the direct transfer of sperm or egg, as he explained (Interview with Ayatollah Sadeqi Tehrani, 19 December 2006, Qom):

> The transfer of sperm or egg alone as *nutfah* is not allowed. However,
> the procedures involving the fertilization of a wife's egg with her hus-
> band's sperm, and then transferring the resulted embryo [*janin*] to
> the uterus of another married woman is *halal* and permissible [*ja'ez
> ast*], whether among siblings or among strangers [*qaribeh*].

Here again, in Ayatollah Sadeqi's view, embryo transfer among siblings is allowed. A sister, for example, is permitted to bear and deliver the child of her brother or her sister. This permissibility quoted
here is similar to that of Ayatollah Yousef Sane'i. One principle is of
central importance: The definition of the act of incest or adultery
does not depend on the transfer or contact of bodily substances. It
depends on the physical act of illicit sexual intercourse, and not on
the act of conception itself.

In the following part of this chapter, I introduce in some detail the
juridical views of one high-ranking Shia cleric regarding the issue of
assisted reproduction and its implication for the use of gestational
surrogacy in infertility treatment.

Ayatollah Mohammad Mo'men Qomi

Ayatollah Mo'men is a learned and very respected high-ranking
seminary cleric, one of the six *faqih* members of the Guardian Council and a member of the Assembly of Experts.[19] He is considered to
be one of the preeminent and notable scholars of the Qur'anic sciences (*'ulum-e qor'ani*) and *fiqh*. His opinions on assisted reproduction are widely recognized among Shia scholars, jurists, and medical
scientists in Iran. He has contributed to a number of articles on assisted reproduction and related topics both in Arabic and Persian,
and is frequently cited in academic publications on assisted reproductive technologies in Iran. I interviewed him on 13 October 2006.
In the same week, his article and an interview that took place with

him that related to cloning (*shabih-sazi*) were published in the journal *Fiqh: kawoshi no dar fiqh-e islami* (*Fiqh*: An Innovative Effort in Islamic *Fiqh*), one of the leading journals in the field of Islamic jurisprudence published in Qom. On the recommendation of Ayatollah Mo'men, I had read another article of his, related to artificial insemination (*leqah-e masnu'i*) in the journal *Fiqh-e ahl-e bayt* before meeting with him.[20]

Ayatollah Mo'men starts his article by referring to the different types of assisted conception and examining the question of *halal* and *haram* in relation to them. Among the many questions he addresses, the following are of utmost importance: the question of the *nasab* of a child by asking who is the father and the mother of the child born through ARTs? Should a child conceived in this way be considered a *walad al-zina*? How should inheritance and marriage rules be applied (Mo'men 1996)? For Ayatollah Mo'men, like the majority of Shia authorities, maternity and paternity are established at conception. In other words, the true mother and father of a child are the woman and the man who have contributed to his conception. According to him, the real father–child relationship is established by ascribing the child to the producer of the *maniyy* (seminal fluid produced by orgasm; here man's sperm),[21] and in an equal way, the true mother–child relationship is established by ascribing the child to the producer of the *tokhmak* (woman's egg).[22]

For many Sunni authorities (see references above and this volume passim), the introduction of other parties into the reproductive process is perceived as analogous to *zina* and comes under the category of *haram;* the resulting child is considered to be an illegitimate child with no paternal relation, although he or she is still related to the mother who bore him or her. However, many Shia authorities do not agree with this position.

For example, Ayatollah Mo'men does not regard assisted conception involving third-party donation as analogous to *zina*, since it does not involve the physical act of sexual intercourse; hence, despite the fact that the act of fertilizing the egg of the woman with the sperm of a man other than her husband (*maniyy-e mard-e namahram*) is *haram*, it creates a paternal relationship between the child and the man who is the originator of sperm (*saheb al-maniyy*). He is responsible for the child's welfare, and they inherit from each other. In other words, the act of injecting the *maniyy* (here man's sperm) of a man other than the husband into the woman's uterus is *haram;* however, the child resulting from such action is not *walad al-zina* and belongs to the producer of the sperm, and all the progeny laws (*ahkam-e nasabi*) are established between them. The mother of the child is the originator of the egg (Mo'men 1996: 70–72).

Here, he clearly separates the acts of insemination (*talqih*) and conception (*en'eqad nutfah*) from the physical and social act of sexual intercourse without a marriage contract (*zina*). Indeed, adultery here should be understood as a physical act of intercourse that occurs between a man and a woman, not as a biological act that occurs between a sperm and an egg. In other words, what is considered to constitute adultery here is not the transfer and contact of bodily substances, but the social act of illicit sexual relationship. Furthermore, he separates sexual intercourse from reproduction and says:

> Sexual intercourse [*ham bastar shodan,* literally "sharing the same bed" in Persian] between husband and wife is one of the regular ways to make children. Artificial insemination is another new way, cloning (*shabih-sazi*) could be also another way. Thus, the act of fertilizing the wife's ovum outside the body with the husband's sperm and then transferring the fertilized egg into the wife's or another woman's uterus or even into an artificial uterus in order to conceive a child have the same legal implication like sharing the same bed on which legal intercourse takes place between a woman and her husband. (Interview with Ayatollah Mohammad Mo'men, 13 October 2006, Qom)

Turning to the notion of maternity, Ayatollah Mo'men, like the majority of Shia authorities, ascribes maternity to the producer of the egg. According to him, being the gestational carrier and giving birth does not create maternal relatedness. The Qur'anic verse (58:2), "Their mothers are only those who gave them birth," is used by many Islamic legal authorities, particularly among Sunni scholars to argue that it is the gestational carrier and deliverer of the child who should be considered the mother (see e.g., Houot and Eich, this volume). In disagreement with these authorities, Ayatollah Mo'men uses the same Qur'anic verse (58:2) to argue that maternity should not be established by birth. The reason for disagreement is that this verse of Qur'an (58:2), according to him, was revealed for those men who compared their wives with their mothers by saying to them, "You are to me as the back (*zihar*) of my mother," implying that they are as untouchable to them as their mothers (Mo'men 2006: 95–96). It should be noted here that *zihar* (literally "back" in Arabic) was a pre-Islamic custom of repudiation or divorce, in which a husband could divorce his wife by verbally declaring to his wife "You are to me as the back of my mother." *Zihar* is rejected by Islam, but sexual intercourse with the wife is prohibited to the man who makes this pronouncement, until he expiates (*kaffara*) for his deed (see e.g., van Gelder 2005: 118–19). However, according to Ayatollah Mo'men, the Qur'anic verse (58:2) "Their mothers are only those who gave them birth" refers to men who pronounce *zihar* and therefore it does not reveal the determination of maternity (*me'yar-e madari*): "Thus, maternity should be assigned to the originator of the egg" (Mo'men 2006: 87).[23] Indeed, what are used in this interpretation are juridical arguments; maternity is established by reasoning and not by referring to biological facts alone.

Furthermore, in the cases of egg donation and gestational surrogacy, which involve one woman's egg and another woman's uterus, Ayatollah Mo'men argues that the child has a *ertebat-e takwini* (a relation through the act of bringing into being and formation) with both women, but only the woman who is the provider of the egg is the true mother of the child. He compares *rahem* (uterus) with *zarf* (a container) and makes it clear that the gestational carrier just provides a place for the *nutfah* (here, "fertilized egg") to grow in. In the course of the interview, I discussed the issue of surrogacy with him. He argues that the practice of surrogacy is allowed, but that it does not establish any filiation (*nasab*) between the child conceived in this way and the woman who carries the child in her uterus (Interview with Ayatollah Mohammad Mo'men, 13 October 2006, Qom). Clearly, he makes a distinction between procedures involving the implantation of the fertilized egg into the uterus of the surrogate woman (gestational surrogacy), and those that involve the injection of the sperm directly into the uterus (traditional surrogacy), which he considers *haram*.

In the case of gestational surrogacy, the surrogate woman just carries the pregnancy and is not the contributor of the female gamete. There is one question that frequently arises: What kind of relationship should be ascribed to the surrogate woman and the child conceived in this way? The issue of *rida'* comes into consideration in this instance, and many Shia authorities and jurists refer to it to constitute their arguments regarding surrogacy. In Islamic legal tradition, the issue of breastfeeding held a special position. The milk bond created between the infant on the one hand and the wet nurse on the other constitutes a basis for kinship relations between people other than those relationships created through ties of marriage and descent. Although foster relationship was a pre-Islamic custom, Islam accepted it and laid down rules (*ahkam*), conditions, and even ethical codes (*adab*) to regulate it. The milk bond constitutes a marriage prohibition and establishes permanent legal relations between the child and the milk mother—who suckles the child—and subsequently between all the other members of the milk mother's kin, including the milk mother's husband and his kin, with no inheritance rights. Marriage prohibition with the milk mother and the milk sister is laid down in the Qur'an (4:23).

However, following the hadith "whatever is forbidden by *nasab* is forbidden by *rida'*," ascribed to Prophet Mohammad, the marriage prohibition was also extended to other milk relations. The Shia position, which is codified in Book 7 of the Iranian Civil Code (Article 1046), deals with the issue of milk kinship and stipulates that kinship relations created by the "act" (and not "milk" as substance, my emphasis) of suckling (*qerabat-e rida'i*) is equivalent to kinship relations created by *nasab* (*qerabat-e nasabi*) as far as impediments to marriage are concerned. Furthermore, Shia scholars add many more conditions and rules, which are very detailed and complex arguments in their own right. For example, two of the prevalent opinions among Shia scholars, which are also part of abovementioned Article 1046, is that the milk of the woman takes its source from a "legitimate conception (*haml-e mashru'*)"; and the milk must be received directly from the breast and it should not be taken, in particular, from a bottle, which implication might be that of the importance of the physical act of suckling (physical connection between milk mother's nipple and child) in the constitution of milk relations rather than purely the transmission of bodily substances or the "reinforcement of agnatic relationship" that Hèritier tries to argue (1999: 276). What is perhaps more important is the implication of the matrimonial union and the legitimacy of sexual relations in the constitution of such an elective kinship. However, milk kinship is another complex legal and cultural means of creating ties of relations in Muslim societies, and the subject of many debates and varied opinions in the context of Islamic jurisprudence. Further discussions are, nonetheless, beyond the scope of this chapter (see, e.g., Clarke 2007 for full references).

Thus, I was interested in Ayatollah Mo'men's viewpoint and whether he considered the gestational carrier (*zan-e hamel*) as analogous to the milk mother (*madar-e rida'i*). Answering my questions, Ayatollah Mo'men first started to briefly address the rulings and conditions of milk relationship in Shia Islamic jurisprudence, briefly discussed above. The practice of gestational surrogacy, according to him, is allowed but should not be considered as analogous to milk kinship. Gestational surrogacy does not establish any filiation (*nasab*) and marriage prohibition (*mahramiyat*) between the children conceived in this way and the surrogate woman and her husband, if she has any. Furthermore, even when the surrogate woman suckles the child, this suckling institutes no marriage prohibition, since her milk originates not from her "husband" (not as "man" per se, and therefore "male substance"—rather, legitimate conception, my emphasis), but from the physical act of pregnancy (Interview with Ayatollah Mo'men, 13 October 2006, Qom).[24]

Even so, the permission given to gestational surrogacy by Ayatollah Mo'men makes the practice of embryo donation (*ehday-e janin*) possible, too. In this case, according to him, the true parents of the child are the providers of the egg and sperm. In other words, in the case of embryo donation, the true parents of the child are the donors of the embryo and not the recipients of the embryo (infertile parents), and the child inherits only from the provider of the embryo. Furthermore, according to Ayatollah Mo'men, embryo donation between siblings is allowed and does not constitute incestuous adultery (*zina-ye ba maharem* or incest). In fact, the contact and transfer of bodily substance is not important in the definition of incest or adultery. What is considered to be incestuous adultery here is the physical act of illicit sexual intercourse that occurs between unmarriageable members of kin.[25]

"The Child Is Like a Deposit [*Amanat*] to Me": Gestational Surrogacy in Practice

Let me turn now to the way in which Iranian gestational surrogates talk about their experience of surrogacy. What drives a woman to carry another couple's embryo for nine months, give birth, and surrender the baby to his/her legal parents? What is the reaction of the family members of potential surrogates when presented with the idea? Does giving birth to a child entitle the person to motherhood? Is motherhood a "biological" or "legal" determination? Here, I would like to focus on the gestational surrogates' narratives I have recorded to illustrate how they conceptualize their experience of gestational surrogacy. They address a set of cultural assumptions about reproduction and relatedness embedded in a legal and social context, assumptions that enable them to bear and deliver a child, whom they do not consider to be their own.

Many gestational surrogates I interviewed had financial motives that explained their acts of carrying another couple's child. Additionally, another reason was one of emotions either between relatives

or friends. Anthropologist Soraya Tremayne (2009) also discussed
exactly these two reasons in some length in her study of third-party
donation in Iran. Women in both groups emphasized the altruistic aspect of the process, helping a woman to become a mother as
well as preventing a marriage from falling apart because of infertility
problems. However, all of them, no matter their personal reasoning,
referred to one commonality: The resulting child does not belong
to the gestational surrogate, but belongs to the true parents of the
child, the contributors of the embryo who are together through legal marriage.

Shabnam[26] has volunteered for surrogacy for the first time. She
is thirty-five years old and it has been four months since she has
divorced from her husband of sixteen years. She has a fifteen-year-
old daughter who lives with her. She explains her motivation after
divorce:

> It is almost four months since I have started thinking about surrogacy
> ... pretty much since I have divorced. It is a considerable amount of
> money. I don't think any pain can sum up to delivery pain. If I had
> not divorced, I wouldn't think about it, but when I think about the
> money involved. ... Well, I told myself I could buy a house and pay its
> mortgage later when I get a job. I want my daughter to feel comfort-
> able in my house. She doesn't like her father.

Although she speaks of her financial needs to undergo surrogacy,
she doesn't eliminate the altruistic aspects of such an arrangement.
Furthermore, her belief that the child she carries is not hers is central to her decision to participate in surrogacy arrangement:

> Although the financial need is a strong drive in this case, I am cer-
> tain that I am doing a *savab* [God-loving deed]. This is not something
> everyone can do, even if they have severe financial needs. I have
> met the woman for whom I'll carry the baby. The egg and sperm had
> been taken from them but since her womb cannot hold the embryo,
> I'll carry it for her. ... Every time we talk, it makes me feel good and
> I become glad of my decision. ... Sometimes I ask myself if I had this
> problem, would I have had such money to give another person to
> carry the baby for me. When I see these things, I thank God for being
> able to carry my own child.

Another gestational surrogate spoke of her financial needs as well
as her altruistic intentions to help an infertile couple:

> It is a God-loving deed, I have been a surrogate mother once, you
> have no idea how happy they got [to have a child] especially the wife;

she loved her husband very much and feared he might divorce her. That is why she insisted on having a baby of their own. ... Well, being pregnant is not easy for everyone, you experience hell while being pregnant, I have already given birth to five kids of my own, it is not that hard for me and I need the money too. We haven't paid off our house yet. ... This way, we were able to pay it off and they became parents as well. God is pleased with both of us. We haven't done anything wrong. It is not like I have slept with her husband. I carried her baby just like my own in my belly. ... I will do it in a heartbeat. I enjoy child-bearing, I don't feel any pain. ... I love babies. (Farideh, 32 years old, married for 19 years,[27] mother of 5 boys, housewife)

As I argued above, the Shia notion of adultery is not established by the biological act of the contact of bodily substances; it is established by the social and physical act of the illicit sexual intercourse. The distinction that Farideh makes here between the act of gestation and the physical proximity through the (illicit) sexual act is a further reinforcement of this Shia thought. In other words, there is also a fundamental difference between reproduction and sexual intercourse in her thinking. Almost all the informants I interviewed referred to this distinction.

Sometimes, gestational surrogacy can also be an act of love toward another woman. Afsaneh is a twenty-six-year-old homemaker who has been married for six years. She is content with her marriage and has a four-year-old daughter and a three-year-old son. She has decided to become a gestational surrogate for her friend. Her friend Akram is thirty-seven years old and works as a driving instructor. She has been married for twenty years, and her uterus had been diagnosed as not appropriate for pregnancy; therefore, the physicians have offered her surrogacy as a reproductive option. Afsaneh and Akram's friendship became tighter while Afsaneh took driving lessons with her. During this time, Akram talked about her infertility problem with Afsaneh; after consulting her husband, Afsaneh decided to be a surrogate for Akram. She says of her decision: "I am only doing this for God's sake; only for Him, my heart and hers. ... It is not her fault. I want her to experience motherhood after all these years. ... She told me about her complications. I offered to be her gestational surrogate to her child. I am really fond of her. I want her to become a mother, just like me."

As seen in the first part of this chapter, according to many Shia scholars the practice of embryo transfer and gestational surrogacy between siblings is allowed and is not considered to constitute incestuous adultery (*zina-ye ba maharem*) or incest. Indeed, the prohibition of incest is social and juridical rather than biological and psychological, as stands in various classical and recent theories of incest.[28] So, as we have seen, a woman is religiously *(shar'i)* allowed to deliver the child of her sister or carry the child of her brother. The two cases I present here will illustrate the social implication of this juridical permissibility. These ethnographic examples also show how the power of sibling intimacy reinforces the affinal bond between spouses as the basis for legitimate offspring reproduction; "alliance" and "descent" combine in the dual roles of spouses and siblings and regulate *nasab*. Here the sibling relations appear foundational.

Taraneh is a forty-year-old woman who wants to act as a surrogate for her brother's wife. Her brother has been married for eight years; his wife cannot bear a child since her uterus is too small.[29] Taraneh says:

> Well, he is my brother. What is he supposed to do? He loves his wife. Well, my kids are older now. I have given birth three times, all of them natural birth. ... When my sister-in-law approached me, I said to myself that I have been pregnant three times, I could do it one more time for my brother. It will be his child! I am forty years old and thank God, my uterus is still healthy; the doctors said they don't see any problem with it. ... It is better not to involve a stranger. My sister-in-law did not want to involve a stranger either. It would have been very expensive. ... I ask God to help us.

Sara is another gestational surrogate who has given birth to her sister's baby. She is a twenty-nine-year-old and has a six-year-old son. She has a BA in business management and, currently, is a housewife. Sara explains:

> My sister is few years older than me. She got married before me but it wasn't in her faith to get pregnant. Her husband is a relative; he is our cousin. They did everything they could to get pregnant but it didn't happen. ... The doctors told her that her uterus could not hold the baby and they recommended surrogacy to her. She talked to me first and asked me if my husband agreed whether I could do it for her. I talked to my husband and he said if I could tolerate the pregnancy and not traveling, not going to parties, he had no objection. ... After this, I was up for it. ... Well, I felt closer to my sister and loved her dearly. I hope God gives her a child this time.

She continues:

> During pregnancy, my mother and sister were around me. My sister didn't let me do anything at home. ... My son is still very young but

he understands a lot of things. He used to tell me "Are you bringing me a sister?" ... I explained to him: "It is auntie's baby that I am carrying. ... Since auntie's belly is small mommy is carrying the baby for her. When the baby arrives, we have to give it back to auntie." ... He had gone to my sister and told her that if his mom's tummy was small, who was supposed to hold him in her tummy.

Thus, without making any connection to incest or incestuous adultery, as we have seen, it is possible for a woman to bear and deliver the child of her brother or her sister. Again, this leads us to the fact that also in social actors' understanding, incest is defined not through the sharing and contact of bodily substances. Indeed, any explanation for the incest prohibition here should take into account the social and legal order of things rather than the biological one. To come to another point: The conceptual understanding of family members of gestational surrogates—their husbands and children in particular, and their reaction toward the subject—can be understood from different points of view.

It is noteworthy that the pattern in all of the cases is the same and none of the families involved considered the engagement in the gestational surrogacy arrangement as a *haram* or illegal act. Since the fertilization of the sperm and egg of the infertile couple, in which the wife is suffering from a lack of uterus or complications in her uterus, happens outside of the surrogate's uterus and later the embryo is transferred to the surrogate's uterus, no legal (e.g., through temporary marriage) or illegal sexual relation can be implied between the legal father (sperm donor) and the gestational surrogate (the woman offering her uterus). On the other hand, the embryo carried by the gestational surrogate is the result of a legal union of an infertile couple, the legal union between the contracting husband's sperm and the contracting wife's eggs, and not the result of an illicit sexual union. In this regard, Shabnam speaks of her experience talking to her daughter:

My daughter was opposed to it in the beginning. I had to tell her. ... There was no way I could hide it from her. ... The belly would grow big and show after all. ... But she used to tell me not to do it since she felt embarrassed in front of her friends and classmates. I assured her not to let anybody know about it; instead our life would get better financially. But she said: "What will we say to our family? What are we supposed to do in front of others? Since you and dad are divorced, won't they say whose baby is this?" I sat her down and explained to her that I am only offering my uterus and this is not a sin at all. ... I am only gestating the child of an infertile married couple. After that, she didn't say anything.

Shadi, who has donated eggs several times, is Shabnam's sister.
She is thirty years old and has a ten-year-old son and a five-year-old
daughter. She talks of her sister's decision to become a gestational
surrogate:

> It is very difficult. You have to wait nine months. When she told me
> she was going to be a gestational surrogate, I thought this was not go-
> ing to be easy but I didn't give her any negative energy. I supported
> her. ... Well, she has a better situation compared to me; her daughter
> is grown and she has more free time. But my situation is different. I
> have to take my son to school every day, pick him up, and look after
> my daughter. So I encouraged her to go for it. We'll see the result of
> this experience.

In response to whether she would like to become a gestational surrogate, she says, "I don't like pregnancy in general. I get depressed;
it will last nine months. [In the infertility center] they asked me to
become a gestational surrogate but I didn't accept. I don't like pregnancy time, it limits you, you have to stay home; my kids are very
energetic. There is special care required. ... It is hard, I can't do it."

Mina, a surrogate, had been married for fifteen years. She is thirty
years old and has had a miscarriage when attempting a surrogacy.
She wants to become a gestational surrogate for the second time,
but this time her husband and her ten-year-old daughters are opposed to it. Her husband supports her for egg and embryo donation,
but does not want her to become a gestational surrogate one more
time. When asked the reason of her husband's disapproval, she says,
"He is not happy with it because I get migraine headaches and I have
to take medication for it. If I decide to do surrogacy, I have to stop
taking medication and my headaches will come back. ... This is one
of his reasons for disagreement; on the other hand, my husband
and daughter want me to bear another child for us, and I have been
giving them excuses about my health condition. But they will be
expectant when they see I have been a surrogate for someone else.
... I seriously don't want to have another child to look after." Mina's
husband responded to the same question: "She can't, it is tough for
her, and she'll become ill-tempered. The first time she did it, I didn't
agree with it easily. I was worried for her. I was worried something
might happen to her. But she insisted to do it ... but this time is different, I won't agree to it. ... If she wants to be pregnant again she
should give birth to our own child."

Farideh also talks about her family and her neighbors:

> Everyone knows what I am doing: my husband, children, neighbors.
> ... I am doing something humanistic. ... Do you know how gracious

it is to carry someone else's baby for nine months? God, help us! My sister-in-law couldn't get pregnant. Her husband stayed with her for eight years but he divorced her because of not having a child. She loved her husband very much. She still looks at his pictures. ... Well, in those days such technology was not available. These treatments are new. ... Maybe if it had been available at that time, they would have had kids by now. ... God knows I would offer to surrogate for her.

Farideh gives her opinion about religious aspects of it: "To be assured about surrogacy, I even consulted with some Shia scholars. ... We believe in *haram* and *halal*. ... They assured me that we are not committing a sin. ... They told me that my uterus was like a bowl that the baby grew inside it." Sara, who has given birth to her sister's child, and Taraneh, who has decided to surrogate for her brother, have a similar opinion. They say: "We thought not to tell anyone in the beginning but it didn't work. ... [In the family] they see you, they will figure it out. ... We decided that it was better to tell the truth. ... Those who don't know, might think that we are doing something wrong ... so we told everyone that the baby was actually theirs and we were only carrying the baby for them."

But Afsaneh and Akram have decided not to tell anyone. However, since the body goes through changes during pregnancy, it is not easy to hide Afsaneh's pregnancy from others. In this regard, she says:

> I have told everyone in my family that I couldn't get pregnant anymore since I had closed my tubes. Now they will be suspicious on how I have got pregnant. ... Akram suggested who would know if we had told them that the tubes had opened on their own. ... As for the baby, we won't say anything up to when I am five months pregnant. No one will know. On the fifth month, I will say it is two months and on the ninth month, I will say I am six months pregnant. ... Then, by the due date, my husband and I will go to the hospital. ... Akram and her husband will come to the hospital too. When I delivered the baby, they take it home. We'll say to everyone that the baby was born dead or it was premature. I have two kids already. No one will care.

Discussion

In these narratives we have seen how the social actors themselves understand assisted reproduction.[30] We have seen how surrogates decide to get pregnant and give birth to a child, whom they consider to be the child of an intended couple and not their own. We have learned how surrogates use the grammar of kinship to disconnect themselves from the experience of the surrogate pregnancy in order to provide a way for another woman to achieve maternity. Indeed, the grammar of kinship is used to maintain social order in dealing with infertility—what I consider as social disorder in this account—which implies a form of regulation, and this regulation does not come from "biogenetic reproductive substances," but from the rules of kinship itself and the social actors who play with these rules. As Lévi-Strauss states: "The rules of kinship and marriage are not made necessary by the social state. They are the social state itself, reshaping biological relationships and natural sentiments, forcing them into structures implying them as well as others, and compelling them to rise above their original characteristics" (1969: 490).

The fact that the embryo carried by the gestational surrogate is the result of a legal union between infertile couples exhibits the importance of the matrimonial union and the legal meaning ascribed to the reproductive male and female substance in emic thought—in Lévi-Strauss's view, "the level of perception."[31] We have also seen gestational surrogates consider their act to be doing something, in their words *savab* (divine merit), that will help another woman to become a mother. Some stress their financial need and appreciate the value of payment;[32] others emphasize emotional bonds and enjoy their acts of assistance in creating a child. However, receiving money for what they do does not contradict their understanding of reproduction and their empathic tendencies toward an infertile woman, which in itself creates a form of female power and asymmetrical reciprocity in favor of creating, keeping, and reinforcing ties of kinship, and, thus, the reproduction of society and social relations. Furthermore, in these narratives we repeatedly hear that a child may not come into being without the will and intervention of God (*khoda*). Even in the operating room, when the male doctor begins by inserting a catheter into the female vagina and releases the embryos, both doctor and patient start to recite the name of God. At this moment an intimacy is established between doctor, patient, and God, as I observed many times in the course of my fieldwork. In fact, assisted reproductive technologies do not displace the belief of the creation of man by God in emic thought; rather, they renew and emphasize the connection between the human and the divine in the ongoing process of creation. This fact is understandable if one considers reproduction as a cultural achievement through which the foundational structures and perceptions of a society and its dynamics are reproduced and contested rather than a sexual act or as simply the combination of male and female reproductive substances. Indeed, according to Annette Weiner, we need to think of reproduction "not as a biological construct, but as a cultural concept in which the basic processes for reproducing human beings, social relations, cosmological phenomena, and material resources are culturally defined and structurally interconnected" (1978: 183).

Conclusion

In this chapter, I examined contemporary Shia juridical positions on the new reproductive technologies and their implications for the use of surrogacy arrangements in infertility treatment in Iran. I have tried to give some insight into how Shia scholars employ an ancient religious-legal system to challenge the bioethical dilemmas of the present and future. As we have seen, many Shia scholars approve of the application of third-party donation and gestational surrogacy as a treatment for infertile married couples.[33] However, the opinions are not monolithic and centralized, and Shia scholars respond controversially to the questions posed by assisted reproduction, although certain principles remain the same.

We have seen that: (1) achieving conception and creating a child does not always depend on sexual intercourse; (2) *nasab* can be seen as legitimate relatedness referring to legal filiation, both agnatic (*nasab-e pedari*) and uterine (*nasab-e madari*) and not "biogenetic relatedness"; (3) according to many Shia scholars, both male and female reproductive substances play a symmetrical role in the procreation of a child and in producing the line of descent, ties of agnatic and uterine kinship; (4) stress is laid on the juridical meaning ascribed to bodily substances and not on the "biogenetic principle of descent." This serves to emphasize the legal constructions of relatedness rather than the biological definition of that through ties of substance as material in the Euro-American thought. Indeed, in Shia juridical logic, the structure of kinship ties is not based on the grammar of "genes,"[34] but rather on a grammar of "closeness" (*qa-rabah*)—the equivalent term in Arabic to the English "kinship" and Persian *khishawandi*, a grammar of social proximity; and (5) the use of donor gametes and embryo or surrogacy arrangements, whether they are allowed or not, is not considered as a kind of adultery or *zina*, and the resulting child is not an illegitimate child. This explains why embryo transfer and gestational surrogacy are not forbidden in Shia Islam, and why some scholars even permit the use of donor gametes—either eggs or sperm—in infertility treatment. In other words, the Shia notion of incest and adultery does not refer to the biological act that occurs through the contact and transfer of bodily substances. It depends on the illegitimate physical act that occurs through illicit sexual intercourse between a man and a woman.

The permissibility of donation between siblings is based on the same logic: embryo transfer between siblings is allowed and is not considered to constitute incestuous adultery (*zina-ye ba maharem* or incest). How should the incest taboo be understood by taking the aforementioned perspectives into account? Annette Weiner (1992: 70–71) explains Malinowski's thinking on the question of incest as follows: "For Malinowski, the incest taboo functioned as a socio-logical regulator that divides 'persons of the opposite sex into lawful and unlawful' relationships, which restrains 'intercourse in virtue of the legal act of marriage and which discriminate[s] between certain unions in respect of their desirability.'"

Indeed, considering the jurisprudential assumptions of the *fuqaha* on relatedness, it seems that they may think about the concept of incest in a similar way. In fact, the contact and transfer of bodily substance is not important in the definition of incest or adultery. What is considered to be incestuous adultery here is the illegitimate physical act of illicit sexual intercourse that occurs between unmar-riageable members of kin (*maharem*). The same may be true about gestational surrogacy: the practice of gestational surrogacy, in which the gestational carrier is not the biological contributor of the egg and just carries the fetus (*janin*) of a married couple, is acknowl-edged by the majority of Shia scholars as an accepted form of as-sisted reproduction.

As we have seen, some Shia legal scholars have argued that ges-tational surrogates can be either married or single. She can be either *mahram* (unmarriageable member of kin) or *namahram* (marriage-able member of kin); even the wife's sister and the husband's sister could act as gestational surrogates. I interviewed two similar cases; one of them had gestated and given birth to the child of her sister, and in another case, a woman acted as a gestational surrogate for her brother. And these are, in Shia thought and practice, neither an act of incestuous adultery nor the subject of illegal *nasab*. Once again, one should note the juridical and social considerations of incest pro-hibition rather than the biological or psychological explanations of that. As such, the content of this chapter should help to explain why the rhetoric of incest does not follow a "universal grammar."

Acknowledgements

I would like to thank Marcia Inhorn and Soraya Tremayne for inviting me to the Yale conference, for their support and encouragement, and for their very helpful comments on this chapter. Many thanks also to all my colleagues in the workshop at Yale for their support, excellent company, and profound discussions. The chapter was developed in part under a German Research Foundation doctoral fellowship from the International Centre for Ethics in the Sciences and Humanities (IZEW), University of Tübingen, where I benefited from the generous support of its director, Prof. Dr. Eve-Marie Engels, and staff. I am also very grateful to Thomas Eich, Morgan Clarke, Raoul Motika, Anke von Kügelgen, Willemijn de Jong, and all my colleagues at IZEW for helping me think through earlier drafts of this paper. In Iran, I am deeply grateful to the IVF physicians and staff members at various clinics and hospitals, far too many to thank individually here. Particularly, I wish to thank Dr. Mehdi Akhondi for his helpful support and guidance throughout all stages of my research. I would also like to thank all the Islamic scholars, jurists, and religious authorities in Qom who have guided me through this research. I am very grateful to my friend Azadeh Torabi for her meticulous reading of the manuscript and translating sections of this paper. A final thank goes to Prof. Édouard Conte, who taught me social anthropology, and to all the men and women who spoke to me and shared the intimate details of their reproductive lives with me.

Notes

1. However, a minority of Shia authorities like Ayatollah Tabrizi (correspondence by letter, 9 October 2006, Qom), Ayatollah Nori Hamedani, and Ayatollah Behjat regard it as forbidden (see Akhondi and Behjati Ardekani 2008: 11).
2. However, the notion of *zina* should not be understood only as referring to "adultery." In Islamic family law, *zina* refers to all varieties of illegitimate intercourse between a man and a woman, applicable to married and unmarried persons. It stands also as analogy to "incest" and "incestuous adultery" as well as "rape" (see also Kohlberg 1985).
3. The Iranian law in compliance with the Islamic law acknowledges *nasab* as legitimate (*mashru'*) and lawful (*qanuni*) only if the father and the mother of the child are within a valid marriage contract at the time of conception (*en'eqad nutfah*). Hence, if conception takes place

as a result of *zina*, it is not possible to acknowledge the child's *nasab* as legitimate. According to Article 1167 of the Iranian Civil Code, a child born as a result of the act of *zina* is not attached to the *zani* (fornicator, both man and woman in Shia thought), is not recognized as legitimate, and is the subject of an illegitimate *nasab* (*nasab-e namashru'*). The term *walad al-zina* ("illegitimate child," "bastard") refers to a child who is the result of the act of *zina*. According to the article 884 of ICC, *walad al-zina* does not inherit from the father, the mother, or their relations (see, e.g., Safai and Emami 2007). In other words, the establishment of the legal filiation (*nasb-e mashru'*) and the right of inheritance is based on legal paternity and maternity, and not just a biological bond between parents and children. It should be noted that the law treats legitimate and illegitimate children equally except for when it comes to inheritance; therefore, the rights and obligations remain the same in matters of custody, guardianship, and alimony (Safai and Emami 2007: 342). Also, in order to protect illegitimate children, the uniformity vote of the National Supreme Court in 1997 requires the birth of the child to be reported to the National Organization for Civil Registration and the birth certificate to be issued under the name of the father. According to Ayatollah Khomeini, the fornicator is recognized as the child's "customary father" (*pedar-e 'orfi*) (Safai and Emami 2007: 342). In cases where the mother of the child is known but not the father, it is approved to issue the birth certificate under the mother's name and at the space provided for father's information, it can be stated as "ambiguous" (www.dastour .ir). I thank Alireza Milanifar for drawing my attention to this aspect.

4. This distinction between the physical and the biological act of adultery is exactly the conclusion that anthropologist Susan Martha Kahn (2000) draws from her notable analysis of rabbinic opinions on ARTs in Israel. However, a systematic comparison of these juridical permissibilities is lacking.

5. According to the Ministry of Health and Medical Education (MOHME), approximately 15 percent of couples are infertile in Iran, which translates into nearly 2 million infertile couples at the time (see, e.g., Mirzazadeh 2005).

6. The Guardian Council comprises twelve members of which six are *fuqaha*, appointed by the Supreme Leader (*maqam-e rahbari*), who serves as Iran's head of state; the other six members, who also have to be Muslims, are jurists proposed by the head of the judiciary and approved by parliament (Article 91 of the constitution).

7. Article 94 of the constitution.

8. One of the purposes of the seminar was to pursue the issue of fertility preservation in healthy women who wish to delay childbearing because of a variety of social factors. Currently, in addition to sperm freezing, some IVF clinics in Iran offer egg freezing in order to preserve the ability to get pregnant when the woman is older. One of the relevant issues in this regard concerns possible solutions available to women

who are willing to freeze their eggs without damaging their hymen (Akhondi, personal communication, January 2010). I personally had a discussion with a thirty-seven-year-old academic woman who was interested in freezing her eggs without losing her hymen. It seems the notion of "virgin birth" demands a new rhetoric.

9. During the seminar, there was a report of one hundred births through surrogacy in one of the cities of Iran alone. Currently, there are some well-known infertility clinics in Tehran and other cities in which surrogacy is offered to infertile couples; however, there is no official statistic available from the surrogacy births. Within a few days after the seminar, I met a number of intended mothers who were visiting the clinic and requiring surrogacy. According to one of the social workers in the clinic, the seminar, public awareness via different means of media, and of course, clerical support of surrogacy made all this possible.

10. As of the writing of this paper, no particular law concerning surrogacy has been passed by Parliament, and the proposed bill is under evaluation. In the absence of a codified law, it is possible to seek advice from authentic fatwas (legal opinions) and legitimate Islamic resources (Article 167 of the constitution) as well as the law for embryo donation and other general laws to resolve disputes concerning surrogacy (Milanifar, personal communication, January 2010). Moreover, the clinics where such alternative treatments are offered have their own internal policies, which include mutual consent between the infertile couple and the surrogate. For instance, the website of Royan Research Center includes information on gestational surrogacy: http://www.royaninstitute.org/cmsfa/index.php?option=com_content&task=view&id=17&Itemid=24 (accessed 20 January 2010, translated from Persian by Azadeh Torabi):

> The procedure does not imply any religious (*shar'i*) and legal (*qanuni*) restrictions, and it is being administered in Iran. The [infertile] couple can either introduce a volunteer to the infertility treatment center to carry on with the surrogacy or they can seek help from the center.
>
> In Royan Research Center, there is a list of volunteer women for gestational surrogacy, which upon the need of the couple they will be available to assist.
>
> Considering the fact that the gestational carrier will endure pregnancy hardships, it is customary (*'orfi*) and acceptable for the infertile couple to compensate her financially. From the religious viewpoint (*shar'i*), the gestational carrier is considered like a milk mother (*madar-e rida'i*) since she has blood relation with the baby; hence, issues such as inheritance and mother-child rights do not apply to them [gestational carrier and the child] according to law.

11. However, the correlation between these two modes of power—juridical and biomedical—does not operate solely in the management of ARTs in Iran; rather, it is more exercised within a complex field in which reli-

gious authorities, medical practitioners, would-be parents, and donors all directly or indirectly interact. I discuss this issue in a work in progress (Garmaroudi Naef n.d.).

12. There are two verses in the Qur'an that are used by many religious authorities both Sunni and Shia to argue that artificial insemination by donor sperm (not by the woman's husband) is not allowed. The first is:

> ... and guard their private parts save from their wives and what their right hands own then being not blameworthy (but whosoever seeks after more than that, those are the transgressors. (*Sura* 23:5–7, trans. Arberry)

The second is:

> Say to the believers, that they cast down their eyes and guard their private parts; that is purer for them. ... And say to the believing women, that they cast down their eyes and guard their private parts, and reveal not their adornment save such as is outward. (*Sura* 24:31, trans. Arberry)

The following hadith is a further illustration used by many Shia Islamic scholars to justify the use of artificial insemination using donor sperm:

> Narrated Ali Ibn Salem that Imam Ja'far Sadeq (702–765 AD, the sixth Shia Imam) said: He who will receive the worst tortures on the day of judgement is the man who placed his seed in a womb forbidden to him. (Rezaniya Mo'allem 2005: 175)

The interpretations and commentaries related to these texts are complex and controversial. A further discussion, however, is beyond the scope of this chapter (see, e.g., Rezaniya Mo'allem 2005: 63–198).

13. However, a minority of Shia authorities regard it as forbidden (see footnote 1, this chapter).

14. *Sura* 58:2, Arberry's translation.

15. I have incorporated his view in detail in this chapter.

16. *Sura* 25:54. Arberry's translation with the modification of "by *nasab*" for his "blood."

17. *Sura* 76:2. Arberry's translation with the modification of "*nutfah*" for his "sperm-drop."

18. In Islamic law, social and sexual interaction between the two genders is defined by a division of men and women into two categories of *mahram* (pl. *maharem*) and *namahram*. The rulings of marriage and its prohibition, incest and fornication/adultery, veil and dress code result from such categories. A *mahram* is an unmarriageable member of kin with whom sexual intercourse would be considered *zina-ye ba maharem*, equated with "incestuous fornication/adultery" and "incest." A *namahram* is potential marriage partner with whom sexual relations without having a marriage contract—permanent or temporary—is forbidden. A *namahram* could be either a close relative like a cousin or a stranger (see also van Gelder 2005: 1–6).

19. The Assembly of Experts is a constitutional body of 86 senior clerics (*mujtahids*), elected by the public every eight years. It is charged (theo-

retically) with electing and dismissing the supreme leader of Iran and supervising his activities.

20. *Sokhani darbare-ye talqih* translated by Musa Danesh. This article—in Arabic, *Kalama-ton fi talqih*—is a Persian version of a chapter of his book entitled *Kalamat-on sadidat-on fi masa'il jadid* in Arabic, which was published in Qom in 1994.

21. The maniyy of the man; "*al-rajol saheb al-maniyy*" (in Arabic), see Mo'men 1994: 101.

22. "*al-mar'at saheb al-boyaydat* (in Arabic), ibid., 101. *Boyaydat* means *tokhmak* (egg) in Persian.

23. "*me'yar-e haqiqi-ye madar budan in ast ke nutfah-ye be wojud amadeh az tokhmak-e zan bashad.*"

24. A girl born of gestational surrogacy, therefore, is not forbidden to marry the surrogate's husband and a son to marry the surrogate woman. So, one could say: Marry the woman who bears and delivers you! Marry the girl whom your wife carried in the womb! One should note, however, the difference between the juridical and the ethical implication of the subject.

25. Again, one might say: You are not allowed to marry the sister of your wife, but your wife's sister can bear and deliver your child! You are not allowed to marry your sister, but your sister can bear and deliver your child!

26. All names have been changed to protect the privacy of the participants who shared their stories with me.

27. When I asked Farideh how old she was when she got married, she smiled and said: "Well, we get married soon in our family (*khanewadeh*). ... I was thirteen when I got married."

28. The literature on incest is extensive. A good summary and bibliographies of the main theories exists in Robin Fox's critical account, "The Red Lamp of Incest: An Enquiry into the Origins of Mind and Society" (Fox 1983).

29. By the time of finalizing this chapter, I was informed that Taraneh had given birth to twins of her brother.

30. The viewpoints of the intended couples have not been analyzed in this chapter (it is a work in progress). Generally speaking, most of the intended couples I interviewed expressed their happiness about the religious permissibility of surrogacy as a solution for their infertility, and since they were the embryo owners, they somehow considered themselves parents of the child as well. They were mainly concerned about the high price of the treatment, the failure of the pregnancy, and the possibility of miscarriage. All the intended mothers I interviewed wanted to keep contact with the surrogate and accompany her in ultrasound sessions and monthly check-ups. Elly Teman's (2003a, 2003b) analysis of Jewish-Israeli surrogates and intended mothers has also shown similar results.

31. "An emic model is one which explains the ideology or behaviour of members of a culture according to indigenous definitions. ... A

commonplace assumption about emic models is that they are 'discovered' rather than 'invented' by the analyst. However, emic models, like phonemic ones, are ultimately exogenous constructions, formalized by the analyst on the basis of distinctive features present in indigenous usage. They are not in themselves 'the native model' though anthropologists often loosely identify them in this way" (Barnard 1996: 180–82).

32. Most Shia authorities who regard gestational surrogacy as permissible allow the surrogate to be compensated monetarily (*ojrat*), and the gesture is considered as an appropriate one (see, e.g., Akhondi and Behjati Ardekani 2008: 11). Since the human act is respectable, the woman who endures the hardships of pregnancy is entitled to receive money for her service just like a milk mother who breastfeeds and takes care of a child. Most of the intended mothers I interviewed approved of paying for the service (as a kind of compensation). It is important to point out that some medical ethicists in Iran (see, e.g., Aramesh 2008, 2009) argue over the issue of payment for the surrogacy. According to Aramesh, commercial surrogacy is unethical and contradicts human dignity, and in the absence of appropriate legislation, will constitute the main ethical problem of surrogacy in Iran (2009: 322).

33. The discussion even goes further to the point that some Shia scholars (like Ayatollah Yousef Sane'i, see *Essays on Modern Human Reproductive Techniques from the View of Jurisprudence and Law* 2003: 396) believe that the donor's relinquishment of his/her gamete and donating it in the form of an anonymous donation to a sperm, egg, and embryo bank is an indication of obliterating the ties of *nasab* (kinship relations) from the gamete owners (Garmaroudi 2008a, 2008c). Ayatollah Ma'refat (correspondence by letter, 20 October 2006, Qom) meanwhile compares egg donation with organ donation and states that transferring one woman's egg to another woman's uterus is allowed; and the act of transferring the egg from one woman's body and implanting it in another woman's uterus reassigns the acknowledgment of maternity from the woman who contributed the egg to the woman who gestates and gives birth to the child. In this case, the egg recipient should be considered the mother of the child and not the provider of the egg. This would permit anonymous egg donation as well as egg donation among close kin. Furthermore, the use of temporary marriage to legitimate egg donation is not required.

34. Again quite similar to rabbinic kinship cosmology, as Kahn describes powerfully in her book (2000: 101).

References

Abbasi-Shavazi, Mohammad Jalal, Marcia C. Inhorn, Hajiieh Bibi Razeghi-Nasrabad, and Ghasem Toloo. 2008. "The 'Iranian ART Revolution': Infertility, Assisted Reproductive Technology, and Third-Party Donation in the Islamic Republic of Iran." *Journal of Middle East Women's Studies* 4(2): 1–28.

Akhondi, M. A., and Z. Behjati Ardekani. 2008. "Surrogacy and the Necessity for its Application in Infertility Treatment" (in Persian). *Medical Journal of Reproduction and Infertility* 9(1): 7–13.

Altorki, Soraya. 1980. "Milk-kinship in Arab Society: An Unexplored Problem in the Ethnography of Marriage." *Ethnology* 19: 233–44.

Aramesh, Kiarash. 2008. "Ethical Assessment of Monetary Relationship in Surrogacy" (in Persian). *Medical Journal of Reproduction and Infertility* 9(1): 36–42.

———. 2009. "Iran's Experience with Surrogate Motherhood: An Islamic View and Ethical Concerns." *Journal of Medical Ethics* 35: 320–22.

Arberry, Arthur J. 1981. *The Koran Interpreted.* London, Boston and Sydney: George Allen & Unwin.

Barnard, Alan. 1996. "Emic and Etic". In *Encyclopedia of Social and Cultural Anthropology,* ed. Alan Barnard and Jonathan Spencer. London and New York: Routledge.

Clarke, Morgan. 2007. "The Modernity of Milk Kinship." *Social Anthropology* 15(3): 287–304.

———. 2009. *Islam and New Kinship: Reproductive Technologies and the Shariah in Lebanon.* New York and Oxford: Berghahn Books.

Conte, Édouard. 2000. "Énigmes persanes, traditions arabes: Les interdictions matrimoniales dérivées de l'allaitement selon l'ayatollah Khomeyni." In *En substances: textes pour Françoise Héritier,* ed. J. L. Jamard, E. Terray, and M. Xanthakou. Paris: Fayard.

———. 2003. "Agnatic Illusions: The Elements of Choice in Arab Kinship." In *Tribes and Power: Nationalism and Ethnicity in the Middle East,* ed. F. Abdul-Jabbar and H. Dawod. London: Saqi Press.

Essays on Gamete and Embryo Donation in Infertility Treatment from Medical, Theological, Legal, Ethical, Psychological, and Sociological Approaches (in Persian). 2005. Tehran: Avesina Research Center and Samt Publications.

Essays on Medical, Legal, Islamic Jurisprudential, Ethical-Philosophical, Sociological, and Psychological Aspects of Surrogacy (in Persian). 2007. Tehran: Avesina Research Center and Samt Publications.

Essays on Modern Human Reproductive Techniques from the View of Jurisprudence and Law (in Persian). 2003. Tehran: Avesina Research Center and Samt Publications.

Fortier, Corrine. 2007. "Blood, Sperm and the Embryo in Sunni Islam and in Mauritania: Milk Kinship, Descent and Medically Assisted Procreation." *Body and Society* 13(3): 15–36.

Fox, Robin. 1983. *The Red Lamp of Incest: An Enquiry into the Origins of Mind and Society.* Notre Dame, IN: University of Notre Dame Press.

Garmaroudi, Shirin.. 2008a. "Verwandtschaft zwischen Unfruchtbarkeit und Religion. Assistierte Reproduktionstechnologien in Iran". In *Bioethische und gesundheitliche Herausforderungen für die islamische Welt: Aids, Drogen und Reproduktionsmedizin,* ed. Raoul Motika and Christian Meier. Available at: http://www.heceas.org/publications_dt.html.

————. 2008b. "Gestational Surrogacy in Iran" (in Persian). *Medical Journal of Reproduction and Infertility* 9(1): 50–64.

————. 2008c. "Sibling Intimacy in the Age of Assisted Reproduction: An Ethnography of New Reproductive Technologies in Iran." Master's thesis. Institute of Social Anthropology, University of Berne.

————. N.d. *"M like Mother": The Enigma of Assisted Reproduction in Iranian Infertility Clinics.* IZEW, University of Tübingen.

Héritier, Françoise. 1999. *Two Sisters and Their Mother: The Anthropology of Incest,* trans. Jeanine Herman. New York: Zone Books.

Inhorn, Marcia C. 2003. *Local Babies, Global Science: Gender, Religion and In Vitro Fertilization in Egypt.* London: Routledge.

————. 2006. "'He Won't Be My Son': Middle Eastern Muslim Men's Discourses of Adoption and Gamete Donation." *Medical Anthropology Quarterly* 20(1): 94–120.

Kahn, Susan Martha. 2000. *Reproducing Jews: A Cultural Account of Assisted Conception in Israel.* Durham, NC: Duke University Press.

Kohlberg, Etan. 1985. "The Position of the walad zinā in Imāmī Shī'ism." *Bulletin of the School of Oriental and African Studies* 48(2): 237–66.

Lévi-Strauss, Claude. 1969. *The Elementary Structures of Kinship,* ed. Rodney Needham, trans. James Harle Bell, John Richard von Sturmer, and Rodney Needham. Boston: Beacon Press.

Milanifar A. R., M. A Akhondi, Z. Behjati Ardekani, and A. Abdolahzadeh. 2008. "Issuing Birth Certificates and ID Cards for Newborns Following a Surrogate Birth and the Legal and Ethical Responsibilities of the Medical Team" (in Persian). *Medical Journal of Reproduction and Infertility* 9(1): 82–88.

Mirzazadeh, Sh. 2005. "A Bank for Embryos: A Report about Sperm, Egg and Embryo Donation in Iran and the World" (in Persian). *Zanan* 117: 68–75.

Mo'men (Ayatollah), Mohammed. 1994. *Kalamat-on sadidat-on fi masa'il jadid* (in Arabic). Qom: Nashr-e Islami.

————. 1996. "Sokhani darbare-ye talqih" [A Debate on the Insemination], trans. Musa Danesh (in Persian). *Fiqh-e ahl-e bayt* 1(4): 49–76 (published in Qom).

————. 2006. "Shabih-sazi" [Cloning] (in Persian). *Fiqh—kawoshi no dar fiqh-e islami* 12(46): 8–14 and 40–136 (published in Qom).

Musavi Bojnurdi (Ayatollah), M. 2007. *Hoquq-e khanewadeh* [Family Law] (in Persian). Tehran: Majd Publications.

Parkes, Peter. 2005. "Milk Kinship in Islam: Substance, Structure, History." *Social Anthropology* 13(3): 307–29.

Rezaniya Mo'allem, M. R. 2003. "Wad'iyat-e hoquqi-e (nasab) nashi az enteqal-e janin." In *Essays on Human Reproductive Techniques from the View of Jurisprudence and Law* (in Persian). Tehran: Avesina Research Centre and Samt Publications.

————. 2005. *Barvarihay-e pezeshki az didgah-e fiqh va hoquq* [Medical Reproduction from the View of Jurisprudence and Law] (in Persian). Qom: Busatn-e ketab.

Sadeqi Tehrani (Ayatollah), M. 2005. *Resale-ye tudih al-masa'l-e nowin* (in Persian), 3rd ed. Tehran: Omid-e Farda.

Safai, S. H., and A. Emami. 2007. *A Concise Family Law* (in Persian). Tehran: Mizan Publication.

Samadi Ahari, M. H. 2004. *Nasab-e nashi az leqah-e masnui dar hoquq-e Iran wa Islam* [Kinship Relations Resulting from Artificial Insemination in Iranian and Islamic Law] (in Persian). Tehran: Ganj-e Danesh.

Sane'i (Ayatollah), Y. 2006. *Resale-ye tudih al-masa'el* (in Persian). Qom: Parto-ye Khorshid.

Teman, Elly. 2003a. "The Medicalization of 'Nature' in the Artificial Body: Surrogate Motherhood in Israel." *Medical Anthropology Quarterly* 17(1): 78–98.

———. 2003b. "'Knowing' the Surrogate Body in Israel." In *Surrogate Motherhood: International Perspectives,* ed. Rachel Cook and Shelley Day Sclater. Oxford: Hart Publishing.

Tremayne, Soraya. 2006. "Not All Muslims are Luddites." *Anthropology Today* 22(3): 1–2.

———. 2007. "Whither Kinship?—New Procreative Practices, Authoritative Knowledge and Relatedness—Case Studies from Iran." In *Essays on Gamete and Embryo Donation in Infertility Treatment from Medical, Theological, Legal, Ethical, Psychological, and Sociological Approaches.* Tehran: Avesina Research Centre and Samt Publications.

———. 2009. "Law, Ethics, and Donor Technologies in Shia Iran." In *Assisting Reproduction, Testing Genes: Global Encounters with New Biotechnologies,* ed. Daphna Birenbaum-Carmeli and Marcia C. Inhorn. New York and Oxford: Berghahn.

Van Gelder, Geert J. 2005. *Close Relationships: Incest and Inbreeding in Classical Arabic Literature.* New York and London: I. B. Tauris.

Weiner, Annette B. 1978. "The Reproductive Model in Trobriand Society." *Mankind* 11(3): 175–86.

———. 1992. *Inalienable Possessions: The Paradox of Keeping-While-Giving.* Berkeley: University of California Press.

Chapter 7

HUMAN EMBRYONIC STEM CELL RESEARCH IN IRAN
THE SIGNIFICANCE OF THE ISLAMIC CONTEXT

Mansooreh Saniei

Introduction

The novel ideas for future remedies to degenerative and thus far incurable diseases that have become related to human embryonic stem cell (ESC) research have been embraced with great enthusiasm around the world. Some medical scientists have concentrated their research on human ESCs, as they believe that these cells offer the greatest prospect both for the better understanding of human development and for their potential to treat human diseases such as Alzheimer's, Parkinson's, heart disease, diabetes, and spinal cord injuries. At the same time, stem cell (SC) research using human embryos raises new, previously unimaginable ethical issues posing a dramatic challenge to humankind. As noted by Beatrix P. Rubin, "This field of research and its therapeutic hope has particularly rendered the human embryo accessible as an object both of experimental manipulation in SC research and of ethical debates" (2008: 13). This newly emerging innovation in biomedical science and technology has, however, caused moralists as well as theologians to review its values.

There exists a range of views on the use of human embryos for research, from those who maintain that it is morally wrong to use embryos for research that later involves destroying them to proponents who hold that it is a moral obligation to help the millions of patients who are suffering and desperate for a cure. These proponents believe that embryos at the early stage of development, which are usually leftover from in vitro fertilization (IVF) procedures, can rightly be used in this research. However, as Cynthia B. Cohen (2007) states, the moral significance of human embryos has been the focus of ethical and policy discussion of SC research since Thompson and his colleagues successfully developed human ESCs in a laboratory dish in 1998.

Religious groups have generally been in the forefront of those speaking out publicly for or against embryo research. The conservative Christian view is that human life is created at conception and embryos should therefore be treated as living human beings. They state that no research-related use of embryos, which is not for the benefit of those particular embryos, should be allowed. In contrast, the Jewish faith holds that an embryo does not become human until 40 days after conception, and Muslim scholars consider human life to begin when the soul enters the developing embryo or fetus, which occurs between 40 and 120 days after conception. This range of views likely accounts for different levels of acceptance for ESC research, which is supported in the Jewish community and is accepted in many Muslim countries, yet is opposed by the Roman Catholic Church and some Protestant denominations (Guinn 2006).

Although different religious traditions exhibit varying levels of plasticity as to when life begins, human ESCs are generally accepted as a source of great potential for human welfare, and have also been recognized as a key scientific, political, social, and economic achievement among many nations. However, there is a need to address the question of whether human embryos are of such immense moral significance that we should never destroy them, even in research that might treat and perhaps save the lives of human beings. As such, the central thesis of this chapter is to present the scientific and moral-religious position of human ESC research in Shia Iran, which has taken the lead in this type of research among Muslim countries since 2003. It will then explore the moral controversy surrounding human ESC research in the Islamic tradition and the ways in which Muslims solve their ethical debates in this field of biomedicine, moving on to describing ethical positions and practical regulations applied in some Muslim countries with diverse traditions, forms of government, and social structures.

The Development of Human ESC Research in Iran

Iran has a long history of scientific achievement. In ancient times, its geographical location between Greece and India placed it at the crossroads of medical developments in the Eastern and Western worlds. Prior to the advent of Islam, Iran was a leader in mathematics and astronomy. However, like the rest of the Middle East, its scientific power declined as Europe entered the Renaissance period in the early 1300s. Over the next several hundred years Iran developed slowly and was unable to reach its full potential scientifically (Morrison and Khademhosseini 2006). Iran is now starting to invest heavily in science, and major developments are occurring in SC science, particularly human ESCs, with the full support of the government.

In 2002, Iran's supreme leader, Ayatollah Khamene'i, publicly supported human embryo research and congratulated the scientists who work on SCs. Iran's clerics and political leaders have also actively promoted science and technology in an attempt to enhance the country's global status (Saniei and De Vries 2008). According to Iran's Shia religious authorities (the grand ayatollahs), embryo research and SC technology for therapeutic purposes is permissible with full consideration and all possible precautions only in pre-ensoulment stages of fetal development (Larijani and Zahedi 2007). Due to the positive decrees (religious opinion about whether or not an action is permissible) on the use of human embryos for SC research and therapeutic goals, Iran is one of the first Muslim countries to produce human ESCs (Larijani et al. 2005). Following this approval, the Royan Institute, one of the leading institutes for SC research in Iran, has expanded its work on investigating the potential for human ESCs to differentiate into various cell types, including cardiomyocytes, beta cells, and neural cells (Baharvand et al. 2004). Other research institutes have been involved in regenerative medicine. These include the Iranian Molecular Medicine Network (with thirty-four research institutes and centers joined as members), the Iran Polymer and Petrochemical Institute, and Shaheed Beheshti University of Medical Sciences (Kinkead 2003). The main goal of this research is to understand human cell specialization and developmental biology as well as to create specialized cells to treat a wide range of diseases and conditions (Baharvand et al. 2006a).

In 2003, the Royan Institute reported the establishment of Iran's first human ESC line named Royan H1 (*royan* in Persian means "embryo") from a blastocyst (Baharvand et al. 2004). With this achievement, Iran became the tenth country in the world capable of producing, cultivating, and freezing human ESCs (Atighetchi 2007). Since 2004, scientists of the Royan Institute have also established five human ESC lines, named Royan H2 to Royan H6. Royan H2, H5, and H6 had the normal (46,XX and 46,XY) and Royan H3 and H4 had the triploid (69,XXY) karyotypes that can differentiate in vitro to a variety of cell types (Baharvand et al. 2006a). This success, although not a breakthrough on its own, has enabled Iranian scientists to pursue many avenues of research into methods of generating therapeutic cells from these cells (Morrison and Khademhosseini 2006). Recent activities include: the differentiation of human ESCs into endocrine pancreatic-like cells and hepatocyte-like cells (Baharvand et al. 2005, 2006b, 2008); the potential therapeutic applications of SCs for multiple sclerosis (Mohyeddin-Bonab et al. 2007a); advanced liver cirrhosis and myocardial infarction (Mohamadnejad et al. 2007; Mohyeddin-Bonab et al. 2007b); as well as bone marrow transplants for the hematopoietic disorders chronic myelogenous leukaemia and thalassemia major (Ghavamzadeh et al. 2003; Ramzi 2009). They are the result of the activity and collaboration of the research centers where the SCs are prepared and clinical centers where the patients are selected and treated. Other landmark achievements include coaxing human ESCs to become mature, insulin-producing cells in 2004 (Baharvand et al. 2006b); cloning the country's first sheep (Ilic 2006) and the first goat (Royan Institute 2008); and conducting the world's first human ESC proteomics study (Baharvand et al. 2006c). In 2008, Royan Institute scientists claimed that they had also succeeded in reprogramming human skin cells to an embryonic-like state to create so-called iPS cells (Iran Daily 2008).

Regulation and Control of Human ESC Research in Iran

The rapid progress in SC science led the Iranian government to put in place appropriate ethical and scientific supervision of this scientific field and its therapeutic applications. The aim was to promote responsible, fair, and humane research. The compilation of the specific National Ethical Guidelines for Biomedical Research was developed as an important effort in Iran in recent years (Larijani and Zahedi 2007). It is noteworthy that Ethical Guidelines for Research on Gametes and Embryos, drafted in 2005, is one of the topics in which the use of human embryos for SC research and therapy is addressed along with the general guidelines (Larijani and Zahedi 2007; Aramesh and Dabbagh 2007). The codes are in accordance with the international declarations and have been customized based on Islamic codes and Iranian culture. National and Regional Ethical Committees in universities and research centers should supervise human ESC research and therapeutic cloning adhering to these guidelines (Larijani and Zahedi 2007). The principles behind the Ethical Guidelines for Gamete and Embryo Research are given in brief below:

1. Respect for human dignity and human rights

2. Voluntary and informed participation in research that will not affect the patient's treatment

3. Respect for privacy and confidentiality

4. Equitable distribution of benefits and harms, especially in research, includes clinical treatment

5. Minimization of risk for the embryo or the future child and maximization of benefit for individuals and society

6. Prohibition of the production of hybrids using humans and animals

7. Prohibition of eugenics

8. Prohibition of the production of human embryos for research purposes

9. Use of only surplus IVF embryos, less than fourteen days old, for research that includes destruction of the embryo

10. Responsible persons for the embryo are the donor, her partner, and recipients

11. Availability of all information regarding research and clinical care of the embryo to responsible persons

It is noteworthy that Iran's approach is currently based on ethical guidelines rather than any parliamentary legislation (Aramesh and Dabbagh 2007). Shia Iran, with respect to Islamic law, extensively allows scientists to use spare IVF and affected preimplantation genetic diagnosis (PGD) embryos for SC research. In respect to the adoption of technology, Iran presents an interesting example. As noted by Soraya Tremayne, "while the Sunni follow the Qur'anic tradition closely, the Shia, especially the Iranian Shia, try to accommodate innovations. *Ijtihad*[1] allows adjustments to accommodate change within Islamic beliefs and *fatwas* follow from such interpretations" (2006: 1). Therefore the rules, regulations, and practice in Iran are mainly based on fatwas, which are not the result of public and secular debate (Aramesh and Dabbagh 2007). Once approved by clergy, new technologies do not tend to require the extensive moral and legal deliberations by other bodies, such as ethics committees (Tremayne 2006). What follows is not a detailed legal report covering all aspects related to embryo issues but a brief overview of the main arguments of Muslim scholars about research using the human embryos at the early stage of development.

Human ESC Research in the Context of Islamic Law

Since human ESC research has begun to be used in many countries, its potential to offer new forms of treatment and insights into human development has come up against serious moral and religious questions. Human embryo research is being carried out in a few Muslim nations in the Middle East, such as Iran (Baharvand et al. 2004) and Turkey (Findikli et al. 2005) where, for some time now, human ESC research programs have been successfully established. These developments raise the question of how embryo research is viewed by Islam. In the national and international Islamic law councils, a positive view of embryo research prevails. While fatwas according to sharia permit human embryo research, this does not, however, mean that there are no restrictions (Saniei 2010).

In Islam, as noted by Ilkilic, "a broad range of arguments is developed in dealing with complex ethical debates, based on the specific nature of Islamic legal and ethical deliberation processes, linked to specific local culture and traditions" (2010: 151). Therefore, the major moral-religious question, which is fundamental, can be formulated thus: Do human embryos at the early stage of development have the same moral status as living human beings and deserve the same protections? This section will depict Muslims' understanding of the moral status of the embryo according to the Qur'an and the tradition of Prophet Muhammad, as well as the view of Islamic scholars on human embryo and SC research and the diverse legislation that exists among Muslim nations. This will be followed by a

discussion of the influence of Islam on national embryo-related legislation, with a digression on the debate on the UN Declaration on
Human Cloning.

The Moral Status of the Human Embryo

Islam always encouraged scientific research, particularly research
directed towards finding cures for human disease. The Prophet (Muhammad) very clearly commanded humans to seek cures, for God
Almighty did not create a disease without creating its cure (Translation of Sahih Bukhari, volume 7, book 71, number 582, cited in
Abdur Rab and Khayat 2006). Islam is commonly regarded as a
research-friendly religion, and it supports any research when it is
done with the desire to alleviate human suffering and disease. From
the Islamic viewpoint, the debate on human research and therapeutic cloning should center essentially on key arguments, such as:
At what stage is an embryo considered a human being? And, is any
tampering with the embryo in conflict with Islamic teaching and
therefore *haram*?

The Qur'an depicts in a few places the development of the human in the mother's womb, speaking of the breathing-in of the soul,
although there is no specific definition of the timing of beginning of
life in either the Qur'an or Sunna. Hence, there are opposing views
about the onset of life and the time when the ensoulment—the in-
fusion of the soul into the body of the fetus, followed by the conferring of moral status on the fetus—occurs. These differences in the
points of view in relation to the interpretation of the Qur'anic verses
concerning this point create a division among Muslim jurists as they
rule on this and related issues. Determination of the time of ensoulment is based upon an interpretation of the Qur'anic scripture: "He
Who created all things in the best way and He began the creation of
man from clay; then made his progeny from a quintessence of de-
spised liquid; then He created him in due proportion, and breathed
into him of His spirit. And He gave you [the faculties of] hearing
and sight and hearts. Little thanks do ye give!" (Qur'an 32:7–9). Another verse passage informs us about the stage of ensoulment during
the intrauterine life: "We created man [*khalaqna*] of an extraction
of clay, then We set him, a drop [*nutfa*] in a safe lodging [i.e., the
womb], then We created of the drop a clot (*'alaqah*), then We created of the clot a tissue [*mudgha*], then We created of the tissue
bones (*'azm*), then we covered the bones in flesh [*yaksu lahman*];

thereafter We produced it as another creature [*khalaqan akhar*]. So blessed be God, the Best of creators [*khaliqin*]" (Qur'an 23:12–14).

This verse of the Qur'an grades inception into three clear phases. The first stage of inception is the time of fusion between the sperm and ovum into a zygote. This stage, as the drop phase (*nutfa*), establishes the genetic code for the individual that will be created out of the zygote as it develops. The second stage, as the blood phase ('*alaqa*), begins when it settles inside a woman's body (assuming here, the womb). And the third phase, as the flesh phase (*mudhga*) ends when the spirit (*ruh*) is embedded into the fetus. The Qur'an itself does not give any concrete indication as to the exact point in time when the ensoulment occurs. However, it has almost been found in the hadith the following indication:

> Verily your creation is on this wise. The constituents of one of you are collected for forty days in his mother's womb; it becomes something that clings ['*alaqa*] in the same [period] [*mithla dhalik*], then it becomes a chewed lump of flesh [*mudgha*] in the same [period] [*mithla dhalik*]. And the angel is sent to him with instructions concerning four things, so the angel writes down his provision [sustenance], his death, his deeds, and whether he will be wretched or fortunate. Then the soul is breathed into him (Al-Bukhari 1979).

According to this hadith each of the first three stages (lodging *nutfa* in the woman's womb, '*alaqa*, and *mudgha*) is assigned a time period of forty days, which makes a total of 120 days. Another hadith shows how on the forty-second night from ejaculation in the uterus, an angel sent by God begins to differentiate the organs of the fetus, but the text does not make any mention of ensoulment.[2] Other *ahadith* (singl. hadith) differ and give forty days as the total of the four stages (Al-Bukhari 1979).[3] However, by a clear majority of scholars, ensoulment is viewed as occurring at the 120th day of pregnancy (Hathout 2006; Hedayat et al. 2006).

The Qur'anic position on the embryological development and the creation of humans presents a focal point connected with embryonic sanctity. Also, reasoning from different *ahadith*, some schools of jurists determined that until the stages were complete, the fetus had no soul, or God had not breathed His spirit into the fetus, and therefore it had not been created yet (Saniei 2010). In other words, the new creation (the person) exists only after some stage of embryonic development and not at the time of fertilization. Moreover, many scholars described early life as occurring in two phases: biological and human. They generally agree that ensoulment differentiates biological life that begins at the moment of fertilization from human life (Fadel 2010). In the Islamic tradition, ensoulment is, therefore, assumed as a central value in the discourse about the moral status of a human embryo or even fetus. Hence, the ensoulment gives the human embryo an exceptional moral status, which is decisively applied to the ethical evaluation of any medical intervention affecting the embryo (Ilkilic and Ertin 2010).

When assessing ethical issues according to Islamic law, Muslim scholars use case-based reasoning. They then draw on the fundamental principles of sharia and also take into consideration similar and related cases. Therefore, before dealing with the debate over embryo research it is necessary to say something about relevant subjects that have already been ruled upon, e.g., IVF and clinical abortion (Fischer 2009; Saniei 2010). For instance, tampering with an embryo, in abortion, at any stage after conception is considered unlawful by many Muslims. Some scholars, nevertheless, believe that abortion before ensoulment, particularly when there is a justification, is lawful. In other words, there should be good reason for an abortion (Bowen 2003). In Islam, abortion is, however, considered to be absolutely forbidden after ensoulment and to be limited to certain circumstances, including when the mother's life is in grave danger (Atighetchi 2007).

All Muslim jurists agree that embryonic life is entitled to respect even before ensoulment, becomes progressively more deserving of rights as development proceeds, and definitely acquires full rights after ensoulment. Generally, most of the verses of the Qur'an quoted against destruction of an embryo or fetus actually deal with life's sanctity.[4] Although the tradition explicitly mentions the beginning of human creation at the zygotic stage, the verses only cover gestation stages from fertilization to personhood. Nonetheless, they do not in any way explain the nature of the zygotic stage, in terms of whether it holds life or carries pluripotent SC with a potential to generate all the cells of the human body (Sachedina 2009). As Abdulaziz Sachedina points out, in Islamic jurisprudence there is an assumption that the term *nafs* self-evidently stands for personhood whose life must be protected through a detailed penal code rather than a theory of inherent dignity of the fetus. Any argument to assert the fetal inviolability at all stages of its journey towards the status of full human being would have required the jurists to seriously engage the Qur'an in deriving an ethical framework to define human personhood in order to affirm the inherent dignity of the pre-ensoulment fetus. The juridical trend is simply to deny personhood to the pre-ensoulment fetus because it does not have full moral status in the absence of differentiated organs to indicate human shape; and, as a consequence, to permit derivation of human ESCs from "spare" frozen embryos (Sachedina 2009).

However, for those Muslim jurists who wanted to provide moral-legal justification for the use of "spare" embryos as the source for derivation of human ESCs for research, juridical solutions were not hard to deduce when legal principles like *maslaha*, which promotes what is beneficial for the public, and necessity (*darura*) that overrules prohibition, could provide religious-legal justification and legitimization (Sachedina 2009).

The Crux of Human ESC Research

Scientific advances and the increasing availability of IVF have resulted in an increasing number of frozen embryos, which are in excess to what a couple needs in the case that they have a successful IVF treatment. If couples have no further desire to reproduce, they face difficult choices about their frozen embryos, which include either discarding them or donating them for infertility treatment or for research (Dickens and Cook 2008). It is noteworthy that Sunni Islamic law prohibits surrogate parenting and the adoption of human embryos due to the importance of determining a child's true parentage and inheritance right (Inhorn 2006). Accordingly, donating embryos to other couples is out of the question in Sunni Islamic tradition. In addition, there would be cases in which couples cannot use their own frozen embryos for religious reasons. In sharia, for instance, any form of IVF implying procreation outside of the framework of an existing legal marriage would be forbidden. Therefore, the embryo could not be implanted after divorce or if the donor of either the oocyte or the sperm had died. In other words, those embryos would suffer no legal harm by their destruction, because according to sharia they could not have developed legally into a human being anyway (Serour 2005). Hence, this would free up "spare" frozen embryos either for research (Weckerly 2002) or discarding.

As mentioned earlier, there are issues other than lineage regarding embryo donation, which are related to when life begins and "ensoulment" happens. Consequently, the moral significance of the early embryo remains at the center of the controversy associated with the permission to use it, while its destruction for harvesting SCs is incompatible with the notion of embryonic sanctity and the respect to the preimplantation embryo (Sachedina 2006). There is also an absolute moral obligation (*fard kifayah*) in Islam for the physicians and scientists to undertake biomedical research that may result in beneficial treatments for thus far incurable diseases (Siddiqi 2002). Nonetheless there is an equally valid concern as to whether the potential benefits of the human ESC research can certainly be translatable into therapy. This requires Muslim scholars to provide evidence related to the standards of the ethical and scientific oversight. They therefore need to assess the potential risks and benefits of human ESC research in light of Islamic values and embryonic sanctity. As Abdulaziz Sachedina (2000) points out, the ethical-religious assessment of research using human embryos for derivation of SCs in Islam can be inferentially deduced from the rulings of sharia that deal with fetal viability and embryonic sanctity in classical and modern juristic decisions. Sharia treats a second source of cells, i.e., fetal tissue following abortion, as analogically similar to cadaver donation for organ transplantation in order to save other lives, and hence, the use of cells from that source is permissible.

In the context of IVF technology, some scholars hold the distinction between the "implanted" embryo that is developing in the uterus and the "spare" embryo that exists outside of the woman's body and has never reached the stage of ensoulment. As discussed earlier, the moral significance of the fetus in Islam has been connected with its development to a particular point when it gradually attains human personhood with full moral rights. Based on Qur'anic passages,[5] the implanted zygote is considered a rights bearer. Consequently, many Muslim jurists do not treat the embryo outside of the uterus as a right bearer (Sachedina 2009). In addition, on the basis of the concept that human life does not start until ensoulment, the great majority of Muslim scholars agree that research on the preimplantation embryo—as it cannot grow independently outside the uterus—is permissible, provided that these embryos were legitimately developed. The permissibility is also conditioned on the fact that these embryos are not produced specifically for research. They then apply to the principle of *maslaha* to permit human ESC research, which gives hope to provide the cures for debilitating conditions. Therefore, as stated by Abdulaziz Sachedina, "It is correct to suggest that a majority of the *Sunni* and *Shia* jurists will have little problem in endorsing ethically regulated research on the SCs that promises potential therapeutic value" (2000: G3).

In 1989, the issue of surplus IVF embryos was discussed by a committee of international Muslim religious scholars and physicians of the Islamic Organization of Medical Science (IOMS). The committee consequently issued a recommendation that explicitly allowed the use of the frozen embryos for research purposes according to Islamic law (Eich 2006). One of the main statements for this recommendation was: "According to the opinion of the majority (with which some disagreed) that the destruction of fertilized egg[s] before their nidation in the uterus is allowed, no matter how this destruction is brought about—according to this opinion there is no reason to forbid scientific experiments in accordance with the *sharia*. During these experiments the egg cells must not be multiplied. Some disagreed entirely with this view" (Al-Awadi 1995,cited in Eich 2006: 7). Hathout also states that "it [a fertilized ovum] cannot produce a human being unless implanted into the uterus, and so implantation was taken to herald the sanctity of human life" (2006: S25).

Following the IOMS recommendation, the Islamic *Fiqh* Council (IFA, *majma' al-fiqh al-islami* in Arabic) organized a similar meeting in 1990. They reviewed several studies about frozen embryos that are almost identical with the studies examined at the IOMS meeting in 1989. The IFA, to the contrary, opposed the scientific use of frozen embryos. In their decree, they emphasized: "In view of what has become reality concerning the possibility to store nonfertilized oocytes for later use, it is necessary to restrict the number of fertilized eggs to the number necessary for a single treatment, in order to avoid a surplus of fertilized eggs. If for any reason such a surplus of fertilized eggs is brought about, they are supposed to be left without medical help, so that the life of this surplus may end in a natural way" (IFA 1990).

The reason for this argument is based on the fear of the misuse of embryos rather than on theological or philosophical reasoning. It is apparent from the argument that allowing the embryo to die on its own is not refuted because this constitutes killing the potential human being. However, allowing the embryo to die also constitutes killing the embryo, but this time by means of not taking any steps to save the potential human being (Aksoy 2005). As noted by Hathout, a fertilized egg in storage does not possess the same rights as a fertilized ovum, which is implanted in a woman's uterus and may be used if the purpose is to protect human life. Moreover, frozen embryos will acquire genetic anomalies and will, sooner or later, die (2006).

The Muslim World League's Islamic Jurisprudence Council conference in December 2003 held in Mecca, Saudi Arabia, issued this fatwa: "It is permissible to use stem cells for either legitimate scientific research or for therapy as long as its sources are legitimate, for example, adults if they give permission as long as it does not inflict harm on them; children with their guardian's permission for a legal benefit without inflicting harm on them; placenta or umbilical cord blood with the permission of the parents; spontaneously aborted embryos or those aborted for a legally acceptable cause and with the permission of the parents; excess fertilized eggs produced during the course of IVF and donated by the parents with assurance that they are not to be used to produce an illegal pregnancy. It is forbidden to obtain or use stem cells if its source is illegitimate as, for example, intentionally aborted fetuses (abortion without a legal medical reason); intentional fertilization between a donated ovum and sperm; and therapeutic cloning" (Muslim World League 2003, cited in Ilkilic and Ertin 2010).

IOMS, in their later meeting held in Cairo in 2006, included presentations by physicians who concluded that embryonic research for therapeutic purposes, including nonreproductive cloning,[6] is Islamically permitted and encouraged (Nordin 2006, cited in Fadel 2010). Moreover, both the Islamic Institute of Turkey (Turkmen and Arda 2008) and the Malaysian National Fatwa Council (Fadel 2010) also supported hESC research. Shia clergy also generally support and encourage SC research including hESC research. As mentioned above, in 2002 Iran's supreme leader Ayatollah Khamene'i publicly supported human embryo research (Saniei and De Vries 2008; Saniei 2010). In 2004, the World Health Organization–Regional Office for the Eastern Mediterranean (WHO-EMRO), recalled all Muslim nations in its statement to make a consensus on "development of a regional position on human cloning" before voting on a United Nations convention to address human cloning (WHO-EMRO 2004). Although this statement positively considered cloning for research into its therapeutic applications, many Muslim countries voted for a ban on all forms of human ESC research in the UN General Assembly for the United Nations Declaration on Human Cloning in 2005 (See Table 7.1). However, at this moment, some member states as well as some other Muslim countries outside of the region are fast developing their scientific infrastructure, within which research and development for health figures prominently and is gradually taking center stage.

The overarching challenge is, therefore, to find a balance between the need to avoid the trampling of human dignity that may possibly be induced by human ESC research, and the need for continued improvement in the quality of human life through research

Table 7.1. Votes from countries from the Regional Office for the Eastern Mediterranean (EMRO) and other countries from the Organization of the Islamic Conference (OIC) on the United Nations Declaration on Human Cloning (Resolution adopted by the General Assembly in March 2005) (Abdur Rab and Khayat 2006)

In favor		*Against*		*Abstained*		*Absent*	
OIC	*EMRO*	*OIC*	*EMRO*	*OIC*	*EMRO*	*OIC*	*EMRO*
Albania	Afghanistan	Gabon	–	Algeria	Egypt	Chad	–
Bangladesh	Bahrain			Azerbaijan	Iran	Gambia	
Benin	Iraq			Cameroon	Jordan	Guinea	
Brunei	Kuwait			Indonesia	Lebanon	Kyrgyzstan	
Comoros	Qatar			Malaysia	Oman	Mali	
Côte d'Ivoire	Libyan Arab			Burkina Faso	Pakistan	Guinea-Bissau	
Djibouti	Morocco			Maldives	Syria	Mauritania	
Guyana	Jamahiriya			Turkey	Tunisia	Mozambique	
Kazakhstan	Sudan				Yemen	Niger	
Sierra Leone	Saudi Arabia				Somalia	Nigeria	
Suriname	United Arab					Senegal	
	Emirates						
Tajikistan						Togo	
Uganda						Turkmenistan	
Uzbekistan							

and development. While the position of many countries remains unchanged, there are others that, increasingly, consider the need for research in therapeutic cloning to outweigh the dangers that it poses and that are creating favorable environments to support research and development in this field of science and technology. In the following section, I shall briefly overview the ethical and legal framework for human embryo and ESC research in selected Sunni Muslim countries.

Status of Embryo and SC Research in Selected Muslim Countries

Although positive attitudes toward scientific research and development seem to prevail in Muslim states in general, this does not mean that there are no significant differences between individual Islamic scholars. In the early part of this chapter, I explained the status of human ESC research and its regulation in Iran. The following is a short presentation of the legal and ethical situation of SC science and embryo research in selected Muslim states.

Turkey

Turkey, whose population is over 95 percent Muslim, is one of the few secular countries among the Muslim nations. However, Islamic approaches play a significant role in defining its people's opinion on controversial issues in the modern world (Ilkilic and Ertin 2010). Turkey mostly concentrates on adult SC research, although it has been reported in some relevant studies about human ESC research (Findikli et al. 2005; Candan and Kahraman 2010). The country adopted a permissive approach to allowing researchers to work on the existing human ESC lines as well as to create embryos via IVF specifically for research purposes (International Society for Stem Cell Research). They have also recognized national policies related to this field of research, while some other Muslim nations use decrees or fatwas to guide this research (Flynn and Matthews 2010). Moreover, the Turkish Ministry of Health as well as their Bioethics Association prepared several guidelines and reports on various aspects of ESC research (Arda and Acıduman 2009). In 2008, the Turkish Academy of Sciences (TÜBA) published the report "Current Concepts in Stem Cell Research," which was prepared by a multidisciplinary Stem Cell Working Group constituted under the auspices of TÜBA. According to this report, human cloning could only be performed under the umbrella of SC research and its regulation (TÜBA 2008, cited in Ilkilic and Ertin 2010).

The Turkish Religious High Council under the Directorate of Religious Affairs issued a series of opinions on IVF, SCs, and the rights of the fetus, which emphasized that the number of embryos produced during IVF treatment should be kept at a minimum level, as the destruction of surplus embryos, which can be regarded as human beings, raises serious doubts from the religious point of view. Based on this report, "spare" IVF embryos should be reserved for SC research rather than be destroyed. However, the use of embryos at the early stage of development is permissible if it is not possible to obtain SCs with the characteristics of ESCs from differentiated adult cells (Yeprem 2006, cited in Ilkilic and Ertin 2010).

Egypt

Egypt has a significant influence on the entire Sunni Muslim world through its Islamic institutions as well as its leading role in organizing international conferences. Moreover, the main Sunni religious authorities reside there, whose decrees are said to be respected by most Sunni groups (Al-Sayyari 2005).

In Egypt the private IVF centers in Cairo mainly use umbilical cord blood (UCB) for SC research rather than human ESCs, as the Egyptian Medical Syndicate opposes the use of embryos for experimentation (Fadel 2010). Indeed, most of the debates in this country concentrate on human cloning, which is not permitted in the rest of the Muslim world. The mufti of Egypt states that cloning contradicts Islamic legislation and is prohibited in all its forms (Al-Sayyari 2005). However, authorities in Egypt tend to accept therapeutic cloning and ESC research. Along similar lines, the Academy of Scientific Research and Technology as well as Gamal Serour, the director of the International Islamic Center for Population Studies and Research at Al Azhar University, support the use of surplus IVF embryos for SC research. It seems that they look forward to deriving a possible approach that might adopt human ESC research in the future (Ilkilic and Ertin 2010). Presently, there is no official policy on human ESC science in Egypt (Boustany 2008).

Arab Gulf States

In the Arab Gulf states, Saudi Arabia is the most prominently involved in SC science and technology. Saudi Arabia opened the Stem Cell Therapy Program at King Faisal Specialist Hospital and Research Center in 2007. Later, Saudi Arabia invested many billions of dollars to establish King Abdullah University of Science and Technology in 2009. At the moment, the main sources for SC research are provided by UCB as well as aborted fetuses; and the use of surplus IVF embryos is still being discussed (Fadel 2010). Saudi Arabia has successfully established reproductive medicine and regulated it by the In-vitro Fertilization Act (No. 2870/1/12) in which they provided a framework for the supervision of clinics. The act also regulates embryo research indirectly and allows storing embryos and gametes with couples' permission (Fischer 2009). However, there are different views on using a human embryo for research proposes. The decree issued by the International Islamic *Fiqh* Academy (IIFA) in Jeddah allows the usage of embryos for research on the condition that they not be implanted for impermissible pregnancies. Similarly, in 2003 a fatwa of the *Fiqh* Council for the Muslim World League permitted researchers to use SCs for therapeutic reasons; another decree of IFA in Mecca prohibits it. Based on the IFA fatwa, the creation, storage, and use of human ESCs for scientific research is not allowed under sharia (Atighetchi 2007; Al-Sayyari 2005). Nonetheless, Saudi Arabia now plans to establish human ESCs.

Qatar has also decided to launch research on human ESCs. It has recently set up Cornell Medical College to establish a SC research laboratory that will be able to expand, maintain, and validate currently available human ESCs and develop new SC lines, signaling that its scientists are ready to work on ESCs (Voice of America 2009).

Conclusion

The use of human embryos has been one of the most controversial and scrutinized aspects of this field, and receives ongoing ethical, social, legal, and religious attention. The process of adoption of the United Nations Declaration on Human Cloning in 2005 demonstrates the polarization of worldviews on this controversial topic. It would seem that individual countries have taken up different policies on the use of the embryo for SC research based on their sociocultural, political, and even economic backgrounds. As Isasi and Knoppers (2006: 9) note, "The historical, cultural and sociological context, the institutional framework, and the mobilization of stakeholders are factors that help explain why countries that seemingly share similar socio-religious beliefs [and perhaps scientific interest] have adopted diametrically opposite public policies."

Iran, as a Shia Islamic country, is influenced by the Islamic faith, which is culture based. Iran has resorted to the extensive use of the mechanisms available to Islam, such as *ijtihad,* to legitimize some matters in hand, e.g., embryo donation to research purposes. All of these have been justified through interpretations and independent reasoning, which the Sunni do not use as much as the Shia. Consequently, there are additional factors influencing the ways in which new knowledge is taken up in countries with the same religious background and scientific interests. For Iran, the introduction of an Islamic system forced religious scholars into an unprecedented role of responsibility and involvement in social planning and public health. Being faced with health crises on a large scale may be partially responsible for scholars invoking *maslaha* and *istihsan* in their rulings on medical and health affairs, rather than considering a question in an isolated or theoretical sense as was done in the past. It seems that the financial burden of debilitating diseases also plays an important role in decision making regarding human ESC research in Iran. This may have given scholars the impetus to reconsider the public health ramifications of degenerative and incurable disorders or the financial hardships that those serious, long-term illnesses have on individuals, families, and society.

Moreover, scientists' technological innovations and achievements hold the hope of a "golden age" that will benefit both Iran and its people intellectually and materially, as is often rhetorically used by Iran's supreme leader, Ayatollah Khamene'i, in justifying Iran's position in the Muslim world. Indeed, the consensus of scientists, physicians, and religious leaders in Iran has paved the way for an evolution in nationwide biotechnology, such as human ESC research and therapies.

Acknowledgments

The author warmly thanks Professor Clare Williams, Director, at the Centre for Biomedicine and Society, Brunel University London for her insightful and constructive comments. She also acknowledges the collaboration established with Dr. Hossein Baharvand, head of the Department of Stem Cell Biology and Technology, Royan Institute, Tehran, whose work she refers to in this chapter. The work upon which this chapter is based is funded by a Wellcome Trust Biomedical Ethics Developing Countries Studentship (grant no. 086072).

Notes

1. *Ijtihad* ("effort"): in Islamic law, the independent or original interpretation of problems not precisely covered by the Qur'an, hadith (traditions
   concerning the Prophet's life and utterances), and *ijma'* (scholarly consensus). In the early Muslim community every adequately qualified jurist had the right to exercise such original thinking, mainly *ra'y* (personal
   judgment) and *qiyas* (analogical reasoning), and those who did so were
   termed *mujtahids*. The Shia, unlike the Sunni, have a series of scholars,
   ayatollahs, who are the most senior and high-ranking Usuli Twelver Shia
   clerics qualified to make new rulings on issues of contention when they
   attain the level of *ijtihad*. For issuing new rulings based on the Qur'an,
   ahadith, and logic, they go through a standard and rigorous training last-
   ing more than thirty years and receive letters of attestation from other
   ayatollahs on their qualifications for issuing new rulings (see Hedayat et
   al. 2006).
2. When forty-two nights have passed over the sperm drops, Allah sends an
   angel to it, who shapes it and makes its ears, eyes, skin, flesh, and bones.
   Then, he says, "O Lord! Is it a male or female? And your Lord decides
   what He wishes and the angel records it." In Ebrahim 1988: 115–16.
3. For instance, the following hadith says:
   "After the zygote [*nutfa*] has been established in the womb for forty or
   forty-five nights, the angel comes and says: 'My Lord, will he be wretched
   or fortunate?' And both these things would be written. Then the angel
   says: 'My Lord, would he be male or female?' And both these things are
   written. And his deeds and actions, his death, his livelihood; these are
   also recorded. Then his document of destiny is rolled and there is no addition to and subtraction from it." (See Al-Bukhari 1979.)
4. For instance, one of these oft-quoted verses in this section declares: "If
   anyone slays a human being unless it be [in punishment] for murder
   or for spreading corruption on earth—it shall be as if he had slain the
   whole of humankind" (Qur'an 5:32). Another verse forbids killing of
   children: "Slay not your children for fear of poverty; We will provide
   for you and them. Surely the slaying of them is a grievous sin" (Qur'an
   17:31). Still another verse forbids the pre-Islamic practice of *wa'd*—a
   practice of burying of live female infants for fear of poverty or disgrace:
   "And when the female infant, buried alive is questioned for what crime
   was she killed…" (Qur'an 81:8). None of these verses deal with abortion
   per se; nor do they define or deal directly with the ontological or legal-
   moral status of the fetus or the religious-legal consequences of expelling
   it before complete gestation.
5. The Muslim jurists have mostly regarded implantation of the zygote in
   the uterus as the determining stage of fetal life when any infliction of
   harm to it requires compensation. In case of abortion, the rule is extrap-
   olated from the interpretation of the following verse in the Qur'an that
   reads: "It is He who produced you from one living soul [*nafs wahida*],

and then a lodging-place [*mustaqarr*] and then a repository [*mustawda'*]"
(Qur'an 6:98). "A lodging place" is the uterus, whereas "a repository" is
the loins in which specific characteristics are preserved for future generations. Obviously these rulings in no way suggest an endeavor to define
the beginning of fetal life in the womb. (See Ibn Kathir 1966: 3:70.)

6. It is therefore useful to note the distinction between human ESC research
and reproductive cloning, which is mostly blurry among both supporters of and those against one of these two techniques. The creation of the
first cloned mammal at the Roslin Institute in 1997 demonstrated that it
is possible to clone a whole mammalian genome, i.e., reproductive cloning. The technique involves using an egg, e.g., from mammal A, which
has had its nucleus removed, and the nucleus from a cell obtained from
mammal B, which is then inserted into the egg. A small electric current
is passed through the egg to stimulate cell division with the aim of forming an embryo that contains the whole genome of mammal B (with a
small amount of DNA carried in the egg's mitochondria from mammal
A). This has been called the somatic cell nuclear transfer (SCNT) technique. When combined with the findings of Thomson's work in isolating
and culturing the first human ESC lines in 1998, this indicated the possibility of applying the SCNT to create patient-specific human ESC lines
that could be used for therapeutic purposes, i.e., therapeutic cloning.
However, therapeutic cloning allows the cloned embryo to develop for
six to eight days to obtain SCs, whereas reproductive cloning would involve placing the embryo into a woman's uterus in an attempt to create
a baby (see Sparrow 2009).

References

Abdur Rab, Muhammad, and M. Haytham Khayat. 2006. "Human Cloning:
Eastern Mediterranean Region Perspective." *Eastern Mediterranean Health
Journal* 12(2) (Supplement): S29–37.

Aksoy, Shaheen. 2005. "Making Regulations and Drawing Up Legislation in
Islamic Countries under Conditions of Uncertainty, with Special Reference to Embryonic Stem Cell Research." *Journal of Medical Ethics* 31(7):
399–403.

Al-Awadi, Abd al Rahman et al. 1995. Al-Ru'ya al-islamiya li-ba'd al-
mumarasat al-tibbiya. 2nd ed. Kuwait.

Al-Bukhari, Sahih. 1979. *Al-Sahih, kitab bad' al-Khalq*, vol. 4. Istanbul: Al-
Maktaba al-Islami.

Al-Sayyari, Rehab A. 2005. "Ethical Aspects of Stem Cell Research." *Saudi
Journal of Kidney Diseases* 16: 606–11.

Aramesh, Kiarash, and Soroush Dabbagh. 2007. "An Islamic View to Stem
Cell Research and Cloning: Iran's Experience." *Amerian Journal of Bioethics* 7(2): 62–63.

Arda, Berna, and Ahmet Acıduman. 2009. "An Evaluation Regarding the Current Situation of Stem Cell Studies in Turkey." *Stem Cell Reviews and Reports* 5: 130–34.

Atighetchi, Dariusch. 2007. *Islamic Bioethics: Problems and Perspectives.* Netherlands: Springer.

Baharvand, Hossein, Saeid K. Ashtiani, Mojtaba R. Valojerdi, Shahverdi Abdolhossein, Adeleh Taee, and Davood Sabour. 2004. "Establishment and In Vitro Differentiation of a New Embryonic Stem Cell Line from Human Blastocyst." *Differentiation* 72(5): 224–29.

Baharvand, Hossein, Saeid K. Ashtiani, Adeleh Taee, Muhammad Massumi, Mojtaba R. Valojerdi, Poopak E. Yazdi, Shabnam Z. Moradi, and Ali Farrokhi. 2006a. "Generation of New Human Embryonic Stem Cell Lines with Diploid and Triploid Karyotypes." *Development, Growth & Differentiation* 48(2): 117–28.

Baharvand, Hossein, Hanieh Jafary, Muhammad Massumi, and Saeid K. Ashtiani. 2006b. "Generation of Insulin Secreting Cells from Human Embryonic Stem Cells." *Development, Growth & Differentiation* 48(2): 323–32.

Baharvand, Hossein, Mohsen Hajheidari, Saeid Kazemi Ashtiani, and Ghasem Hosseini Salekdeh. 2006c. "Proteomic Signature of Human Embryonic Stem Cells." *Proteomics* 6, no. 12: 3544–49.

Baharvand, Hossein, Seyed Mahmoud Hashemi, and Mansoureh Shahsavani. 2008. "Differentiation of Human Embryonic Stem Cells into Functional Hepatocyte-like Cells in a Serum-free Adherent Culture Condition." *Differentiation* 76(5): 465–77.

Baharvand, Hossein. 2009. "Preface". In *Trends in Stem Cell Biology and Technology,* ed. Hossein Baharvand. New York: Humana Press, Springer.

Boustany, Fouad N. 2008, *Final Report of Mapping Bioethics Regulations in 16 Arab Member States in the UNESCO.* Paris: UNESCO, 40–41.

Bowen, Donna Lee. 2003. "Three Contemporary Muslim Ethics of Abortion Fiqh." In *Islamic Ethics of Life: Abortion, War, and Euthanasia,* ed. Jonathon E. Brockopp. Columbia: University of South Carolina Press.

Candan, Zafar N., and Semra Kahraman. 2010. "Establishment and Characterization of Human Embryonic Stem Cell Lines, Turkey Perspectives." *In Vitro Cellular and Developmental Biology.* 46: 345–55.

Cohen, Cynthia B. 2007. *Renewing the Stuff of Life: Stem Cell, Ethics, and Public Policy.* New York: Oxford University Press.

Dickens, Bernard M., and Rebecca J. Cook. 2008. "Multiple Pregnancy: Legal and Ethical Issues." *International Journal of Gynecology & Obstetrics* 103(3): 270–74.

Eich, Thomas. 2006. "Decision-making Processes among Contemporary Ulama: The Example of Frozen Embryos." Paper presented in the conference on Islam and Bioethics: Concerns, Challenges and Responses. USA. 27–28 March.

Fadel, Hossam E. 2010. "Developments in Stem Cell Research and Therapeutic Cloning: Islamic Ethical Positions, a Review." *Bioethics* 26(3): 1–8.

Findikli, Necati, Semra Kahraman, Oya Akcin, Semra Sertyel, and Zafer N. Candan. 2005. "Establishment and Characterization of New Human Embryonic Stem Cell Lines." *Reproductive BioMedicine Online* 10: 617–27.

Fischer, Nils. 2009. "Embryo Research in the Middle East." *Journal of International Biotechnology Law* 6: 235–41.

Flynn, Jesse M., and Kirstin R. W. Matthews. 2010. "Stem Cell Research in the Greater Middle East: The Importance of Establishing Policy and Ethics Interoperability to Foster International Collaborations." *Stem Cell Reviews and Reports* 6: 143–50.

Ghavamzadeh, Ardeshir, Masoud Iravani, Pejman Jabehdar-Maralani, AmirReza Hajrasouliha, and Sina Tavakoli. 2003. "Allogenic Peripheral Blood and Bone Marrow Stem Cell Transplantation for Chronic Myelogenous Leukemia: Single Center Study from Iran." *Haematologica* 88(4): ELT13.

Guinn, David E. 2006. *Handbook of Bioethics and Religion.* New York: Oxford University Press.

Hathout, Hassan. 2006. "An Islamic Perspective on Human Genetic and Reproductive Technologies." *Eastern Mediterranean Health Journal* 12(2) (Supplement): 22–28.

Hedayat, Kamyar M., P. Shooshtarizadeh, and M. Raza. 2006. "Therapeutic Abortion in Islam: Contemporary Views of Muslim Shiite Scholars and Effect of Recent Iranian Legislation." *Journal of Medical Ethics* 32(11): 652–57.

Ibn Kathir, *Tafsir.* Beirut: Dar al-Andalus, 1966, 3:70.

IFA. 1990. "Majallat majma' al-fiqh al-islami." 3: 2151f (cited in Eich 2006).

Ilic, Dusko. 2006. "Latest Developments in the Field of Stem Cell Research and Regenerative Medicine." *Regenerative Medicine* 1(6): 757–62.

Ilkilic, Ilhan, and Hakan Ertin. 2010. "Ethical Aspects of Human Embryonic Stem Cell Research in the Islamic World: Positions and Reflections." *Stem Cell Reviews and Reports* 6: 151–61.

Inhorn, Marcia C. 2006. "Making Muslim Babies: IVF and Gamete Donation in Sunni versus Shia Islam." *Culture, Medicine and Psychiatry* 30(4): 427–50.

Iran Daily. 2008. *Iran First Mideast Producer of iPS Cells.* http://www.iran-daily.com/1387/3191/pdf/i8.pdf (accessed August 19, 2009).

Isasi, Rosario M, and Knoppers, Bartha M. 2006. "Mind the Gap: Policy Approaches to Embryonic Stem Cell and Cloning Research in 50 Countries." European Journal of Health Law 9: 9–26.

Kinkead, Gwen. 2003. "Stem Cell Transplants Offer New Hope in Some Cases of Blindness." New York Times. http://query.nytimes.com/gst/fullpage.html?res=9907E7DE103BF936A25757C0A9659C8B63 (accessed August 19, 2009).

Larijani, Bagher, and Farzaneh Zahedi. 2007. "Biotechnology, Bioethics and National Ethical Guidelines in Biomedical Research in Iran." *Asian Biotechnology and Development Review* 9(3): 43–56.

Larijani, Bagher, Farzaneh Zahedi, and Hossein Malek-Afzali. 2005. "Medical Ethics in the Islamic Republic of Iran." *Eastern Mediterranean Health Journal* 11(5–6): 1061–72.

Mohamadnejad, Mehdi, Kamran Alimoghaddam, Mandana Mohyeddin-Bonab, Mohamad Bagheri, Maryam Bashtar, Hossein Ghanaati, Hossein Baharvand, Ardeshir Ghavamzadeh, and Reza Malekzadeh. 2007. "Phase 1 Human Trial of Autologous Bone Marrow-Hematopoetic Stem Cell Transplantation in Patients with Decompensated Cirrhosis." *Archives of Iranian Medicine* 10(4): 459–66.

Mahmood, K. *Malaysia Taking Steps to Ban Reproductive Cloning: Report.* http://www.islamonline.net/english/news/2003–01/11/article06.shtml (cited in Fadel 2010).

Mohyeddin-Bonab, Mandana, Sepideh Yazdanbakhsh, Jamshid Lotfi, Kamran Alimoghaddom, Fatemeh Talebian, Farnaz Hooshmand, Ardeshir Ghavamzadeh, and Behrouz Nikbin. 2007a. "Does Mesenchymal Stem Cell Therapy Help Multiple Sclerosis Patients? Report of a Pilot Study." *Iranian Journal of Immunology* 4(1): 50–57.

Mohyeddin-Bonab, Mandana, Kamran Alimoghaddam, Hamid Mirkhani, Massoud Eslami, Mahmood Ghasemi al-Mohamad, and Ardeshir Ghavamzadeh. 2007b. "Autologous In Vitro Expanded Mesenchymal Stem Cell Therapy for Human Old Myocardial Infarction." *Archives of Iranian Medicine* 10(4): 467–73.

Morrison, David W. G., and Ali Khademhosseini. 2006. "Stem Cell Science in Iran." http://isg-mit.org/resource/isgnews/ind. php?id=353 (accessed 9 April 2009).

Muslim World League, Islamic Jurisprudence Council Conference. 2003. *Regarding Stem Cells. Fatwa number 3. Makka, Saudi Arabia.* http://www.themwl.org/Fatwa/default.aspx?d=1&cidi=152&l=AR&cid=12 (cited in Fadel 2010).

Nordin, Musa Mohd. 2006. *Islamic Medical Ethics Amidst Developing Biotechnologies. The Human Genetic and Reproductive Technologies: Comparing Religious and Secular Perspectives. Islamic Organization of Medical Sciences.* Cairo (cited in Fadel 2010).

Qur'an, Al-Mu'minun, 23, 12–14.

Qur'an, As-Sajdeh, 32, 7–9.

Qur'an, Al-An'am, 6:98.

Ramzi, Mani. 2009. "Hematopoietic Stem Cell Transplantation in Southern Iran: History, Current Status and Future Direction." *Iranian Red Crescent Medical Journal* 11(4): 364–70.

Royan Institute. 2008. http://www.royaninstitute.org/cmsen/index.php?option=com_content&task=view&id=165&Itemid=1 (accessed 20 August 2009).

Rubin, Beatrix P. 2008. "Therapeutic Promise in the Discourse of Human Embryonic Stem Cell Research." *Science as Culture* 17(1): 13–27.

Sachedina, Abdulaziz. 2000. "Islamic Perspectives on Research with Human Embryonic Stem Cells." In *Ethical Issues in Human Stem Cell Research*

Religious Perspectives, vol. 3. Rockville, MD: Government Printing Office (National Bioethics Advisory Commission).

———. 2006. "No Harm, No Harassment: Major Principles of Health Care Ethics in Islam." In *Handbook of Bioethics and Religion*, ed. D. E. Guinn. New York: Oxford University Press.

———. 2009. *Islamic Biomedical Ethics: Principles and Application*. New York: Oxford University Press.

Saniei, Mansooreh. 2010. "Human Embryonic Stem Cell Research in Iran: The Role of the Islamic Context." *SCRIPTed* 7: 324–34.

Saniei, Mansooreh, and Raymond DeVries. 2008. "Embryonic Stem Cell Research in Iran: Status and Ethics." *Indian Journal of Medical Ethics* 5(4): 181–84.

Serour, Gamal I. 2005. "Religious Perspectives of Ethical Issues in ART: Islamic Perspectives of Ethical Issues in ART." *Middle East Fertility Society Journal* 10(3): 185–90.

Siddiqi, Muzammil. 2002. "An Islamic Perspective on Stem Cells Research." http://www.IslamiCity.com (accessed 20 August 2009).

Sparrow, Robert. 2009. "Therapeutic Cloning and Reproductive Liberty." *Journal of Medical Philosophy* 34: 102–18.

Tremayne, Soraya. 2006. "Not All Muslims Are Luddites." *Anthropology Today* 22(3): 1–2.

TUBA Stem Cell Research Group. 2008. *Current Issues in Stem Cell Researches*. http://www.tuba.gov.tr/index.php?id=422 (accessed 22 December 2009).

Turkmen, H. Ozturk, and Berna Arda. 2008. "Ethical and Legal Aspects of Stem Cell Practices in Turkey: Where Are We?" *Journal of Medical Ethics* 34: 833–37.

United Nations Declaration on Human Cloning. 2005. *General Assembly Adopts United Nations Declaration on Human Cloning*. http://www.un.org/News/Press/docs/2005/ga10333.doc.htm (accessed 10 November 2009).

Voice of America. 2009. *Virgin Mega-Brand Launches Stem Cell Bank in Qatar*. http://www1.voanews.com/english/news/a-13-2009-03-23-voa50-68636117.html (accessed 19 December 2010).

Weckerly, Michele. 2002. "The Islamic View on Stem Cell Research." http://org.law.rutgers.edu/publications/law-religion/new_devs/RJLR_ND_56.pdf (accessed 24 August 2009).

World Health Organization—Regional Office for the Eastern Mediterranean. 2004. *Development of a Regional Position on Human Cloning*. http://www.emro.who.int/rpc/pdf/RC51-INF-DOC-11.pdf (accessed 20 December 2010).

Yeprem, Saim. 2006. *İslâm'ın kök hücreye bakışı*. Diyanet Aylık Dergi 191: 25–29.

Part III

Islamic Biopolitics and the "Modern" Nation-State
Comparative Case Studies of ART

INTRODUCTION TO PART III

P. Sean Brotherton

In order to contribute to creating a nuanced discussion of laws, states, and Islamic biopolitics, I would like to offer here some brief comments that are directed toward highlighting the significance of each chapter in this section, and their interconnections.

To begin, I borrow from Clarke's innovative application of Latour's notion on the "work of purification," that is to say, the insidious way in which the notion of Western modernity is predicated on the maintenance of neatly compartmentalized—and separate spheres— of everyday life. Working against this conceptual trope, collectively, these chapters offer ethnographic accounts of the manifest ways the spheres of the juridical, religious, social, political, ethical, scientific, and, at times, pragmatic become "hybridized" and intimately inter- woven through the lived experiences, practices, and discourses of couples seeking out ARTs.

These chapters speak directly to what anthropologist Anna Tsing refers to as the metaphor of friction. "Friction," Tsing (2005: 5–6) notes, "reminds us that heterogeneous and unequal encounters can lead to new arrangements of culture and power" and, importantly, inflect "historical trajectories, enabling, excluding, and particular- izing them." Such an approach importantly addresses the articula- tion between what scholars hastily gloss over as the "local" and the "global" in order to enrich our understanding of local and transna- tional connections that enable and constrain flows of ideas, tech- nologies, bodily parts, knowledge, funding, and people.

In the chapter on "Third-Party Reproductive Assistance around the Mediterranean: Comparing Sunni Egypt, Catholic Italy, and Multisectarian Lebanon" by Inhorn, Patrizio, and Serour, the authors provide an ethnographic lens to highlight how itinerant biomedical technologies take shape, are practiced, and are rationalized in different political-religious contexts. Through a comparison of Sunni Egypt, Catholic Italy, and multisectarian Lebanon, the paper genealogically traces the establishment, institutionalization, and differing regulatory practices of ARTs in these three countries. Through mapping out couples' "therapeutic itineraries" in search of reproductive success, or through a terrain Inhorn terms "reproscapes," the authors demonstrate how regimes of knowledge and the biomedical practices they inspire circulate, transgressing political, geographic, and religious boundaries. These ebbs and flows of people and technology, or what Inhorn further characterizes as "reproflows" is, in part, influenced by changing religious and political discourses.

Whether analyzing Sunni Muslim bans on all forms of third-party assistance, changes in Italian parliamentary law (vis-à-vis Vatican edicts) or Iran's Ayatollah Khamene'i's fatwa permitting both egg and sperm donation, it becomes clear that all of these disparate events quickly translate into material outcomes on how ARTs are conceptualized and practiced. The rich ethnographic vignettes of this chapter provide a refreshing account of the interplay between the discursive domain of religious restrictions enacted through formalized and informal laws and the pragmatic behavior of individuals in pursuit of ARTs. Often times, within this messy interplay, the apparent "rules of law" become flexible and are transformed in creative and unexpected ways.

In Morgan Clarke's chapter on "Islamic Bioethics and Religious Politics in Lebanon: On Hizbullah and ARTs," Clarke highlights how biomedical expertise and discourses of scientific innovation, specifically in the arena of ARTs, are marshaled as key areas in order to index what he tentatively terms "Islamic modernity." Rather than eschewing "religion," "politics," and "science" as discrete domains of analysis, Clarke begins the laborious task of cultivating a theoretical and epistemological lexicon in which to tackle the overarching questions that animate the debates in the broader field of "Islamic bioethics." This chapter provides an excellent corollary to the other chapters in this section in that it "unpacks" how political discourses come to stand for biomedical inquiry and technological advancement, and vice versa. Importantly, Clarke directs our analytical gaze to the processes through which itinerant biomedical technologies operate under the guise of different frameworks that are supported by ostensibly competing religio-scientific rationalities.

The third chapter by Gürtin is another excellent example of how seemingly secular constitutional law becomes "hybridized" through the practice of ARTs in Turkey. Similar to Inhorn et al., this chapter is keen on highlighting these tensions through, in Gürtin's words, "recognizing and engaging with the discord between public discourses and private behaviors regarding the acceptability and demand for various ART procedures." On the one hand, the Turkish state has made access to ARTs a kind of "positive right," thereby reflecting what Gürtin terms a "progressive and liberal stance." On the other hand, however, the contingencies for eligibility are quite "restrictive," reifying a heteronormative, conservative stance to the definition of the "family."

In concluding her analysis, Gürtin argues against the ardent desire of many scholars to "construct one coherent narrative regarding Islam and the Turkish experience of assisted reproduction." As the other authors in this publication echo in their respective works, it is impossible to construct, more generally, a monolithic portrayal of Islam and biotechnologies that will address the heterogeneity of this region.

References

Tsing, Anna Lowenhaupt. 2005. *Friction: An Ethnography of Global Connection.* Princeton, NJ: Princeton University Press.

Chapter 8

THIRD-PARTY REPRODUCTIVE ASSISTANCE AROUND THE MEDITERRANEAN
COMPARING SUNNI EGYPT, CATHOLIC ITALY, AND MULTISECTARIAN LEBANON

*Marcia C. Inhorn, Pasquale Patrizio,
and Gamal I. Serour*

Introduction: The Case for Comparisons

In 2008, the world celebrated the thirtieth anniversary of in vitro fertilization (IVF) with a conference—both scientific and celebratory—in Paris, the "City of Lights." However, the world's first IVF baby, Louise Brown, was not a Parisian. Rather, she was born in England in 1978 to a working-class father and his wife, whose fallopian tubes were blocked, thus necessitating the IVF procedure. The Anglican Church ardently opposed the creation of "test-tube babies" at the time. Hence, the two English reproductive scientists who helped to conceive Louise Brown—Patrick Steptoe and Robert Edwards—were severely criticized, and baby Louise had to be delivered in secrecy. Nearly thirty-five years later, in November 2010, Robert Edwards won the Nobel Prize for his invention of IVF. Religious opposition was still registered—this time by the Catholic Church, which criticized the Nobel Prize committee for its decision.

Religious moralities have clearly played a major role in decisions surrounding the acceptance or rejection of IVF and related practices of assisted conception. One major area of rejection has been third-party reproductive assistance. In many countries where IVF is legally practiced, third-party reproductive assistance with gamete donors and surrogates is nonetheless legally or religiously restricted. This "ban" on third parties provides the focus of our comparative study.[1]

Comparisons, we argue, are quite useful, but are relatively infrequent in the scholarly literature on assisted reproductive technologies (ARTs). Despite more than thirty years since the introduction of IVF, only three edited volumes have adopted an explicitly comparative perspective. Eric Blyth and Ruth Landau's early seminal volume, *Third Party Assisted Conception across Cultures: Social, Legal and Ethical Perspectives* (first issued in hardback in 1988 and reissued in paperback with updates in 2004), provides a thirteen-country comparison. Most of the countries represented are either in Europe (e.g., Finland, Germany, Poland, United Kingdom), North America (Canada, United States), or Southeast Asia (Australia, Hong Kong, New Zealand, Singapore). However, Argentina and South Africa are included as examples from the global south, and Israel is the topic of a chapter by Landau, who practices as a social worker there. Quite strikingly, no Muslim-majority country is included in the anthology, including in the second paperback edition. In August 2009, Blyth and Landau—both practicing social workers who are concerned with ART in clinical practice—have published a new edited volume, called *Faith and Fertility: Attitudes towards Reproductive Practices in Different Religions from Ancient to Modern Times.* Islam is included in the comparison of eight world religious traditions. However, the focus of the volume is on religious law and jurisprudence at the theological/clerical level. Thus, attitudes of patients and practitioners (including clinical social workers) engaged in the on-the-ground *practice* of IVF, as well as the local moral decision-making incumbent in this realm, are largely missing from the new volume.

Another new edited volume, *Assisting Reproduction, Testing Genes: Global Encounters with New Biotechnologies,* has recently been published by Berghahn Books (Birenbaum-Carmeli and Inhorn 2009). *Assisting Reproduction* contains ten ethnographic case studies from three Muslim countries (Iran, Lebanon, and Turkey), three Catholic countries (Argentina, Ecuador, Brazil), one Hindu country (India), one Jewish country (Israel), and two postsocialist societies where religion has been suppressed (Bulgaria, Vietnam). Unlike *Third-Party*

Assisted Conception across Cultures, which focuses on national law, or *Faith and Fertility*, which focuses on religious law, *Assisting Reproduction, Testing Genes* is ethnographic, prioritizing the *practice* of assisted reproductive and genetic technologies within local cultures, as these cultures are embedded within specific political histories and moral economies.

Such ART comparisons—based on law, religion, culture, politics, and economy—are useful for several reasons. First, they can demonstrate the timeline of ART invention, establishment, and diffusion, and the astounding rapidity with which ARTs have globalized. This global metric has been accompanied by what David Harvey (1990) has called "time-space compression": namely, the global spread of ART technologies and techniques is constantly escalating, such that the "lag period" between ART invention (usually in Euro-America, Australia, or Japan) and diffusion to the global south is diminishing. To take but one example, eight years elapsed between the birth of the first European IVF baby and the first Middle Eastern one, but only two years elapsed between the birth of the first European ICSI baby (a later variant of IVF) and the birth of the first Middle Eastern one. Such rapidly converging chronologies—facilitated by other global technologies, such as the Internet—demonstrate the importance of studying the global history of IVF, an endeavor that has yet to be systematically undertaken on a scholarly level.[2]

Second, such comparisons can help to delineate the similarities in clinical ART practice around the world. Although IVF clinics in Bogota, Colombia, and Timbuktu, Mali, may lack the glamour of IVF performed in Beverly Hills, California, they may nonetheless perform ART procedures with the exact same technologies and techniques as clinics in Euro-America. Such clinical consistencies serve to demonstrate the scientific "literacy" and "modernity" of physicians and patients living in nations on the receiving end of global ART transfers (Inhorn 2003). For example, Ecuador, a resource-poor, high-altitude Catholic country in South America, is proud of its thriving IVF industry, in which third-party donor programs are flourishing and IVF physicians, most of them Catholic, see themselves as purveyors of high-tech biomedicine in "God's laboratory" (Roberts 2009).

Third, global comparisons may also indicate the ways in which societies differ in their practice of ART, differences that are most often based on social, cultural, legal, religious, and bioethical norms. Such ART diversity is strikingly apparent in the twenty-seven member states of the European Union. Whereas "progressive" Scandinavian countries such as Norway and Sweden have enacted "restrictive" legislation against both third-party donation and surrogacy, "traditional" Catholic Spain (with its large and growing Muslim Andalusian population) is now the European epicenter of so-called reproductive tourism, because of its "liberal" policies allowing third-party reproductive assistance, especially egg donation (Matorras 2005).[3] Denmark, on the other hand, is the hub for the global export of sperm, because of liberal guidelines and a well-regulated sperm donation industry. Indeed, the striking degree of heterogeneity across Europe has led to recent calls for international guidelines—even laws—to coordinate ART practices across the continent (Deech 2003).

Fourth, comparisons can suggest the similarities and differences in moral and legal reasoning that have led to ART heterogeneity. In "Compatible Contradictions: Religion and the Naturalization of Assisted Reproduction," a group of religious studies scholars and anthropologists (Traina et al. 2008) trace the divergent moral discourses that have led to both consensus and disharmony in ART practices among the monotheistic traditions of Christianity, Judaism, and Islam. Whereas ARTs are allowed, with some limitations, in both Islam and Judaism, the Vatican still prohibits all forms of reproductive intervention, including ART. However, Catholicism is the only branch of Christianity to disallow ART altogether; as shown in this comparative essay, Eastern Orthodox and Protestant traditions allow various forms of ART. Islam, too, has permitted IVF since its inception; however, the Sunni and Shia branches of Islam have diverged considerably in the moral discourse surrounding third-party reproductive assistance, as described in other chapters in this volume. Judaism shows similar strands of divergence, based on levels of religious orthodoxy (e.g., Orthodox Judaism versus Reform Judaism) (Weitzman 2009; Washofsky 2009). Nonetheless, as shown in Susan Kahn's *Reproducing Jews: A Cultural Account of Assisted Conception in Israel* (2000), Judaism is among the most "ART-friendly" of all the religions, encouraging assisted reproduction based on Israeli-Jewish pronatalism and the relative openness of rabbinical interpretation.

The Case for a Mediterranean Comparison

This chapter attempts to examine some of the convergences, divergences, and moral nuances occurring around the Mediterranean. Specifically, Egypt, Italy, and Lebanon have been chosen as comparative case studies. Why the Mediterranean, and why these three countries in particular? For one, the Mediterranean region is the birthplace of the three major monotheistic traditions, Judaism, Christianity, and Islam (in chronological order). Italy is home to Rome and the Vatican, the birthplace of Catholicism. Al Azhar University, which is the world's oldest and most important religious university in the Sunni Islamic world, was built in the center of Cairo, Egypt, where it remains today. Lebanon, where much blood has been shed over religion, nonetheless is *the* most religiously diverse (and some would argue, tolerant) society in the Mediterranean region and in the Middle East more generally. As the "meeting place" of all three monotheistic religions, Lebanon currently hosts eighteen recognized religious sects, including Sunni, Shia, Druze, Catholic Maronites, Roman Catholics, Greek Orthodox, various Protestant sects, and even a remaining Lebanese Jewish population.[4]

Second, the relative geographic proximity of the Mediterranean countries has led to what has been termed "reproflows" (Inhorn 2010): namely, the cross-regional flows of people (e.g., physicians, patients, pharmaceutical representatives, embryo carriers), technologies (e.g., micromanipulators, cryopreservation tanks, 4D ultrasound machines), "body bits"[5] (e.g., donor sperm, embryos, human hormones), and ideas (e.g., implanting six IVF embryos is clinically risky, paid surrogacy is immoral), which are abundantly apparent in the actual practice of ART. Such reproflows exist within a larger "reproscape," or a complex, transnational, reproductive health landscape characterized by circulating peoples, technologies, body parts, media, finance, and ideas (Inhorn 2010). A "Mediterranean reproscape" clearly exists; for example, Moroccan physicians send patients to Southern France; the Italian company Serono (now a subsidiary of Merck) ships hormones to Egypt; Syrian IVF patients cross the checkpoint into Lebanon in order to obtain ARTs forbidden in Syria. Such Mediterranean circulations—across borders and across the sea—have existed for centuries, as in the case of Moorish Spain (Rogozen-Soltar 2007, 2010).

Here, we want to compare Mediterranean attitudes toward third-party reproductive assistance. We argue that the Mediterranean, as a region, boasts some of the most stringent "anti-third-party-ART" sentiment in the world. Namely, the Vatican holds the position that life begins at conception and bans *all* forms of reproductive assistance (including contraception, abortion, in vitro fertilization, third-party gamete donation, and surrogacy), while the Sunni world allows ART but bans third parties altogether (including egg donors, sperm donors, embryo donors, ooplasm donors, and surrogates, including family members). We want to examine these bans in Egypt and Italy—in theory and in practice—and suggest how Italy has become more like Egypt in recent years. Furthermore, we examine the case of Lebanon to show how a multisectarian Muslim-Christian country grapples with the complexities of these bans. Namely, what is a Sunni-Hizbullah-Maronite-Greek Orthodox-Druze-Armenian-Protestant-etc. country to do? How do Lebanese Catholic Maronite IVF physicians justify their practice of ARTs, including gamete donation? Or Lebanese Shia Muslim physicians for that matter? The answers, we argue, are not easy—not only for the Lebanese, but also for Italian Catholics, Egyptian Sunni Muslims, and all those other patients who do not want to abide by religious bans, for one reason or another. In the second half of this chapter, we provide a series of ethnographic case vignettes to hear the voices and examine the reasoning of a number of "reproductive tourists," all from the Mediterranean region. We argue that reproductive bans have led to so-called reproductive tourism, which might be more accurately defined as "reproductive exile" (Inhorn and Patrizio 2009). But before we examine their experiences of travel, we compare the religious and legal situation in the three countries, spelling out the similarities, differences, and resulting moral quandaries for physicians and patients.

Sunni Egypt

By 1980, only two years after Louise Brown's birth, the Grand Shaikh of Egypt's Al Azhar University had issued the first fatwa[6] permitting IVF to be practiced by Muslims. By 1986, the first IVF center had opened in Egypt, with the first Egyptian IVF baby, Hebbatallah Mohamed, born in 1987. By 1990, Egypt's first experiment in state subsidization of IVF for the poor came to fruition with the birth of a full-fledged IVF clinic—and then the first IVF baby—in a public maternity hospital in Alexandria (Inhorn 1994). Following the 1991 Belgian invention of intracytoplasmic sperm injection (ICSI), this variant of IVF—designed to overcome male infertility—spread in 1994 across the Mediterranean to Egypt, where it was introduced in an IVF clinic in Cairo (Inhorn 2003). By 1996, Egypt already hosted ten private IVF clinics in major cities. By the year 2003, the Egyptian IVF industry had truly blossomed, with approximately fifty clinics, five of them at least partially state subsidized (Inhorn 2010). In 2003, Al Azhar University itself, through its Department of Obstetrics and Gynecology and International Islamic Center for Population Studies and Research, had opened a state-subsidized IVF clinic to serve the Cairene poor, and to provide training for physicians and embryologists.[7]

Similar stories of diffusion and expansion were found throughout Muslim countries during this period. In 1997, a global survey of ART clinics in sixty-two countries was published; eight Middle Eastern Muslim countries (Egypt, Iran, Kuwait, Jordan, Lebanon, Morocco, Qatar, and Turkey) and three South and Southeast Asian Muslim countries (Indonesia, Malaysia, and Pakistan) were represented. None of these Muslim countries practiced donor insemination (or any other form of third-party reproductive assistance). As noted by the study authors, "AID [artificial insemination with donor sperm] is considered adultery and leads to confusion regarding the lines of genealogy, whose purity is of prime importance in Islam" (Meirow and Schenker 1997: 134).

This ban on sperm donation—and all other forms of third-party assistance—has been clearly spelled out multiple times in fatwas and bioethical decrees issued in the Sunni Muslim countries. Follow-ing the issuance in 1980 of the original Al Azhar fatwa, the Islamic *Fiqh* Council issued a nearly identical fatwa banning all forms of third-party assistance in its seventh meeting held in Mecca in 1984. Subsequently, fatwas supporting ART but banning third-party assis-tance have been issued in Kuwait, Qatar, and the United Arab Emir-ates (Serour 2008). In 1997, at the ninth Islamic law and medicine conference, held under the auspices of the Kuwait-based Islamic Organization for Medical Sciences (IOMS) in Casablanca, a land-mark five-point bioethical declaration included recommendations to prevent human cloning and to prohibit all situations in which a third party invades a marital relationship through donation of re-productive material (Moosa 2003). As noted by Islamic legal scholar Ebrahim Moosa (2003: 23): "In terms of ethics, Muslim authorities consider the transmission of reproductive material between persons who are not legally married to be a major violation of Islamic law. This sensitivity stems from the fact that Islamic law has a strict taboo on sexual relations outside wedlock (*zina*). The taboo is designed to protect paternity (i.e., family), which is designated as one of the five goals of Islamic law, the others being the protection of religion, life, property, and reason."

Such a ban on third-party reproductive assistance of all kinds is effectively in place in the Sunni world, which represents approxi-mately 80–90 percent of the world's more than 1.5 billion Muslims (Inhorn 2003; Meirow and Schenker 1997; Serour 1996; Serour and Dickens 2001). In Sunni Egypt, as well as the Sunni-dominant Mid-dle Eastern nations of North Africa (Algeria, Libya, Morocco, Tuni-sia), the Arab Gulf (Kuwait, Oman, Qatar, Saudi Arabia, United Arab

Emirates, Yemen), and the Levant (Jordan, Palestine, Syria), third-party assisted reproduction is *not* practiced—at least knowingly—in IVF clinics. In the Sunni countries, this ban on donors and surrogacy has been instantiated through antidonation bioethical codes, antidonation professional codes for obstetricians and gynecologists, and antidonation laws that specify the punishments that will ensue if an IVF practitioner wrongfully undertakes any form of third-party assisted conception. Such punishments range from permanent clinic closing to confiscation of all profits derived from donation to physician imprisonment and even the death penalty (although this has never happened and is not bound by legislation).

Yet, the ban in the Sunni world seems to derive less from the threat of legal punishment than from the force of Islamic morality. Namely, the majority of Sunni Muslims—both physicians and their patients—ardently support the Sunni ban on third-party donation, for three important reasons: (1) the moral implications of third-party donation for marriage; (2) the potential for incest; and (3) the moral implications of donation for kinship and family life.

With regard to marriage, Islam is a religion that can be said to privilege—even mandate—heterosexual marital relations. As is made clear in the original Al Azhar fatwa, reproduction outside of marriage is considered *zina*, or adultery, which is strictly forbidden in Islam. Although third-party donation does not involve the sexual "body contact" of adulterous relations, nor presumably the desire to engage in an extramarital affair, it is nonetheless considered by Sunni Muslim religious scholars to be a form of adultery, by virtue of introducing a third party into the sacred dyad of husband and wife. It is the very fact that another man's sperm or another woman's eggs enter a place where they do not belong that makes donation of any kind inherently wrong—or *haram*, religiously forbidden—and hence threatening to the marital bond.

The second aspect of third-party donation that troubles marriage is the potential for incest among the offspring of unknown donors. Moral concerns have been raised about the potential for a single anonymous donor's offspring to meet and marry each other, thereby undertaking an incestuous union of half-siblings. In a small country such as Lebanon, with only 4 million inhabitants, such unwitting incest of the children of an anonymous donor is a real possibility, a moral concern that has also been raised in neighboring Israel (Kahn 2000).

The final moral concern voiced by Sunni Muslims, including clerics, IVF physicians, and patients themselves, is that third-party donation confuses issues of kinship, descent, and inheritance. As with marriage, Islam is a religion that can be said to privilege—even mandate—biological inheritance. Preserving the biological "origins" of each child—meaning its relationship to a known biological mother and father—is considered not only an ideal in Islam, but a moral imperative. The problem with third-party donation, therefore, is that it destroys a child's *nasab*, lineage or genealogy, which is immoral in addition to being psychologically devastating to the donor child.

It is important to emphasize that these moral concerns are taken very seriously. To our knowledge, not one single IVF clinic in a Sunni-dominant Muslim country practices third-party assisted conception. Physicians are sometimes asked about gamete donation and surrogacy by IVF patients who cannot conceive a child in any other way. Patients are told that it is "against the religion," and, therefore, not performed in the country. Or, if they are interested in pursuing this option, they are told that they must travel "outside" to Europe, North America, or Asia. Such cases of Sunni Muslim reproductive tourism are certainly beginning to occur, as we shall see in the case vignettes that follow. However, the vast majority of infertile Sunni Muslim couples abide by the religious ban on donation and surrogacy, agreeing with the moral justifications for it. For example, in ethnographic interviews undertaken by the first author with nearly six hundred infertile individuals and couples in Egypt (1988–89, 1996), Lebanon (2003), United Arab Emirates (2007), and "Arab Detroit" (2003–5, 2007–8), only a handful of Sunni Muslim couples (<10) were willing to contemplate any form of third-party donation. Of the few men and women who "approved" of the practice, their approval was most often a "last resort" when no other ART option could be expected to solve the infertility problem. Furthermore, only egg donation was approved of, because it allowed the infertile wife to experience a pregnancy and could be compared religiously to the *halal* (religiously permitted) practice of polygyny. Sperm donation, on the other hand, was not; it was said to confuse patrilineal descent and constitute a form of *zina*, or a wife's "extramarital" acceptance of another man's sperm. Most importantly, men argued that a donor child "won't be my son" (Inhorn 2006, 2012). In their view, sperm donation would be like "raising another man's child."

Catholic Italy

These Sunni Islamic moral injunctions against third-party reproductive assistance are somewhat different from those issued by the Roman Catholic Church. It is fair to state that the Roman Catholic ban on ART is even more restrictive than the Sunni ban on third parties. Indeed, the Catholic Church's doctrine toward all forms of reproductive technology (including contraception and abortion) is *the* most restrictive in the world.

With regard to ART, the Catholic Church disapproves of IVF because it disassociates procreation from sex, both of which are intended to occur only within the holy covenant of matrimony. According to the Catholic doctrine of "natural law," no artificial barriers or aids to conception are to be used during the procreative act. Replacing loving intercourse with the masturbation and surgical procedures required in IVF will necessarily erode marital unity (Traina et al. 2008). A life that is created by medical practitioners—rather than through an act of conjugal love between two married people—"establishes the domination of technology over the origin and destiny of the human person" (Catechism 2002: 509, as cited in Richards 2009). The technology of IVF, therefore, threatens the unity of marriage; IVF physicians themselves become "third parties" to a marriage, intruding into the marital functions of sex and procreation. Similarly, all forms of third-party donation—of eggs, sperm, embryos, or uteruses, as in surrogacy—are seen as "offenses" to the conjugal unity of the couple, introducing an "emotional and spiritual wedge between husband and wife both symbolized by and enacted in sexual infidelity" (Traina et al. 2008: 38). In this regard, the association of infidelity with third-party donation is similar to one of the moral justifications undergirding the Sunni ban on this practice.

But perhaps even more important to Roman Catholic doctrine is the threat that ART poses to human life in the form of the embryo. The Catholic Church considers life to begin at the moment of conception; hence, all human embryos created through ART are considered to be sacrosanct. As a form of human life, embryos must never be forsaken. Yet, according to the Church, the processes of ART "destroy" embryos—and hence, human life—in multiple ways. For one, multiple embryos are often transferred to a woman's uterus in a single IVF cycle, without all of the embryos implanting. The high failure rates following embryo transfer are considered to be a loss of potential human life, to which the Catholic Church objects (Richards 2009). Furthermore, the Catholic Church is concerned with the overproduction of embryos in ART, leading to problems of so-called embryo disposition (Nachtigall et al. 2005). Excess or unused embryos that are produced through ART may be cryopreserved, but their "quality," clinically speaking, declines considerably during long-term storage. After five years of cryopreservation, some

IVF clinics routinely dispose of all excess embryos from cold storage. Furthermore, some unused embryos—especially those of poor clinical quality (and, hence, less likely to implant)—are routinely disposed of in IVF laboratories, while others are destined for human research.

The Catholic Church's view is that the destruction of *any* embryo is inherently wrong; such a view underlies the Church's ban on stem cell research as well. This view of the embryo as a human life from the moment of conception is not shared by any of the schools of Islamic jurisprudence. Indeed, embryo disposition is only a problem in Islam if an embryo is donated to a third party. Embryo disposal and even multifetal pregnancy reduction (i.e., a form of selective abortion) in cases of multiple-gestation IVF pregnancies (twins, triplets, etc.) are allowed by the Sunni Islamic authorities, particularly if the prospect of carrying the pregnancy to viability is markedly reduced or the health of the mother is in serious jeopardy (Serour 2008). Embryo research is similarly allowed, if the latter occurs within fourteen days of initial fertilization. This consensus on embryo research—and hence stem cell research—was reached at a conference on the "Dilemma of Stem Cell Research" held in Cairo in November 2007 (Serour 2008). In short, in Islam, the human embryo simply is not sacrosanct as it is in Roman Catholicism. Thus, the ban in place in Sunni Islam takes a somewhat different form from the ban in place in Catholicism, arising as they do from rather different moral principles.

Furthermore, in Sunni Egypt, as in other Sunni-dominant countries, the religious ban on third-party reproductive assistance is adhered to in actual clinical practice. This is not so in the Roman Catholic countries. Despite the Church's clear and forceful opposition to all forms of ART, Catholic infertility physicians and patients around the world have largely refused to abide by the ban, as seen also with the widespread use of contraception (and even abortion) among the world's Catholics. For example, by 1992, most of the Catholic countries of Latin America had begun to perform IVF and had joined a Latin American registry of IVF clinics (Nicholson and Nicholson 1994). Ahead of Egypt with its 10 IVF clinics, Argentina by that time had 16 clinics, performing 1,416 IVF cycles annually. This was followed by Brazil (7 clinics), Chile (6 clinics), Mexico (4 clinics), Venezuela and Colombia (3 clinics each), with solo clinics in Bolivia, Ecuador, Guatemala, Panama, Paraguay, and Uruguay. Because of Catholic sensitivities toward embryo preservation and disposal, Latin American IVF clinics at that time were reporting high-order embryo transfers (five or more at a time), resulting in high levels of risky multiple-gestation pregnancies.

Just as with the Catholic countries of Latin America, Italy refused to abide by the Vatican's ban on ART (Bonaccorso 2008).[8] The first IVF clinic in Italy was established by Professor Ettore Cittadini in Palermo, Sicily, in 1982, and the first birth occurred in 1984, a baby girl named Eleonora. By the late 1980s, Italy had developed one of the most "cutting-edge" IVF industries in the world, earning Italy the moniker of "the Wild West" of Europe. Serono—one of the world's two major multinational ART pharmaceutical firms (along with Organon, now Schering-Plough)—was started and headquartered in Italy. IVF centers multiplied in all of Italy's major cities (e.g., Rome, Milan, Naples, Florence). In 1994, an Italian IVF physician helped a sixty-three-year-old postmenopausal woman conceive a child through the use of donor eggs and hormonal stimulation. Italian reproductive scientists were also at the forefront of egg freezing, which first occurred in an IVF center in Bologna. In 1999, Italian IVF researchers developed genetic screening tests of IVF embryos that could help to boost the fertility rate of older women. Together, the Italian developments in egg freezing, egg donation, and genetic testing of embryos heralded the beginning of an ART industry intended for career women who had delayed conception into their forties and beyond.

Furthermore, in 2001, teams in both the United States and Italy announced that they were working on producing the first human clone, following the cloning of Dolly the Sheep in 1997. By 2002, the "maverick" leader of the Italian team, Severino Antinori—who happened to be the same Italian physician who had helped the sixty-three-year-old postmenopausal woman to conceive—claimed that he had already cloned a small number of human infants outside of Italy, for infertile couples living in Russia and "an Islamic country." The births of these children were said to be impending.

Perhaps the announcement of human cloning was the "straw that broke the Italian camel's back." Only one year later, on 11 December 2003, the Italian senate passed a bill introducing tight restrictions on ART, which were subsequently signed into law by the prime minister of the Republic of Italy, Silvio Berlusconi, on 19 February 2004. Indeed, in 2004, the political majority in Italy was "center-right" under Berlusconi, who was, at that time at least, "pro-Vatican."[9] Thus, both politicians and the Vatican were strongly in favor of the law; it was quickly presented and approved by the branches of the Italian government without any chance for amendments (i.e., the law was considered "sealed"). The passing of this legislation turned Italy overnight from Europe's most progressive to most restrictive ART regime—second only to the tiny Latin American country of Costa Rica, which outlawed all forms of ART in 2000, after ARTs had been deemed constitutional there in 1995 (Benagiano and Gianaroli 2004).[10] The restrictive Italian legislation emerged after ten years of heated parliamentary debate on the subject of ART, accompanied by a scientific study by the Italian Health Commission. The resulting "Medically Assisted Reproduction Law," known in Italy as "Law 40/2004," was championed by the Vatican and conservative politicians in the Italian parliament and was far more restrictive than anticipated.

The major features of the ART-restrictive Law 40 included: (1) the use of ARTs only among "stable heterosexual couples who live together and are of childbearing age" and are "clinically infertile"; (2) the prohibition of embryo cryopreservation; (3) the prohibition of third-party gamete donation (eggs, sperm, embryos) and surrogacy; (4) the prohibition of embryo research; (4) the prohibition of ART use for single women or same-sex couples; (5) the fertilization of no more than three oocytes (i.e., eggs) at any one time; (6) the simultaneous transfer to the uterus of all fertilized eggs; and (7) the prohibition of preimplantation genetic diagnosis (PGD) and prenatal screening for genetic disorders among human embryos (Benagiano and Gianaroli 2004).

The law provided absolute protection to the human embryo: no donation to research, disposal in the laboratory, or destruction of any kind. However, as pointed out by scientific critics, the embryo benefits from this "protection" only while it is in the laboratory. As soon as the embryo is transferred to a woman's uterus, this protection is lost, because the embryo may fail to implant or, even worse, the mother may still opt for a termination of pregnancy under Italy's intact abortion law (law 194/1978). Indeed, as pointed out by Italian bioethicists, the ART law does not harmonize at all with Italy's abortion law, passed in 1978, which still allows a pregnant Italian woman to request termination within ninety days of her last menstrual period (Benagiano and Gianaroli 2004). In principle, the Italian parliament should have restricted IVF altogether, as in the case of Costa Rica, or revoked its abortion law at the same time the ART legislation was passed.

Not surprisingly, Italy's "pro-life" ART law was immediately condemned by IVF scientists worldwide, and was called "medieval" by Italy's female parliamentarians. Furthermore, the "fallout" from the

Italian legislation has been well documented over the past five years. The success rates of IVF in Italy have fallen considerably, from 25 to 11 percent within the first year of the law's passage. Several Italian IVF physicians have relocated their clinics outside the country's borders, taking their Italian patients with them. Italy now has one of the highest percentages of so-called reproductive tourists, namely, infertile Italian couples who leave the country because they cannot access appropriate care in their own country. Within the first year of the law's passing, clinics in Spain, Austria, and Switzerland reported a 20 percent increase in Italian patients coming for ART treatment, particularly for egg and sperm donation.

Furthermore, the Italian law has shifted the concept of gamete donation as an altruistic "gift" to a pure act of commerce. Before Italy's restrictive law came into being, egg donations occurred as voluntary acts between patients in Italian IVF clinics, without payments to the egg donor. Once the law was passed, however, Italian women needing donor oocytes began having to "buy eggs," often for considerable fees, in foreign IVF clinics that allow egg donation.

The Church's and parliament's justifications for the new ban on gamete donation in Italy in fact tended to mirror most of the moral justifications found in Sunni Egypt and other parts of the Sunni world. According to proponents of the ban, gamete donation is said to: (1) cause the risk of future incestuous relationships among the children of anonymous donors; (2) damage the personal identity of the child, because of lack of knowledge about biological origins; (3) lead to parental rejection of the donor child, especially among infertile men who cannot claim biological paternity and who may therefore abandon the donor child; and (4) cause the risk of "positive eugenics"—i.e., creating a child with sought-after characteristics of a donor (e.g., blue eyes, blonde hair, IQ>130). In laying out these moral justifications for the ban on third-party donation, proponents of the ban—including the Vatican bishops—proved to converge with Sunni clerics in their thinking, even if there were no direct influences from across the Mediterranean.

Indeed, critics immediately charged that the moral principles of the Catholic Church were being transformed into unprecedented legal norms. As such, within the first year of the new law, the Italian reproductive science community and left-wing politicians mobilized to oppose the legislation. Italy's Radical Party, known for its anti-Catholic, anticlerical positions, collected the 500,000 necessary signatures to call for a referendum vote on the new ART law. Furthermore, a number of Italian reproductive scientists staged a hunger strike in the hope of influencing the referendum, which was scheduled to take place through a public vote on 12–13 June 2005. Unfortunately for the Italian opposition, the clerics won. In a Vatican-approved strategy, the Church campaigned against the referendum, and the country's Catholic bishops called upon their parishioners to boycott the vote. As a result Italians "stayed home in droves": i.e., the Italian IVF referendum ended with half the required vote (25 percent rather than 50 percent), leaving the ART restrictions firmly in place.

As of this writing, the law banning most forms of ART in Italy continues. Italian IVF physicians are restricted to performing only IVF and ICSI with a married couple's gametes and without any form of third-party donation. Italian couples continue to leave the country en masse in search of third-party reproductive assistance, and the Italian birth rate continues to decline. As of now, the Italian birth rate is 1.38, well below replacement level and lower than all other Mediterranean countries except Malta (1.37), Croatia (1.35), and Greece (1.33).

Perhaps fearing the slow death of the Italian population, Italian parliamentarians have recently heeded the calls of the Italian progressive party, Italia Dei Valori, to enter into a dialogue over the ART law. In April 2009, the Italian parliament heard scientific evidence—including by one of the authors of this chapter[11]—showing that the ART law has been bad for women's health. In the period since the law's passage, rates of high-risk triplet pregnancies have almost doubled in women younger than age thirty-seven, because, according to the law, all three embryos must be transferred rather than frozen. In addition, women require more IVF cycles in order to become pregnant. As women age, the number of competent oocytes (i.e., able to produce a live birth) decreases. Since, by law, only three eggs can be chosen for in vitro fertilization, it becomes much more unlikely that the most "competent" oocytes will be chosen for fertilization. Quite paradoxically, given the Catholic objections to embryo destruction, this leads to *higher* rates of embryo wastage and the need for repeat IVF cycles. Furthermore, women aged thirty-seven and above have been significantly penalized by the new law, because their chances for an ART pregnancy are worse to begin with. Without the possibility of utilizing all of the eggs produced during normal hormonal stimulation, and without the possibility of embryo screening, egg donation, or embryo cryopreservation (all of which facilitate ART pregnancy rates in older women), their chances of IVF success are, indeed, minimal.

As a result of this evidence, the Italian constitutional court, comparable to the Supreme Court in the United States, has changed some aspects of Law 40. First, the number of ART-created embryos is no longer limited to three, and the decision remains in the hands of the IVF physician. Second, it is possible to freeze the excess embryos. Finally, it is possible to undertake PGD on these ART-created embryos. However, whether these amendments will stand is questionable. Currently, the politically governed Italian Ministry of Health is working vigorously to overturn the amendments.[12]

Italy thus provides an example of the convergence of state religion and state law—largely against the wishes of the mostly Catholic IVF practitioners and infertile Catholic patients who seek IVF. This disharmony between a religiously inspired national law and the wishes of the people is quite different from the case of Egypt, where no national law exists, but where both Muslim IVF practitioners and patients wish to follow the fatwa rulings of the religious establishment.

Multisectarian Lebanon

This brings us to the case of Lebanon, a religiously "mixed" community, with significant populations of Catholics, Sunni Muslims, Shia Muslims, and other minority Muslim and Christian religious sects. A census has not been taken in Lebanon since 1932, before the founding of the Lebanese nation-state, because so-called political demography is a highly sensitive issue in a country without a true religious majority. However, it is widely believed that the Christian population of Lebanon, once the largest single group, has declined significantly during the past thirty-five years of civil war and ongoing political violence. The Shia population during this period has meanwhile increased disproportionately, not only because of higher fertility rates, but also because relatively fewer of the poor Shia Muslims of Southern Lebanon were able to emigrate from the country. Until the Lebanese civil war (1975–1990), Sunni Muslims dominated the coastal cities of Lebanon, such as Tripoli in the north. However, large populations of Shia Muslims fleeing from the South now live in periurban slums surrounding most coastal cities (including Beirut). And the Druze, an offshoot of the Shia, continue to live in pockets in Lebanon's central mountains, as well as in Beirut, the urban hub of the country. In addition, significant refugee populations (Armenians fleeing the Turks, Palestinians fleeing the Israelis, Iraqis fleeing the current war, Syrians fleeing poverty and now war) live in Lebanon, along with minority Christian sects, the largest of which is Greek Orthodox. Indeed, it is fair to say that Lebanon is *the* most heterogeneous Middle Eastern society, and perhaps the most religiously heterodox of all societies in the Mediterranean. Today, demographers agree that Muslims constitute a solid majority—almost 60 percent, with Shia outstripping the Sunni population by several percentage points (approximately 27 percent versus 24 percent, with Druze at 5 percent of the total population). Christians constitute the remaining 40 percent, with the largest group being Catholic Maronites,[13] followed by Greek Orthodox.

Given the multisectarian nature of Lebanese society, it is important to try to understand how the local IVF industry has developed there, and to which religious authorities it has turned for guidance surrounding ARTs and particularly third-party reproductive assistance. First, it is important to note that, compared to Egypt and Italy, Lebanon is a relative latecomer to IVF and related ARTs. The first IVF clinics did not open in Beirut until the mid-1990s, nearly a decade later than in Egypt and nearly fifteen years after Italy's IVF sector began. This relative "Lebanese delay" has everything to do with the fifteen-year civil war: it was not until the early 1990s, after the fighting stopped, that Lebanon was able to begin rebuilding its medical infrastructure, which had been severely damaged during the period of prolonged battle, including in urban centers.

Prior to the civil war, Lebanon was well known in the Middle Eastern region for "3 E's": medical Education, Entrepreneurship, and Excellence. By the mid-1990s, these aspects of Lebanese medical society had begun to return. Local gynecologists began opening their own small hospitals and private IVF clinics. Expatriate Lebanese physicians, trained in the West, returned to the country to start IVF clinics staffed by local doctors. Eventually, several of Lebanon's major private hospitals opened their own IVF centers. By 2003, when two anthropologists reached Lebanon to study ART there,[14] the country boasted between fifteen and twenty clinics, depending upon how "clinic" was defined.

Before the year 2000, it appears that all Lebanese IVF clinics abided by the Middle East regional ban on third-party reproductive assistance. Why would this be true in a "mixed" Muslim-Christian country? First, Lebanese IVF physicians, circulating through regional medical conferences, were clearly aware that the Islamic religious authorities did not approve of any form of donation or surrogacy. They knew that third-party donation was not being practiced in any Muslim country at that time, and they felt obliged, even if they were Christian, to follow the local religious norms. To do otherwise would be to incite potential anger and resistance among Muslim clients of Lebanese IVF centers. Second, some Christian IVF physicians, particularly Catholic Maronites, felt personal moral am-bivalence about practicing third-party donation and cryopreserving human embryos. Thus, they were only too happy to follow the rela-tively restrictive Sunni Muslim guidelines, rather than turning to Christian nations in Europe for guidance.

But the third and most important reason has to do with the Shia Muslim clergy. Namely, before the year 2000—and even today—many Shia Muslim clergy concur with the Sunni ban on third-party reproductive assistance. They do not agree with egg donation, sperm donation, or surrogacy, and they have issued fatwas to that effect, to be adhered to by their followers.[15] Such anti-third-party fatwas have been issued in Shia-dominant Iraq, Bahrain, and Lebanon itself. In Lebanon, the popular local Shia cleric, Muhammad Husayn Fadlal-lah, issued a fatwa decision in the late 1990s banning any form of gamete donation or surrogacy.

The year 2000, however, was a watershed in Lebanon. At a Middle East Fertility Society (MEFS) meeting held in Beirut, the audience of Middle Eastern IVF practitioners literally gasped in incredulity when an Iranian female IVF physician, dressed in a black chador, described her clinic's efforts to overcome age-related ovulatory fail-ure through egg donation. When questioned further, this Iranian physician explained that the supreme leader of the Islamic Repub-lic of Iran, Ayatollah Ali al-Hussein al-Khamene'i, the hand-picked successor to Iran's Ayatollah Khomeini, had recently (1999) issued a fatwa effectively permitting *both* egg and sperm donor technologies to be used (Inhorn 2006). Interestingly, the moral justification for allowing donor technologies was included in the text of Ayatollah Khamene'i's fatwa: preserving the marriage of the infertile couple through the birth of donor children would prevent the "marital and psychological disputes" that would inevitably arise from remaining childless indefinitely. In short, both preservation of lineage *and* pres-ervation of marriage mattered to Ayatollah Khamene'i—an opinion at odds with the majority Sunni thinking on the subject.

This "millennial moment" in Iran had an almost immediate im-pact in Lebanon. Religiously pious Shia Muslims, including members of Lebanon's Hizbullah party, were the first to press for third-party donation, because they followed the spiritual guidance of Ayatollah Khamene'i in Iran. Some Shia IVF physicians began to respond to these requests, developing "informal" egg and sperm donation ar-rangements within their clinics. Sometimes infertile couples were asked to find their own "donors" (e.g., relatives or friends), while at other times Shia female IVF clients were asked to donate their excess eggs to fellow Shia IVF patients (i.e., a kind of within-clinic "egg sharing"). Eventually some clinics were able to find "anonymous" donors—for example, medical students who agreed to donate sperm, young American women who agreed to travel to Beirut for egg donation, and poor Palestinian refugee camp women who became gestational surrogates—all for a sizable fee (Inhorn 2012).

In short, the "door to donation" was opened in Lebanon in 2000, as a direct result of the Iranian supreme leader's allowance of donor technologies. Starting with entrepreneurial Shia IVF physicians who cited the new Iranian guidelines, the local Lebanese Shia clergy soon followed, issuing formal fatwas or informal opinions to their followers about the permissibility of third-party reproductive assistance, especially egg donation, which most agreed was now *halal,* or religiously permitted (Clarke 2009).[16]

In addition, Christian IVF practitioners soon joined the pro-donation bandwagon in Lebanon, setting up informal programs in their clinics. Many Western-leaning Lebanese Christian IVF practitioners had been frustrated by the earlier Sunni-inspired ban on third-party assistance, and were hence glad that Shia clerics had offered new rulings. Being able to provide gamete donation—and even surrogacy—allowed them to offer the "full spectrum" of possible ART services to their IVF patients. Indeed, it is fair to state that Lebanese Christians—both physicians and patients—were as eager as Lebanese Shia to introduce third-party reproductive assistance to Lebanon, even if their own inspiration was European, rather than Iranian. Third-party reproductive assistance in Lebanon could showcase Lebanon's European-style "modernity," while also providing a tremendous source of profit to the local IVF industry. Furthermore, many Lebanese Christians, like their Italian counterparts, did not have any moral qualms about using donor technologies. They considered "donation" to be an act of altruism, similar to child adoption, which most of them condoned on Christian religious grounds.[17]

The lifting of the third-party ART ban in Lebanon has certainly had its detractors, however. It is very important to state that most cycles of IVF occurring in Lebanon do *not* involve gamete donation, embryo donation, or surrogacy, simply because third-party reproductive assistance is widely acknowledged to be an option of "last resort"—a kind of "necessary evil," or "act of desperation" when all else fails. Today in Lebanon, the vast majority of Sunni IVF patients do not accept third-party reproductive assistance, and there are many

Shia patients who do not as well (Inhorn 2012). Furthermore, not all IVF physicians agree with the lifting of the ban in Lebanon. One politically powerful Shia IVF physician has attempted repeatedly to introduce legislation banning all forms of third-party assistance in Lebanon. Despite significant support among Sunni political groups, the bill has never been passed, probably because of a combination of multisectarian resistance and postwar exhaustion and apathy.[18]

It is also important to state that some IVF physicians in Lebanon retain significant moral and medical ambivalence toward the way donation is being practiced in the country. First, there is no local IVF scientific registry of any sort (as in Latin America, mentioned above); thus, there are no reliable statistics on the numbers of IVF cycles with and without donation. Second, there is no reliable regulatory system in the country. As a result, third-party reproductive assistance is being carried out "behind closed doors," in the unregulated, sometimes "secretive" environment of private IVF clinics (Inhorn 2004). As a result of this lack of regulatory oversight, practices that would never occur in Euro-American settings do, in fact, take place in Lebanese IVF clinics. For example, "fresh" sperm samples are used in sperm donation, without any kind of mandatory screening for HIV virus, hepatitis virus, and other sexually transmitted infections. Similarly, no mandatory genetic testing is performed with either donors or recipients. Hence, serious genetic diseases, such as cystic fibrosis, may be perpetuated within the Lebanese IVF population (Inhorn 2012). Furthermore, forms of donation that have been ethically banned in the United States and parts of Europe have been practiced in Lebanon. One such form is ooplasm donation—where the cytoplasm of a younger woman's oocytes is injected into an older woman's oocytes to improve their quality. If these oocytes are subsequently fertilized, transferred to the older woman's uterus, and lead to a successful IVF pregnancy, the child will be born with three types of DNA—one from the reproductively "elderly" mother, one from the father, and one from the young female ooplasm donor. Finally, there is grave potential for exploitation within the Lebanese IVF industry. For example, poor refugees or maids from Africa, Southeast Asia, or war-torn parts of the Middle East may be coerced into serving as egg donors and gestational surrogates because of the lure of payment. According to some Lebanese IVF physicians—both Muslim and Christian—these types of practices should not be occurring in the country, because they jeopardize the reproductive rights of women, as well as maternal and child health.

In this "anything goes" environment, Lebanon has now taken the former place of Italy as the "Wild West" of Mediterranean fertility treatment. Even Spain—the contemporary European hub of egg donation—does not allow surrogacy, whereas Lebanon does. And Israel, always at the cutting edge of ART developments, nonetheless maintains a strict regulatory environment, which is not found in its northern neighbor. Because of travel bans between the two countries, Lebanon and Israel have little in the way of reproductive scientific or technological exchange. Furthermore, Israel does not provide any kind of regulatory model for a neighboring country that it has invaded three times within thirty years, or at a rate of once every decade.

As of this writing, Lebanon and Iran are the only two Middle Eastern Muslim countries where third-party reproductive assistance is practiced. All other Muslim countries, including Egypt, continue to ban third-party donation and surrogacy, based on a moral injunction that is, at once, very strongly felt among most Sunni Muslims and also upheld in clinical practice among the Sunni Muslim countries. Italy, too, has become quite "Sunni"—banning all manner of third-party reproductive assistance and even embryo cryopreservation techniques that are widely practiced in the Sunni world. Although Sunni clerics were certainly not the inspiration for Italy's third-party ART ban, it is noteworthy that similar moral justifications have been used in both cases. As a result, Italy, once incredibly permissive, has become more restrictive than any Muslim country where ART is practiced. Such an irony—one that defies global "East-West" stereotypes—was clearly unanticipated when IVF was born in Europe more than thirty years ago.

From ART Bans to Reproductive "Tourism": Case Vignettes

Where do reproductive bans—some old, some new—leave patients who attempt to solve their infertility problems? Reproductive bans, whether applied by moral force or by law, never produce straightforward outcomes. We would argue that the Sunni ban on third-party reproductive assistance has "held" quite successfully for more than thirty years. For the vast majority of Sunni Muslims, the ban makes moral sense, and hence they are eager to uphold it. However, the lifting of this ban in two Shia-majority countries has had a marked effect. Namely, the strength of the Sunni ban is perceptibly weakening, as at least some Sunni Muslim IVF patients reconsider their own moral stances, especially regarding egg donation. Furthermore, Italian IVF patients—having gone from one "permissive" extreme to another "restrictive" one—have refused to abide by a law that they consider unfair and retrogressive. Italian IVF patients who have the means are traveling abroad for ART services. So are some Sunni Muslim patients who have decided to use third-party reproductive assistance "against the religion," by traveling to Lebanon, Iran, or countries beyond the Middle East.

Reproductive bans, we argue, produce "reproductive resistance." In the case of ARTs, such resistance is seen most clearly in cases of "reproductive tourism," or what is more neutrally being called "cross-border reproductive care."[19] In the final section of this chapter, we tell the stories of real people who have traveled across borders for reproductive care.[20] Through their stories, morality and pragmatism intersect, demonstrating the complexity of the "reproscape" in which infertile couples around the Mediterranean must make their reproductive decisions.

Dalia and Galal: From Egypt to the United States[21]

Dalia and Galal are an internationally sophisticated Egyptian couple who represent the upper crust of Egyptian society—wealthy elites who are able to purchase the fruits of globalization, including high-cost, high-tech medical services such as IVF. Dalia had married Galal four years before their first IVF attempt, knowing that Galal, her first cousin,[22] suffered from a surgically irreparable varicocele, or a cluster of dilated veins in his testicles causing him to have a very poor sperm count. Galal's infertility became known to his extended family when, after fathering one son in his first marriage, he was unable to impregnate his wife again. Galal eventually divorced his first wife and fell in love with his attractive cousin, Dalia. Dalia was also smitten with Galal, a kind, handsome, rich factory owner. However, Dalia's parents were deeply opposed to her marrying a man known to be infertile, even if he was her relative. Dalia recalled, "My mother got sick, crying all the time and making fights with me. She wanted to 'see my children.' My family made a lot of problems, but I loved him so I married him. When I married him, I thought maybe I won't be pregnant. This was something that made it a little easier; I accepted his infertility."

In part to escape family pressure and in part to seek medical advice, Dalia and Galal decided to immigrate to the United States, where Galal, an ex-military man, had once received basic training, and where Dalia now had a sister living in California. Once settled in Pasadena, they sought treatment for Galal's infertility and were told that, given his poor semen profile, they should undergo artificial insemination using donor semen from a sperm bank. Incredulous, Dalia and Galal explained to the American physician, "We are Muslims and this is forbidden." So he referred them to an Egyptian Muslim physician running his own Los Angeles (LA)-based IVF clinic. This was the first time either Dalia or Galal had ever heard of IVF. But once they talked with the Egyptian doctor, they were soon convinced that IVF was allowed within Islam as long as both sperm and eggs came from husband and wife.

Following their consultation with the Muslim doctor, as well as a second opinion from another LA-based, "religious" Lebanese Christian physician, Dalia and Galal decided to go ahead with one trial of IVF, which cost them $16,300 and which they paid for in a series of four installments. When the in vitro fertilization process produced extra embryos that were not to be transferred to Dalia's uterus, the IVF clinic staff gave Dalia and Galal three choices: freezing, destroying, or donating to another couple. As Dalia explained: "We said, 'Destroy! It is our religion.' If it's from the man and his wife, yes, it is okay [in Islam]. But to donate eggs or sperm, this is *haram* [sinful]!"

Galal added,

> There is a fatwa from Al-Azhar about this. If I give someone my sperm, this baby is going to take another [man's] name, and he's going to take [from him] some money, some inheritance, although he's not "from him." Maybe I give another woman my sperm and she gets a son, and another woman and she gets a daughter, and when they grow up, he marries his [half] sister. This [i.e., potential incest] is the main thing [problem].

Although Dalia and Galal acknowledged that laboratory mistakes resulting in "accidental" donation might still be made, even under the best of circumstances, they believed that they had avoided this eventuality by relying on a religiously vigilant, scrupulous, Middle Eastern–born Muslim physician to carry out the actual IVF procedure. However, they were concerned about the general moral decline of American IVF practices, including the frequent donation of sperm, ova, and embryos from third parties. In their view as religiously observant Sunni Muslims, such donation practices would inevitably lead to an immoral and genealogically bewildering "mixture of relations." Furthermore, they had heard that one American doctor made approximately twenty babies "from himself"[23]—probably in an attempt "to become successful and famous." Given the morally questionable nature of American IVF practices undertaken by American physicians, Dalia and Galal concluded that, in retrospect, it was better that their trial of IVF did not succeed in the United States. When Galal's real estate ventures in Orange County, California, also soured, they decided to return to Egypt. There, Dalia opened a successful children's clothing boutique in an affluent suburb of Cairo, where wealthy women clients could purchase the latest children's fashions imported by Dalia from the United States.

But, as expected, Dalia and Galal's return to Egypt also meant increased "family interference." Relatives on both sides of their family began urging them to go to doctors in Egypt, where "science is constantly advancing." However, Galal still maintained serious reservations about the ability of Egyptian doctors to carry out IVF with any hope of success. As Dalia explained, "My husband at first didn't want to do it in Egypt. He thought maybe some mistakes would be made. Plus, we heard a lot [of people] say that they make this in Egypt 'for commerce.'"

It wasn't until they read two news articles, one in the major daily newspaper *Al-Ahram* and the other in the news magazine *Nus id-Dunya*, that Dalia and Galal changed their opinion. The media were covering the advent of ICSI in Egypt, in which men such as Galal with serious male infertility problems could finally be helped to have a child. Dalia and Galal decided that ICSI might be the solution to their childlessness, and they proceeded to the clinics of two physicians offering this new technology. One made Dalia and Galal feel like "he was just in it for the money." So they chose another physician, who they perceived as both a good Muslim and a good doctor. Now, Dalia says,

> Galal is happy to be doing it in Egypt. After what we went through in the United States, we prefer to do it in Egypt—because they're Muslim here. And you must feel comfortable with the doctor. He must feel what you feel. He must not be doing it just for a job. He must like you to have babies. With [this doctor], he shows you his feelings. From the first time we came here, we felt this. He's not doing it just for the money. He pats you and says, "OK, it will be all right."

Dalia needed the doctor's reassurance after her first trial of ICSI was cancelled. After going to great lengths to obtain the hormonal medications necessary to stimulate her ovaries, including having friends and relatives bring the drugs by car and plane from Alexandria and Saudi Arabia, these agents did not succeed in producing an adequate number of ova for retrieval. As Dalia explained, "It costs your body and your feelings and your money. It's not easy. But my husband always supports me. You feel like you're desperate and after that, he says, 'We will try again.'"

When Dalia told the doctor that she did not think she could go through the emotional rollercoaster of another failed trial, he told her to remain hopeful, and this time he provided her with the hormonal medications from his own clinic supply. On their second try, the hormones worked to produce a substantial number of mature ova, and Dalia and Galal were therefore able to go forward with the ICSI procedure. Although ICSI is one of the most expensive assisted reproductive technologies available in Egypt, it cost Dalia and Galal only LE 10,000 ($2,940), or less than one-fifth of what it had cost them to undertake one trial of IVF in the United States.

Luckily for Dalia, she became the mother of a test-tube baby, a beautiful little girl named Deena, and later, a second ICSI son named Muhammad. As Dalia has explained, "Even if they have all these facilities now for IVF and ICSI, after everything, if God wants me to have a child I will, and if not, I won't." Clearly, Dalia is grateful that God has granted her permission to become the mother of two beloved, test-tube babies.

Chiara and Alessandro: From Italy to Spain to the United States[24]

Chiara and Alessandro are an Italian career couple, he an officer in the Italian police force and she a research geologist. This handsome couple had been trying to make a baby throughout their ten years of marriage, eventually turning to ARTs for help. In Rome, where all of the IVF clinics are private and expensive, Chiara and Alessandro undertook two ART cycles, each time without success. As a couple with so-called unexplained infertility,[25] Chiara and Alessandro were frustrated by the absence of a diagnosis, as well as the $16,000 they had spent on two failed procedures.

Chiara and Alessandro also felt stymied by Italy's restrictive legislation. Through research they conducted on the Internet, they realized that preimplantation genetic diagnosis (PGD) might allow them to understand the cause of their infertility. However, PGD was officially prohibited under Italy's Law 40. As Alessandro explained,

> It is not permitted. When you ask the reason for your infertility problems, the doctor just says, "This is something unknown. There is not

a medical reason at the moment. The science doesn't exist to find out the real reasons." But this is not true. We tried to do some research on the Internet, and we find that it is possible, by PGD, to find some of the factors behind this problem. In Italy, "unknown infertility" problems may have a reason.

In Italy, the physicians also told Alessandro that his sperm count was low and that the solution for him would be ICSI. After two failed ICSI trials, Alessandro and Chiara turned to Spain, the European "hub" of reproductive tourism. Despite a one-year wait, the couple managed to get an appointment at an IVF clinic in Barcelona, where an Italian female IVF physician had married a Spanish IVF doctor. In Barcelona, Chiara and Alessandro underwent one more ICSI cycle, again without success, but at a total price tag of $12,000.

"When we went home from Spain, she told me that maybe she did not want to do any more [embryo] transfers," Alessandro explained. "And I tried to convince her—to say that maybe the next time, if we search, we will find the main reason for the infertility. So I tried to make some research on the Internet, and that's where we tried to find [IVF clinic] sites in New York and at the famous research centers, like Yale, Harvard, and Berkeley universities."

Delighted to find an Italian IVF doctor at Yale, Alessandro sent an e-mail, which was answered directly and immediately. Alessandro and Chiara made an appointment, after being assured that PGD could be used in the United States to make a potential diagnosis of their infertility problem.

"It's not so easy to come here [to the United States], to speak another language, especially about medical symptoms," Alessandro explained. "And this [Italian] doctor suggested that we don't try to do more ICSI [cycles] without a firm diagnosis. He told us that it is maybe possible that [Chiara] could have a problem with her oocytes, but that we would have to try PGD to confirm this hypothesis."

In order to save money, Chiara and Alessandro were instructed to undertake the preliminary hormonal stimulation in Rome, before traveling to America. Their physician in Italy e-mailed the Yale Fertility Center, so that the timing of the oocyte harvesting would be precise upon the couple's arrival in the United States.

Settling into a hotel next door to the clinic, Chiara and Alessandro waited patiently for the results of their PGD diagnosis. As the doctor had surmised, Chiara suffered from poor oocyte quality. Although only thirty-two years of age, she had the "old oocytes" of a menopausal woman.

Alessandro explained:

[The doctor] suggested that we don't try to do any more ICSI cycles without donor eggs. Because without a donor, we were just basically wasting our money. So, for the first time, we learned that we needed to do ICSI with donor egg. So, we've been going along, at all of these different places, and we've actually been given the wrong information! This is very frustrating! If we'd had PGD in Italy, we could have discovered this a long time ago.

Chiara was particularly angry with the Italian IVF physician who told her—after her PGD diagnosis in the United States—that she should still use her own oocytes in another ICSI cycle. "After the PGD discovered my problem, in Italy, they continued to say to me, 'But you can try with your own oocytes!' Why would they say this to me? I do not know. This was very risky, because my oocytes, they have this genetic problem."

Angered by their treatment in Italy, the couple contemplated their options. They could try again in Spain, this time with donor eggs. That would have been the cheapest destination, given that clinics in Spain "import" poor women from all over South and Central America to donate their oocytes for very low fees. However, Chiara was uncomfortable with this choice. She explained:

In Spain, they give more human support [than in Italy], but the technical level is better in Italy. However, the laws are not as strict in Spain as they are in Italy, so I could do donor and PGD in Spain. The problem is, Spain is a big center for Europe. All the Europeans are coming to Spain, and especially to Barcelona, to receive donor eggs. The problem in Barcelona is that they put you on a waiting list, and maybe you may stay for one or two years before being called, even though you have to take the medicines in the meantime, just in case. Generally, they don't work with fresh oocytes, only cryopreserved ones.[26] And, even if there are eggs, for the most part, the donors are coming from South America. The clinics are bringing and paying them very, very low amounts, like $1,000. And me, I am blonde and white, so someone from Central America is going to look a little bit different from me. For a girl like me, to get a matching donor, there is going to be a long line. And, we don't know about the health of this donor. Having a healthy and sane donor is the most important thing.

Discouraged, Chiara checked into adoption. But this, too, seemed extremely difficult. "The worst problem in Italy is wanting to adopt," Chiara said.

There are not any Italian children to adopt, so the cost to adopt a child in Italy is very, very high. And if you want to adopt from overseas, the international procedures are very strict and it requires a very long time. They say adoption is easier than it is. In Italy, you have to be observed for twelve hours, and you have to have a room for the child. You cannot put other children in the same bedroom. You also have to stay in the same city to raise the child. But my husband changes cities every three to four years because of his work.

Using the last of their life savings and getting "a little help" from Chiara's parents, the couple made the difficult decision to undergo the $30,000 ICSI-donor egg cycle in the United States.[27] Although the costs were prohibitive and Alessandro had to ask for a special leave permit from his supervisor at work, the couple felt "forced" to pursue third-party reproductive assistance outside their home country. "Maybe if we can do this kind of treatment in Italy, it would be more comfortable for us," Alessandro suggested. "We had some logistical problems coming here. But because this is not permitted in Italy at all, we had to find another solution. We were *forced* to find a solution. So it is like forced travel."

Alessandro continued,

The Italian constitution says that Italy is a *nonreligious state.* But in fact, this is not true. Italian citizens must follow the Italian law, and the Italian law is affected by the association of Italian bishops, who said, "We must respect life." I'm a practicing Catholic, but I wish the Italian Church had a different position so that we could obtain this kind of thing. The official position is always "no." But if you speak face-to-face with some Italian priests, they view this [ART] as "helping nature."

During their fourth and final ICSI cycle in the United States, Chiara and Alessandro remained hopeful. With donor oocytes, the Yale doctor predicted that their chance of pregnancy could be as high as 60 percent. "Yes, we're glad we're here, with an Italian doctor, at Yale, and close to New York," Chiara stated. "We can even make a little 'holiday' while we do the medical treatment, so that we can try to relax and don't think about this problem all of the time. It has been a lot of effort, but we're full of hope."

At the end of their interview with the anthropologist, Alessandro joked, "Are you sure that no names are being used? Because if I go back to Italy, maybe they will handcuff me!" As a police officer, Alessandro was especially concerned about following the law of the land—even if he felt that the restrictive Italian ART law was unfair.

Upon their return to Italy, Chiara's and Alessandro's dreams of having a test-tube baby came to a sudden and tragic end. Alessandro resumed his high-intensity job as a police offer, but was soon killed in the line of duty. Alessandro was forty years old, leaving behind the thirty-two-year-old love of his life, but no children.

Hatem and Huda: From Syria to Lebanon[28]

Hatem and Huda decided to try their luck at IVF in a hospital-based clinic in Beirut, which catered to all of the religious sects found in multisectarian Lebanon. However, Hatem and Huda were not Lebanese, having traveled from rural Syria to Beirut in order to undergo a trial of IVF. Like most Syrian reproductive tourists, Hatem was convinced that Lebanese IVF clinics were superior to the fledgling clinics in neighboring Syria, a Middle Eastern nation-state that has long been isolated from, and even sanctioned by, the West. Thus, he had been bringing his wife to Beirut for IVF since 1997. Hatem had another reason for bringing Huda to Lebanon: There, they could access donor eggs, which were unavailable in the Sunni-dominant country of Syria, where third-party gamete donation is strictly prohibited.

Double first cousins (on both paternal and maternal sides) and married for seventeen years, Hatem and Huda clearly loved each other, despite the perplexing dilemma of her premature ovarian failure. Although Huda was only thirty-six at the time, she had entered menopause in her twenties, and required hormonal stimulation followed by IVF in order to achieve a pregnancy. After five unsuccessful trials of IVF, the IVF physicians in Beirut recommended egg donation as the most likely successful option. As Sunni Muslims, Hatem and Huda knew that egg donation was forbidden in their religion. Yet, as Hatem explained, they rationalized their use of donor eggs in a previous IVF cycle in the following way:

> As long as the donor agrees, then this would reduce the *haram* [forbiddenness] based on our religion. Because she, the donor, is in need of money, she gave nine to ten eggs, and the doctor divided the eggs between that couple and us. We took five, and that couple, who were recently married, took five. And I personally entered into the lab to make sure that *my* sperm were being used. It's okay because it's *my* sperm.

Indeed, Huda became pregnant with donor twins, a male and a female, in 1999. At six months and seventeen days of pregnancy, she began to miscarry, and Hatem rushed her to a hospital in Syria. As Hatem recounts, "They opened her stomach [by cesarean], and there were twins, who still lived for forty-eight hours. They had lung deficiency because they were little and not fully developed. The girl died twelve hours before the boy."

After this traumatic experience, Huda could no longer accept the idea of egg donation. According to Hatem, who spoke for Huda as she sat quietly in the room:

> She was tortured [during the pregnancy]. She stayed four months vomiting whatever she ate, and she lost weight—from 88 kilograms to 55 kilograms. And she was under a lot of stress because of our social environment in Syria. In our [farming] community, they stare at babies and see if they resemble the mother and father. We are not living in a city of 4–5 million. We are in a closed community of 15,000 people. And so, the first time, when we had twins, they did a blood test and everyone was surprised. Their blood group was AB, and it didn't match ours.[29] Now everyone will *really* examine the personal traits of this [donor] baby if we do it again. They will look at us suspiciously. Not the doctors; they keep everything confidential. But people in the community who might come to visit and look at us curiously.

For his part, Hatem is willing to accept donor eggs again and has already made inquiries about finding a willing Shia Muslim egg donor in Syria. On the day of our interview, we also spoke about the possibility of finding a willing donor within the Beirut IVF clinic. Hatem saw no other way to achieve parenthood, given that he loves his wife and refuses to divorce her. Although Hatem is an affluent farmer from a large family of twenty children (by one father and three co-wives), he continues to resist all forms of social pressure to divorce or marry polygynously. His commitment, he says, is based on his deep love for Huda. As he told me:

> Had I not loved her, I wouldn't have waited for seventeen years. I would have married another. By religious law, I can remarry, but I don't want to. She told me I should marry another woman, and she even offered or suggested that she would get me engaged, because we're already old. We've reached middle age without kids. We're living in a large family with six of my brothers, and they all have children. That's why she's feeling very depressed and very angry that she's alone without children, although she's always surrounded by children. But, of course, she keeps these feelings to herself.

> The love between us—I love her *a lot*. I was the one who considered going for IVF, for her sake. But we must keep it secret, because if my parents knew about us having an IVF child, the child would be marginalized and living a lonely life. So we keep everything secret, and we just mention to our families that she's receiving treatment.

As in so many IVF stories, Huda and Hatem were ultimately unsuccessful in their seventh attempted IVF trial. Huda's own eggs failed to mature under hormonal stimulation, and no egg donors were currently available at the clinic. Thus, Hatem and Huda returned home quietly to Syria, with little remaining hope of achieving parenthood, but with the love that had kept them together for nearly twenty years.

Conclusion

In this chapter, we have attempted to compare three Mediterranean countries, examining the evolving religious, legal, and cultural discourses surrounding ART, and particularly third-party reproductive assistance, in each country. ARTs themselves have evolved dramatically over the past three decades, and with this evolution, societies have responded in different ways. Some of these outcomes have been expected, while others have not. For example, few would have predicted that, by the new millennium, Iran and Lebanon would be on the cutting edge of ART development (and, in the case of Iran, a stem cell industry), whereas Italy, initially the Wild West of European ART, would become one of the most restrictive ART regimes in the world through pressures from the Vatican.

Sunni Egypt, meanwhile, has "held steady" over the past twenty-five years, allowing most forms of ART, with the exception of third-party reproductive assistance. This third-party reproductive ban in Egypt is upheld throughout the Sunni Muslim world, for it is based on religious discourses that are strongly felt and clinically upheld within the local moral worlds of Sunni IVF patients and practitioners. The story of the wealthy Egyptian couple, Dalia and Galal, is a case in point. Although they could have defied the reproductive ban through travel to any more "permissive" Euro-American setting, they chose to uphold the ban, even when they were given a choice to use donor sperm and to donate their embryos in the American IVF clinics they visited on their "quest for conception" (Inhorn 1994).

However, for many IVF patients faced with reproductive bans, the moral choices are not so easy. Indeed, reproductive bans have led to interesting outcomes, the main one being increased "reproflows" of IVF patients attempting to escape bans in their home countries. For couples like Chiara and Alessandro or Hatem and Huda, their so-called reproductive tourism to the United States and Lebanon, respectively, could be thought of as "reproductive exile" (Inhorn and

Patrizio 2009). In both cases, they felt severely restricted by their inability to obtain donor eggs within their home countries, and thus "forced" to travel abroad in order to attempt to conceive donor children within the context of long-term, loving marriages. In the case of Chiara and Alessandro, the outcome was truly tragic, for they were unable to bear witness to the fruits of their reproductive labor, which had involved multiple cross-border journeys and the expenditure of hundreds of thousands of dollars.

Italy—the country from which Chiara and Alessandro were escaping—is a particularly interesting example of the "strengthening" of a reproductive ban over time. Indeed, after nearly twenty-five years of open defiance by the Italian IVF community, the Vatican was finally able to assert its religious hegemony over clinical practice, through the imposition of recent anti-ART legislation. In terms of third-party reproductive assistance, Italy has become "more Sunni," justifying its third-party ban in ways very similar to Sunni Muslim discourse on the subject. However, Italy has also become much more restrictive than *any* Sunni Muslim country, in that it also bans cryopreservation, embryo disposal and research, PGD, and other ART technologies that are practiced relatively freely across the Muslim world. In this regard, Islamic attitudes toward reproductive technologies in general show greater tolerance than the Roman Catholic Church's disapproval of *all* reproductive technologies, ART included. As shown in this chapter, Italians are beginning to "fight back." Recent legislative challenges have highlighted the poor clinical outcomes among childless Italian couples, in a country where plummeting birth rates have also become a cause for national concern.

The same may be said of Lebanon, where postwar depopulation, particularly of the Christian population, has raised new concerns about politically sensitive demographic and gender imbalances in the country (Inhorn and Kobeissi 2007). The worrying decline of an already small (pop. 4 million) country has not been raised directly by the Lebanese government in its laissez-faire attitude toward ARTs. However, the resulting lack of any form of legislation or regulation of the local IVF industry may, in fact, stem from the felt need to "birth" new Lebanese citizens by any means possible. As a result, "anything goes" in Lebanese IVF clinics: Christian doctors provide Christian Lebanese sperm donors for Shia couples; Shia couples donate embryos to infertile Christian couples; Syrian egg donors are imported across the border by Lebanese Armenian infertile couples; American egg donors are flown to Beirut for egg harvesting and "donation" to infertile members of Hizbullah; poor Palestinian women donate their uteruses to wealthy Sunni couples who need a gestational surrogate; and Syrians, Egyptians, and couples from Arab Gulf countries travel to Lebanon during "summer holidays" to obtain donor gametes in IVF clinics there. Within Lebanon, gametes and embryos are being passed across sectarian, national, and racial boundaries in ways unprecedented in the Middle East, or the rest of the Muslim world, for that matter.

The very availability of multiple forms of third-party reproductive assistance in Lebanon (and Iran) has led to a concomitant weakening of the Sunni Muslim ban, as patients such as Hatem and Huda reconsider their own moral stances toward donor technologies. However, in the Sunni Muslim world, individual challenges to the reproductive ban occur in secret, as infertile couples travel across national borders in search of gametes prohibited to them by their religion. As of this writing, more direct challenges to the Sunni clerical authorities who have written antidonation fatwas have yet to occur. In this regard, the Sunni ban is quite "Catholic": one antidonation religious opinion initially issuing from Egypt has become the hegemonic authoritative discourse across the Sunni world. Even though there is no central authority in Islam, the Sunni ban on third-party reproductive assistance is strong and binding. It has the force of moral authority that the Vatican has hoped for all along, but has certainly failed to achieve with regard to reproductive technologies.[30]

Such varying ART outcomes suggest the need for three scholarly interventions: (1) careful scrutiny of ART history, most of which has yet to be written; (2) regional comparisons, which are rarely carried out; and (3) understanding of cultural, religious, and legal debates by scholars who are steeped in the languages and cultures of particular societies. As we have shown in this chapter, it is sometimes very important to undertake unlikely comparisons, for example, between a Sunni Muslim Middle Eastern country, a Catholic European country, and a country that is a combination of religious and cultural traditions. At a time in history when the so-called Christian and Muslim worlds are seen as fundamentally different and separate, we have to realize that they are, in fact, inextricably linked, with technologies, peoples, and ideas circulating and influencing one another in various ways. The Islamic world cannot be considered in isolation from the Christian world, a trope of incommensurability that has been too prominent in post-9/11 discourses. Our chapter provides one attempt to bridge this chasm, an intervention that is desperately needed as we enter the second decade of the new millennium.

Notes

1. We are using the term "ban" to mean legal or religious "restrictions" on the practice of third-party reproductive assistance. As authors, we are not intending to pass judgment on the morality or bioethics of such "bans" and "restrictions." Our chapter is meant to be descriptive rather than prescriptive. It is an expanded version of our article by the same title in *Reproductive BioMedicine Online* 21 (2010): 848–53.

2. A comprehensive global history of IVF has yet to be undertaken, as noted by Sarah Franklin (personal communication).

3. The quotations around terms such as "liberal," "restrictive," "progressive," and "traditional" are intended to signal our own understanding of the problematics of ART discourses; namely, it is truly difficult to find the correct "vocabulary" with which to describe ART policies around the world. As with "bans" and "restrictions," our use is intended to be descriptive rather than prescriptive. We are not professional bioethicists or policy makers, although all of us necessarily engage in these global discourses through our ART scholarship. The first author is a medical anthropologist and feminist technoscience scholar who has published extensively on infertility and ARTs in the Middle East. The second author is a professor of obstetrics and gynecology and ART clinician who has dual training in bioethics. The third author is also a professor of obstetrics and gynecology and ART clinician, who is one of the cofounders of the first IVF clinic in Egypt. He publishes extensively on Islamic bioethics and ARTs.

4. There are 18 officially recognized religious sects in Lebanon. Until 1948, Lebanon was also the home of a small population of mostly Beirut-based Jews, who generally left for the nation of Israel upon its founding.

5. This term was suggested by Wendy Chavkin, editor of *The Globalization of Motherhood.*

6. As noted by Iqbal and Noble (2009: 108), "A *fatwa* is a legal pronouncement made by a *mufti*, a scholar capable of issuing judgements on Islamic law (*sharia*). These are neither binding nor legally enforceable, but provide invaluable insight when gauging Islamic opinions on a given topic. Fatwas can be published in daily newspapers and periodicals or broadcast on radio or television."

7. This IVF clinic was founded by Gamal I. Serour.

8. See Bonaccorso 2008 for an anthropological study of Italian ART in practice.

9. During his term of office, Prime Minister Berlusconi shifted from pro-Vatican to anti-Vatican because of numerous scandals, including one involving prostitution, in which he was condemned by the Catholic bishops. We thank Thomas Eich for this insight.

10. The poignant documentary film, *Beautiful Sin,* by Costa Rican-American filmmaker Gabriela Quiroz examines the plight of infertile Costa Rican couples before and after the IVF ban in that country.

11. This was Pasquale Patrizio, who is originally from Naples, Italy.

12. We thank Prof. Carlo Flamigni for the most up-to-date information on the state of the Italian legislative amendments.

13. The Lebanese Catholic Maronites have a long and continuous association with the Roman Catholic Church, but have their own Lebanese patriarch, liturgy, and customs. The president of Lebanon is always Maronite.

14. The first author, Marcia C. Inhorn, and another author in this volume, Morgan Clarke. See Clarke and Inhorn (2011).

15. Unlike Sunni Muslims, Shia Muslims are encouraged to follow particular Shia clerics, who, themselves, are hierarchically ranked according to charisma and religious knowledge.

16. Both Clarke (2009) and Inhorn (2012) provide comprehensive overviews of Lebanon's Islamic debates on this subject. See also Clarke and Inhorn (2011).

17. Christian groups in Lebanon practice adoption; thus, there are Christian-run orphanages with children available to infertile couples. With the exception of Iran, most Muslim countries do not condone adoption, because legal adoption is clearly prohibited in the Islamic scriptures, including the Qur'an. Permanent fostering and guardianship, however, are encouraged.

18. The politics of organizing the necessary sectarian subcommittees to pass the bill is so daunting that it has yet to be undertaken; the political will and organizational finesse is simply not available at this time, as pointed out by Morgan Clarke (personal communication).

19. A special issue on "Cross-border Reproductive Care: Travelling for Conception and the Global ART Market," guest-edited by Zeynep Gürtin and Marcia C. Inhorn, appeared in *Reproductive BioMedicine Online* (November 2011).

20. All names are pseudonyms.

21. This story has been published in chapter 4, "Religion," in Inhorn (2003). It is based on a series of interviews carried out by the first author in Cairo in 1996. This couple has since then permanently settled in the U.S. They remain in contact with the first author.

22. Consanguinity, or cousin marriage, is a common and even preferred form of marriage across the Muslim world. See Inhorn (1996, 2012) and Inhorn et al. (2009) for detailed discussions.

23. In a famous case reported in the American media, an infertility doctor was discovered to have used his own sperm to impregnate patients whose husbands suffered from male infertility. His patients began to suspect this when many of their offspring resembled the physician rather than their own husbands. The doctor was eventually questioned by police authorities and admitted what he had done. He was tried and imprisoned for his medically unethical practices.

24. This story is based on an interview carried out by the first author in New Haven, CT, in 2008. The sad ending to the story was reported to the second author in summer 2009.

25. "Unexplained infertility" is an ambiguous category that is decreasing in prevalence with improvement in diagnosis, especially the advent of preimplantation genetic diagnosis (PGD).
26. Egg freezing is a relatively new technology with uncertain results. If possible, using "fresh" oocytes is preferable in a donor egg cycle.
27. U.S. prices, especially for donor oocytes and surrogates, are the highest in the world.
28. This story has been published in Inhorn (2007, 2012). It is based on an interview carried out by the first author in Beirut in 2003.
29. The premature infants required blood transfusions, which is why the parents' nonmatching blood types became a point of contention.
30. We thank Morgan Clarke for this important insight.

References

Benagiano, Giuseppe, and Luca Gianaroli. 2004. "The New Italian IVF Legislation." *Reproductive BioMedicine Online* 9: 117–25.

Birenbaum-Carmeli, Daphna, and Marcia C. Inhorn, eds. 2009. *Assisting Reproduction, Testing Genes: Global Encounters with New Biotechnologies*. New York: Berghahn.

Blyth, Eric, and Ruth Landau, eds. 2004. *Third Party Assisted Conception across Cultures: Social, Legal and Ethical Perspectives*. London: Jessica Kingsley.

———, eds. 2009. *Faith and Fertility: Attitudes towards Reproductive Practices in Different Religions from Ancient to Modern Times*. London: Jessica Kingsley.

Bonaccorso, Monica. 2008. *Conceiving Kinship: Assisted Conception, Procreation and Family in Southern Europe*. New York: Berghahn.

Clarke, Morgan. 2009. *Islam and New Kinship: Reproductive Technology and the Shariah in Lebanon*. New York: Berghahn.

Clarke, Morgan, and Marcia C. Inhorn. 2011. "Mutuality and Immediacy between *Marja'* and *Muqllid*: Evidence from Male IVF Patients in Shi'i Lebanon." *International Journal of Middle East Studies* 43(3): 409–27.

Deech, Ruth. 2003. "Reproductive Tourism in Europe: Infertility and Human Rights." *Global Governance* 9: 425–32.

Harvey, David. 1990. *The Condition of Postmodernity: An Enquiry into the Origins of Cultural Change*. Oxford: Oxford University Press.

Inhorn, Marcia C. 1994. *Quest for Conception: Gender, Infertility, and Egyptian Medical Traditions*. Philadelphia: University of Pennsylvania Press.

———. 1996. *Infertility and Patriarchy: The Cultural Politics of Gender and Family Life in Egypt*. Philadelphia: University of Pennsylvania Press.

———. 2003. *Local Babies, Global Science: Gender, Religion, and In Vitro Fertilization in Egypt*. New York: Routledge.

———. 2004. "Privacy, Privatization, and the Politics of Patronage: Ethnographic Challenges to Penetrating the Secret World of Middle Eastern, Hospital-based In Vitro Fertilization." *Social Science & Medicine* 59: 2095–108.

———. 2006. "'He Won't Be My Son': Middle Eastern Muslim Men's Discourses of Adoption and Gamete Donation." *Medical Anthropology Quarterly* 20: 94–120.

———. 2007. "Loving Your Infertile Muslim Spouse: Notes on the Globalization of IVF and Its Romantic Commitments in Sunni Egypt and Shia Lebanon." In *Love and Globalization: Transformations of Intimacy in the Global World*, ed. Mark Padilla, Jennifer S. Hirsch, Miguel Munoz-Laboy, Robert E. Sember, and Richard G. Parker. Nashville, TN: Vanderbilt University Press.

———. 2010. "'Assisted' Motherhood in Global Dubai: Reproductive Tourists and Their Helpers." In *The Globalization of Motherhood: Deconstructions and Reconstructions of Biology and Care*, ed. Wendy Chavkin and JaneMaree Maher. New York: Routledge.

———. 2012. *The New Arab Man: Emergent Masculinities, Technologies, and Islam in the Middle East*. Princeton, NJ: Princeton University Press.

Inhorn, Marcia C., and Loulou Kobeissi. 2007. "The Public Health Costs of War in Iraq: Lessons from Post-War Lebanon." *Journal of Social Affairs* 23:13–47.

Inhorn, Marcia C., Loulou Kobeissi, Antoine A. Abu-Musa, Johnny Awwad, Michael H. Fakih, Najwa Hmmoud, Antoine B. Hannoun, Da'ad Lakkis, and Zaher Nassar. 2009. "Male Infertility and Consanguinity in Lebanon: The Power of Ethnographic Epidemiology." In *Anthropology and Public Health: Bridging Differences in Culture and Society*, ed. Robert A. Hahn and Marcia C. Inhorn. New York: Oxford University Press.

Inhorn, Marcia C., and Pasquale Patrizio. 2009. "Rethinking Reproductive 'Tourism' as Reproductive 'Exile.'" *Fertility and Sterility* 92: 904–6.

Iqbal, Mohammad, and Ray Noble. 2009. "Islamic Identity and the Ethics of Assisted Reproduction." In *Faith and Fertility: Attitudes towards Reproductive Practices in Different Religions from Ancient to Modern Times*, ed. Eric Blyth and Ruth Landau. London: Jessica Kingsley.

Kahn, Susan Martha. 2000. *Reproducing Jews: A Cultural Account of Assisted Conception in Israel*. Durham, NC: Duke University Press.

Matorras, Roberto. 2005. "Reproductive Exile versus Reproductive Tourism." *Human Reproduction* 20: 35–71.

Meirow, Dror, and Joseph G. Schenker. 1997. "The Current Status of Sperm Donation in Assisted Reproduction Technology: Ethical and Legal Considerations." *Journal of Assisted Reproduction and Genetics* 14: 133–38.

Moosa, Ebrahim. 2003. "Human Cloning in Muslim Ethics." *Voices across Boundaries* (Fall): 23–26.

Nachtigall, Robert D., Gay Becker, Carrie Friese, Annaliese Butler, and Kristin MacDougall. 2005. "Parents' Conceptualization of Their Frozen Embryos Complicates the Disposition Decision." *Fertility and Sterility* 84: 431–34.

Nicholson, Roberto F., and Roberto E. Nicholson. 1994. "Assisted Reproduction in Latin America." *Journal of Assisted Reproduction and Genetics* 11: 438–44.

Richards, Jim. 2009. "A Roman Catholic Perspective on Fertility Issues: Objective Truths, Moral Absolutes and the Natural Law." In *Faith and Fertility: Attitudes towards Reproductive Practices in Different Religions from Ancient to Modern Times,* ed. Eric Blyth and Ruth Landau. London: Jessica Kingsley.

Roberts, Elizabeth F. S. 2009. "The Traffic between Women: Female Alliance and Familial Egg Donation in Ecuador." In *Assisting Reproduction, Testing Genes: Global Encounters with New Biotechnologies,* ed. Daphna Birenbaum-Carmeli and Marcia C. Inhorn. New York: Berghahn.

Rogozen-Soltar, Mikaela. 2007. "Al-Andalus in Andalusia: Negotiating Moorish History and Regional Identity in Southern Spain." *Anthropology Quarterly* 80: 863–86.

———. 2010. "Andalusian Encounters: Immigration, Islam, and Regional Identity in Southern Spain." PhD diss., University of Michigan.

Serour, Gamal I. 1996. "Bioethics in Reproductive Health: A Muslim's Perspective." *Middle East Fertility Society Journal* 1: 30–35.

———. 2008. "Islamic Perspectives in Human Reproduction." *Reproductive BioMedicine Online* 17 (suppl. 3): 34–38.

Serour, Gamal. I., and Bernard M. Dickens. 2001. "Assisted Reproduction Developments in the Islamic World." *International Journal of Gynecology & Obstetrics* 74: 187–93.

Traina, Cristina, Eugenia Georges, Marcia C. Inhorn, Susan Kahn, and Maura A. Ryan. 2008. "Compatible Contradictions: Religion and the Naturalization of Assisted Reproduction." In *Altering Nature—Volume II: Religion, Biotechnology, and Public Policy,* ed. B. Andrew Lustig, Baruch A. Brody, and Gerald P. McKenny. New York: Springer.

Washofsky, Mark. 2009. "Faith and Fertility in Reform Jewish Thought." In *Faith and Fertility: Attitudes towards Reproductive Practices in Different Religions from Ancient to Modern Time,* ed. Eric Blyth and Ruth Landau. London: Jessica Kingsley.

Weitzman, Gideon. 2009. "'Give Me Children or Else I Am Dead': Orthodox Jewish Perspectives on Fertility." In *Faith and Fertility: Attitudes towards Reproductive Practices in Different Religions from Ancient to Modern Times,* ed. Eric Blyth and Ruth Landau. London: Jessica Kingsley.

Chapter 9

ISLAMIC BIOETHICS AND
RELIGIOUS POLITICS IN LEBANON
ON HIZBULLAH AND ARTS

Morgan Clarke

Introduction

The supreme leader of the Islamic Republic of Iran, Ayatollah 'Ali al-Khamene'i, is politically a conservative, and indeed in the eyes of many, a highly repressive figure.[1] He is, however, most unwilling to restrict the use of advanced fertility treatments. Like a number of other Shia clerics, he does not prohibit the use of donor eggs or donor embryos, nor that of surrogacy arrangements; more unusually, he also finds no reason to prohibit the use of donor sperm (see this volume passim; Clarke 2007a). Secondly, within the wider Middle East it is only in predominantly Shia Iran and in Lebanon, which has a sizeable (Twelver) Shia community in which Iran has an important stake through the Lebanese Hizbullah, that donor gamete procedures and surrogacy arrangements can be undertaken (Inhorn et al., this volume). It has proved tempting to understand these seemingly related, but in fact distinct phenomena in terms of a contrast between "Sunni" and "Shia" religious opinion (see, e.g., Clarke 2009). Here I want to reinsert these instances—and "Islamic bioethics"[2] more generally—into their larger context, focusing on the example of Lebanon, where I carried out field research on the Islamic legal debates over in vitro fertilization (IVF) and related technologies, as well as their medical application, in 2003–2004. I worked primarily with Sunni and Shia Muslim religious specialists, but also interviewed medical specialists working in the fertility sector (see Clarke 2009); I have been back to Lebanon since (2007–2008), looking at sharia discourse more widely (see, e.g., Clarke 2010). Attention to the political, I will argue, may be a better guide to understanding medical ethics in Middle Eastern contexts than a narrow focus on the "religious."

In Lebanon's multiconfessional setting, medical ethics become, among other things, an arena for competition between religious authorities and traditions: some claim a privileged relationship to the "contemporary" (*mu'asir*), of which advanced biomedicine is an important component; to restrict its possibilities can appear retrograde. That is especially the case among Lebanon's Shia communities, where important social and political movements have emerged such as Hizbullah, for which a claim to what one might call an Islamic modernity is a defining feature (Deeb 2006). I would in fact prefer to call this project one of "contemporaneity": it is "keeping up with the times" (*muwakibat al-'asr*) rather than the radical break with tradition that modernity implies that is more often stressed (and see below). Nevertheless, the notion of "alternative modernities" (Gaonkar 2001) is both well enough established and flexible enough to allow a certain laxity in this regard. Islamic modernities are presented as morally superior to the hegemonic Western liberal paradigm; an "Islamic bioethics" would seem integral to the larger project; some hold Shia jurisprudence, in the hands of "contemporary" scholars at least, to be particularly well equipped.

Assisted reproduction is a particularly potent trope for such intercivilizational (and sectarian) comparisons, combining as it does the moral, more especially sexual morality, with the medical and scientific. The restriction (or otherwise) of certain procedures, paradigmatically those involving donor gametes, can of course, one should say, be read in various ways and from different perspectives.[3] What may be gratefully perceived as "open-minded" (*munfatih*) by a needy patient might be deemed dangerous for "society" or even "religion" by those without such a stake. Not to obstruct the therapeutic possibilities of medical science may seem admirably contemporary to some, while a needless concession to the prevailing materialism of the age to others. In the Lebanese context, opinions such as Khamene'i's on fertility treatment can be mobilized to argue for a Shia modernity, or for a critique of its pretensions.

I begin by sketching this Lebanese scene and presenting some examples of the mobilization of biomedical concerns and imagery by Hizbullah personalities in the public sphere. I go on, however, to probe a little more deeply into the structures of religious authority that underpin this project. In addition to thinking through Khamene'i's role in the Lebanese context, I bring in the further example of Lebanon's own Ayatollah Fadlallah, who died in the summer of 2010. Historically close to Hizbullah, Fadlallah was nevertheless a distinct figure with his own agenda, who styled himself as especially "contemporary." The relationship between such religious authorities as Fadlallah and Khamene'i and their lay Shia followers is not, in Lebanon at least, the bureaucratized, impersonal relation of authority between the rationalized state and its legal citizens that Weber (1978) proposed as the ideal type of modernity (Clarke 2010). Pronouncements by such authorities on medical ethical issues take the form of responses to personal, individual requests for guidance: that is, fatwas, expert "opinion," which may be informed by informal consultation with trusted associates with, in this case, medical expertise. These authorities are not specialists, except in the wider sense of being comprehensive scholars of Islamic law: in this context, "Islamic bioethics" has no separate existence as a discipline in its own right, and could indeed be regarded as a rather questionable category for just these reasons. This is not, then, an equivalent to the dedicated, interdisciplinary committees convened to inform professional medical and state policy, which have arguably been the fundamental driver for the new discipline of bioethics.[4] In this exact form, we should note, this constellation of authorities and practices is particular to these pious Shia communities in Lebanon: Khamene'i's role and the structures for the generation of regulation and legislation in Iran—nominally an Islamic state—are different again from the Lebanese case.

The reasons why there is no ban on donor procedures and surrogacy arrangements in Lebanon and Iran are thus very different, and turn not on "religion" per se, nor on how "contemporary" one or another religious authority might be, but on how their respective states are organized and laws and regulations are generated. If we wish to perceive clearly how medical ethical issues play out in Middle Eastern contexts, then we need to look beyond the rhetoric of religious discourse to the ways in which religious opinion and medical practice are related, articulated through varying regimes of religious and state legal authority (Brockopp and Eich 2008: 1). This has larger consequences: we will come to see that "Islamic bioeth-

ics"—and, more especially, contrasts such as those between Sunni
and Shia positions—may be as much a function of national and indeed international politics as of theology. Just as idealized Islamic
visions of modernity (or "contemporaneity") may differ from hegemonic Western liberal ones, so the articulation of those visions
with the institutions of modern Middle Eastern states takes multiple
forms. I thus conclude by arguing that a focus on religious opinion alone would in several respects be insufficient for an accurate
understanding of what an "Islamic bioethics" might be—either as
an independent phenomenon in its own right, or as the object of
Western academic and clinical desire. Religio-legal positions are situated within wider intellectual and political projects; the possibility
of isolating bioethics as a distinct institution and practice implies
a particular assembly of relations of authority; the topography of
such relations in the Middle East is more varied than is sometimes
implied.[5]

Assisted Reproduction and Religious Discourse in Lebanon

Lebanon has a vigorous fertility treatment sector and striking religious diversity: Catholic, Orthodox, and other visions of Christianity are set alongside Sunni, Shia, Druze, and other Muslim ethical
traditions. While such diversity is hardly unique to Lebanon, no one
community predominates demographically over the others. Further, much, although certainly not all, in Lebanese politics turns on
the mobilization of communitarian identities.[6] Religious discourse
and debate are thus conspicuous in the public sphere and very far
from homogeneous. The necessity of gaining a consensus between
these "communities," at least as mediated by professional politicians
and religious specialists, frequently paralyzes the legislature, and in
the case of proposed regulation of assisted reproductive technology
(ART) such a consensus has indeed proved elusive: Catholic and Orthodox Christian, as well as Sunni and Shia Muslim opinions in these
matters, are far from easily reconciled (Clarke 2009: 161–65; Inhorn
et al. this volume).[7] As one of the doctors most closely involved in
a proposed draft law told me, "Some ministers said that it might
contravene the positions of some of the religious communities, and
we would have to get their opinions. Eighteen committees!"—that
is, one for each of Lebanon's official religious communities (Clarke
2009: 163). These techniques thus remain (to the best of my knowl-

edge) unregulated, by parliament at least, and many controversial procedures such as those involving donor gametes are indeed available in Lebanon as they are not elsewhere in the Middle East, with the notable exception of Iran (see this volume passim).[8] Doctors by and large perceive ethical decisions as their patients' responsibility, although may themselves choose not to provide certain services on ethical grounds (Clarke 2009: 152–77; and see Inhorn 2004, 2006).

Regarding religious discourse on assisted reproduction, the most frequently drawn comparison, among medical practitioners at least, is between the "Christian," paradigmatically Catholic position—under which any medical intervention in human reproduction is, broadly speaking, forbidden—and the "Islamic" one, which allows such intervention as contraception and IVF, albeit within variously defined limits. As one pious Shia practitioner put it to me, she had seen "in the debates, the round tables that the Christians are behind here;" and as a Christian doctor had it, "There are two religions here. Islam allows everything—whatever medicine can do to help, you can do it. Christianity—they don't allow IVF, so how can they allow egg donation?!" As the latter indicates, this motif can be as much as an internal, Christian plea that the Church "keep up with the times" as an external critique: "Let the Church accept contraceptive pills and then we'll talk about IVF," as another doctor put it to me.

Between the Islamic communities, a similar subrivalry then plays out, where (Usuli Twelver) Shias may claim a greater rationality and flexibility in their school's jurisprudence, due to the greater prominence given to reason (*'aql*) as a source of religious law and to the relative freedom of their religious specialists to exercise their own independent reasoning (*ijtihad*) in interpreting scripture. This latter has become something of a cliché of this discourse of religious rivalry, although it should be heavily qualified: Sunni Salafism, whether in "modernist" guise as bequeathed from Muhammad 'Abduh or in the "conservative" Wahhabi tradition, equally privileges *ijtihad*.[9] But in Lebanon at least many religiously conscious Shias see their religion as excelling in a dialectic of "contemporaneity" versus being "stuck in the past."

A Pious Contemporary

Within the Shia clerical class itself, enthusiasm for scientific and medical advance is thus one of the ways in which religious specialists can portray themselves as especially able to "keep up with the times." In Shia Lebanon, the revolutionary strand of this tradition is represented preeminently by Hizbullah, whose leaders "emphasize the importance of techno-economic knowledge and scientific developments, which acquire legal justification in Shi'i society through the process of *ijtihad* ... essential to revolutionary progress," as reflected in the curriculum taught in Hizbullah's seminaries (Abisaab 2006: 233, 249). Dominating the Shia public sphere through its satellite television channel al-Manar and radio station al-Nur (91.9 FM), Hizbullah wages an insistent war on a stereotype of Shia "backwardness" (*takhalluf*) held by some sections of Lebanese society: the country's Shia communities were long stigmatized as impoverished peasant and manual workers. Medical institutions and concerns are central to the construction of what Deeb (2006) terms "an enchanted modern" and the underpinning of Hizbullah's popular appeal: the Hizbullah-linked Martyrs' Association runs a major hospital, Al-Rassoul al-'Azam, in Beirut's southern suburbs, for instance, where women are required to wear *hijab* (modest apparel, "the veil") (Deeb 2006: 115).[10]

One of the key battlegrounds for Shia reformists has been over the symbolically crucial arena of Ashura, the annual commemoration of the martyrdom of Imam Husayn at Karbala, Iraq, in 680 CE, emblematic of the Shia faith and a core resource for the mobilization of Shia identity as most powerfully demonstrated during the Iranian revolution itself (Fischer 1980). Nominally "traditional" practices of self-mortification during the commemorations, such as flagellation and the cutting of the head with razors or swords, have long been the target of reformists.[11] Ayatollah Khomeini was known to have been against such practices; his successor Khamene'i came out with an explicit authoritative statement of opinion (fatwa) in 1994 condemning them, which, mediated through Hizbullah, had a considerable effect on practice in Lebanon (Shaery-Eisenlohr 2008: 135–36). Khamene'i further encouraged the substitution of this bloodletting with blood donation,[12] which has become a highly popular alternative in Lebanon, also as presenting a preferable image to "non-Shi'ites to whom the images of Shi'ites covered in their own blood with swords drawn are hardly comprehensible, represent signs of exaggerated religiosity and backwardness and reinforce ... stereotypes;" the Hizbullah-run Islamic Health Committee collects the blood donated during Ashura and forwards it to various hospitals in Lebanon (Shaery-Eisenlohr 2008: 136, 247n27; see also Deeb 2005: 28).

A sermon given during Ashura in 2008[13] by Sayyid Hasan Nasrallah, secretary general of Hizbullah—a powerful orator and a revered figure for many in Lebanon and beyond for his leadership of "the resistance" (*al-muqawamah*) to Israeli occupation—gave another distinctively "contemporary" twist to the established theology of death and martyrdom central to the commemorations.[14] Nasrallah's theme was, as fitting, the "culture of Karbala" and what it tells us about the nobility of martyrdom; discussion of martyrdom would inevitably lead, he promised, to a discussion of the mundane world (*al-dunya*) and the next (*al-akhirah*), life and death. Death is not annihilation (*fana'*), but a door and a bridge to the next life. But there are different forms of death: one man dies on his bed, in his sleep; another in an accident; another killed as a martyr. Whatever the case, at the fatal moment the angel of death comes and pulls out (*tanza'*) the soul from the body. During this process, the person suffers from "the agonies of death" (*sakarat al-mawt*), a terrible pain. "Let me," Nasrallah elaborated, "explain this through a simple example, one all of you except save the very youngest perhaps will have experienced. When you go to the dentist to have a tooth removed or treated, the first thing the dentist has to do is take out the nerve. How much you suffer from the top of your body to the very bottom from this one little nerve! So how do you think it is when the soul has to be pulled out from all the cells and nerves, bone and muscle of the person?" But the martyr, however they died, enjoys a gentle, even a happy transfer to the next world. The biomedical imagery—the simile of the dentist stripping out the nerve from a troublesome molar, and the image of the angel of death stripping out the soul from every cell (*khaliyah*) of the body—was striking, a harnessing of scientific to religious imagery in the pursuit of political rhetoric that was in this instance, according to my clerical sources, all Nasrallah's own.

For a rather more homely example, take a radio program on Hizbullah's radio station al-Nur featuring Shaykh Muhammad Tawfiq al-Muqdad, Ayatollah Khamene'i's "general jurisprudential representative" (*al-wakil al-shar'i al-'amm*) in Lebanon, authorized to answer people's queries about the ayatollah's position on various points of the sharia and a passionate advocate of his take on fertility treatment.[15] Shaykh Muqdad has a twice-weekly show on al-Nur, "The Jurisprudence of the Sharia" (*Fiqh al-shari'a*), a comprehensive guide starting, as in the legal handbooks (*risalat*) that are its model, with matters of worship (*'ibadat*) and moving on to social transactions (*mu'amalat*).[16] Shaykh Muqdad instructs the audience in the relevant rulings, and they can phone in with questions. Here I wish to highlight the conversations that took place during one show (Wednesday, 2 April 2008) that continued the previous program's discussion of ritual pollution and ablution. Shaykh Muqdad moved onto the topic of the toilet functions (*takhalli*): evacuation of bodily waste is entirely natural—the Prophet, as every one else, did so— but should be performed in private; certain parts of the body (the *'awrah*) should never be revealed; not even other women should see a woman's *'awrah* for instance. "What about the ruling of the doctor [*hukm al-tabib*]?" asked the presenter, alluding to an important issue as regards the practice of fertility treatment: medical examinations and procedures may require the doctor to view and manipulate the private parts. "Yes," said the shaykh, "the female doctor can look at the *'awrah* of the woman.[17] ... Of course, female doctors are common: it is not allowed to go to a male doctor."

This broached a theme that was to dominate the rest of the show: while in an earlier age for a woman to submit to such an examination by a man would be a scandalous breach of Islamic morality, the overwhelming prestige of modern medical science has led many to cast such scruples aside. However, the more recent advent of female education and labor, vital to "Islamic modernists" for the putative creation of a properly gendered public sphere, has led to the widespread availability of female doctors at the service of Muslim women. The sexist, and in this context un-Islamic, prejudices of yesteryear endure, however, much to Shaykh Muqdad's disgust: "Regrettably," he continued, "some of our married sisters [i.e., in Islam] are taking things lightly in this matter. So many people are asking us, you know, 'By God, I don't have trust in women doctors! I want to go to a male doctor.' That's not on." A series of callers, however, only confirmed his analysis. One man called in to say that he needed to take his wife to the doctor, and, "she will have to undress, but the thing is, not all the women doctors are as good: it is just that in our region there aren't any." Shaykh Muqdad broke in, "That's not right sir, not right!" The presenter tried to moderate his flow, but the shaykh ploughed on: "To go to your current [male] doctor is not permissible. You can go to a second [female] doctor, a third. Just as there are faults with women doctors so there are with male doctors too." And the shaykh went on after the call: "I want to pause on this, because, as I said, we have seen so much of this in the office, people not trusting women doctors." He went on:

> This talk which I am hearing, that "By God, women doctors don't have skill and proficiency and perspicacity in their profession like men"—this is superstition, it's, I mean, heresy [*hartaqah*], with no basis in truth. It's not acceptable, not in the sharia, nor in custom nor

socially, not at all. The woman must go to one female doctor, then a second, third, fourth, fifth until her mind is at rest.

Further calls continued in a similar vein, however, until the shaykh ended the program with a final tirade: "What I am saying, some people are satisfied with it, some not; some accept it, some not. As for me, between God and myself I just want to absolve myself of my responsibility [as a scholar] before God by announcing what God's ruling is in this matter, and who accepts it accepts it, and who doesn't accept it. ... I say he's a sinner!"[18]

Personalized Authority

Islamic contemporaneity, politics, and medical ethics can be tightly bound up together, then. But as the final quote illustrates, while the opinions being promulgated may be contemporary, the relationships of religious authority they are based in are not, in Lebanon at least, the bureaucratized, rationalized "governmentality" of bourgeois modernity.[19] Muslims are responsible for their actions before God, but nonspecialists cannot be expected to know the details of the sharia, God's right "way" through life: they should consult an expert. It is the specialist scholar's duty to share that knowledge with them, knowledge that is developed by the very highest ranks of the Shia clerical hierarchy, the *mujtahids*, those recognized by their peers as capable of exercising their independent reasoning (*ijithad*) in interpreting scripture. Of these *mujtahids*, a limited number, by popular demand, serve as a *marja'* (pl. *maraji'*), a "source" of authoritative legal opinion. Scholars such as Shaykh Muqdad are then bound to transmit those opinions, in this case those of Ayatollah Khamene'i, to the masses.

Hizbullah supports the Iranian revolutionary model of an Islamic state, governed by Islamic laws and principles under the ultimate authority of a guardian religious scholar (*al-wali al-faqih*)—now Khamene'i, Khomeini's chosen successor—although it acknowledges that this is not a realistic ambition in multiconfessional Lebanon, for the present at least. The Islamization of the state would require a total realignment of relations of power and authority, a "work of purification"[20] that would render the domination of the bureaucratic state apparatus properly "Islamic." Without such a state, as in Lebanon, relations of religious authority must remain personal in form: thus Hizbullah also acknowledges Khamene'i as *marja'*,[21] although his claim to this, the highest rank in the Shia clerical hierarchy, is highly controversial. For many, he was elevated to the position as a purely political move beyond his scholarly achievements and over those of others (Clarke 2007a: 288–93), and Khamene'i is in fact, within Iran and clerical circles beyond Iran, not of special prominence as an expert scholar of religious law despite his political preeminence. In Lebanon, however, he does enjoy a considerable popular following, as heir to the tremendous prestige of Khomeini and as the foremost patron of Hizbullah.[22]

Such figures are not, within their field, specialists, as a fully developed Weberian vision of rationalized authority might require; as "bioethicists," for example—their orientation towards the sharia is comprehensive. Their pronouncements on such matters arise, just as the answers of Shaykh Muqdad, in response to queries of all sorts from the laity, nowadays in fact mostly received through electronic media, as e-mails to their websites (Clarke 2010). These are particular responses to particular questions and cases, often elliptical, sometimes frustratingly so: never programmatic, comprehensive presentations of "policy."

Khamene'i's fatwa on the use of donor sperm is a case in point. Asked by an anonymous petitioner, "Is it allowed to fertilize the wife of an infertile man with the sperm of a stranger [*rajul ajnabi*, i.e., a man other than her husband], by placing the sperm in her womb?" he replies:

> There is no legal obstacle [*la mani' shar'an*] to the fertilization of the woman with the sperm of a stranger in itself, but forbidden preliminary actions such as prohibited looking and touching and so on must be avoided. And in any case if a child is born in this way, it is not related to the husband, but to the producer of the sperm and to the woman, who is [here] the owner of the egg and the womb. (Khamene'i 2006: part 2: 70; and see Clarke 2007a and 2009: 117–25)

This is terse, to say the least—the expert spares the layperson the details of the debate, of which there are, one should say, a very great many (see, e.g., Sistani 2004 and Clarke 2009 passim). But we will surely struggle to perceive such a statement as an instance of "Islamic bioethics," if by that we mean a separate discipline instituted to generate an intellectual framework ultimately for the generation of policy recommendations.

Let me take up another example. One of my richest sources here is a selection of correspondence to the website of Lebanon's own Ayatollah Muhammad Husayn Fadlallah (d. 2010), kindly passed on to me by the staff of the ayatollah's offices. A controversial figure, Fadlallah was often thought of as Hizbullah's "spiritual guide." However, although instrumental in the education of a generation radicalized by civil war and Israeli occupation who flocked to the emergent Hizbullah in the 1980s, Fadlallah put considerable distance between himself and Hizbullah and its Iranian backers in later years, carving out a distinct role and abandoning an earlier commitment to Khomeini's "guardianship of the jurist" (Clarke 2010: 357–67; n.d.). He stood at the head of his own important network of charitable and educational institutions that includes a major hospital and several other clinics, as well as a radio station and a busy website (www.bayynat.org.lb).

Fadlallah was widely, if not universally, recognized as a *marja'*, popular in Lebanon and further afield (especially in the West) for his preeminently "contemporary" and "open-minded" views, particularly with regard to women's rights (Hamiyah 2004), views that also attracted a fair measure of controversy (Aziz 2001b). Central to this contemporary image was his enthusiastic embrace of science and technology, exemplified by his famously ready permission of research into human cloning, a totemic topic (Clarke 2009: 66, 85n21).[23] His opinions on assisted reproduction have, like those of Khamene'i, had a real impact on practice in Lebanon: he allowed the use of donor eggs, for instance, even if not donor sperm (Clarke 2009: 125–33; Clarke and Inhorn 2011; Inhorn 2006: 112).

One correspondent to the website[24] talks of looking for a "legal loophole" or "way out" (*manfadh shar'i*) of his dilemma: after divorcing his first wife, he married again and had a daughter, but then suffered from the atrophy of one of his testicles. He traveled abroad and married another woman, telling his new wife that he could no longer have children, which she accepted. But then they came to Lebanon and, "she began to suffer from the story of her husband not being capable of begetting children and started saying that she couldn't live without offspring." As Fadlallah did not, unlike Khamene'i, allow the use of donor sperm, the response is that:

> The problem will not be solved except by her divorce from you, and her marriage to someone else after the end of her *'idda* [waiting period before remarriage after divorce], and the placing of the sperm of that person in her womb by insemination, then her divorce from him, waiting until the delivery of the pregnancy so that her *'idda* from the second man is finished so that her marriage to you a second time is licit. And although the child will be of this second husband, its mother will be your wife, the source of the egg, and it will be a ward [*rabib*]

to you,[25] but will not inherit from you, nor you from it, but will be an heir to its father, the source of the sperm, and its mother, namely, your wife.[26]

These sorts of "ruses" (*hiyal shar'iyah*), a casuistry addressing individual dilemmas, are paralleled in the use of temporary marriages to facilitate egg donation or surrogacy arrangements and "milk kinship" (*rida'*) to institute forms of kinship relatedness subsequent to such procedures.[27] But again, they are clearly not designed as policy recommendations to shape the regulation of medical practice, even if Fadlallah was famously ready to engage with medical audiences (e.g., Fadlallah 1995).[28]

Genre Trouble

The preceding should, I feel, force us to think carefully about what is sometimes a little too loosely referred to as "Islamic bioethics" or "Islamic medical ethics." This latter is more, I would argue, an object of academic desire than a distinct reality. At its very most basic—as an answer to a question of the form "Is X allowed in Y?" where X stands for a controversial medical procedure such as, for instance, abortion, and Y for a religious or cultural tradition, as for example "Islam"— that desire is readily satisfied in what is most commonly labeled "the jurisprudence of medicine" (*fiqh al-tibb*): not a separate discipline in its own right but a subgenre of Islamic legal discourse, albeit a rapidly burgeoning one. This is of course a very crude, and inadequate, characterization of what bioethics has become as an academic and practical discipline (as indeed it is also of Islamic jurisprudence).

It also very obviously represents an appeal for an impossible simplicity in its address: what is this "Islam" and where is it to be found? Who speaks for it? That is not to say that to ask such questions would be merely naïve: we will need answers to them if suitable policies are to be evolved; and the need for policy, clinical or state legal, was after all, by some lights, the fundamental driver for the formation of an institutionalized bioethics in its original American forms.[29] Farouk Mahmoud (this volume) is right to urge those who pretend to some expertise in this area to recognize and respond to that need. But the problem is that we can so readily obtain such answers, and in quantity: one can, for one thing, simply send an e-mail to a recognized scholar—and there are a very great many.

Further, there are a multiplicity of genres of Islamic legal expression (Clarke 2009: 67–68; Hamdy 2008: 84), and we should be careful that we are comparing like with like. Specialists express their thoughts and opinions on such matters in a variety of settings, from informal consultations held sitting against the wall on the floor of mosques, over the telephone, or between court sessions to blog postings, newspaper articles, and book-length monographs. For the social scientist all of this material is of interest; but the more policy oriented should beware: one wants unambiguously authoritative statements from recognized authorities—technically, fatwas, for which read "expert opinion," not "law"—and deciding what is and is not to be considered as such, let alone which are of genuine significance, poses its own problems (Clarke 2010; Tappan, this volume).[30]

To develop the point, it has become conventional in our field to distinguish the "Sunni" and "Shia position" on assisted reproduction (as admittedly I myself have done repeatedly): a Sunni consensus allows procedures involving just a husband and (one) wife and forbids those involving third parties as in some sense akin to adultery (*zina*); Shia authorities are varied in their opinions, but frequently allow donor procedures, especially those involving eggs and embryos. It is precisely this simplicity that practical considerations demand; and, I should say, this characterization is broadly correct on the evidence we have (see this volume passim). But, besides its unfortunate sectarian overtones, it conceals something important: a varied terrain of religious and state authority. One can find any and every permutation of opinion among the innumerable multiplicity of voices within "Sunni Islam," which includes more than a billion Muslims and a very considerable proportion of the World Wide Web's domains. On a recent trip to Lebanon, for instance, I was chatting about my research with a Sunni sharia court judge, a distinguished and respected scholar. To my surprise, he told me that he himself found the use of donor sperm unexceptionable, akin to "adoption," that is, in its Islamic form where a child does not take the name of the adopting father (Clarke 2009: 72–74). This is diametrically opposed to the public "consensus." But he is not alone in standing apart: Al Azhar University in Cairo bubbles with opinions allowing surrogacy; distinguished authorities see no problem with exploiting Islam's permission of polygyny to allow a man to use the eggs of one wife to fertilize the womb of another; Syrian Shaykh al-Buti finds the likening of third-party donation to adultery "fantastic" and admits himself forced to find other means to ban it (Clarke 2009: 104, 106–7, 113nn30–31, 114n45).

This vast domain of opinion and debate notwithstanding, an "official" opinion has nevertheless emerged, official enough to be reflected in a uniform ban, parliamentary or clinical, on the practice of third-party donor procedures and surrogacy arrangements throughout the Sunni-majority Middle East (see Inhorn et al., this volume). Two factors need to be considered here: the different patterns of religious authority prevailing and national politics. Emblematic of the Ottoman regime, state muftis (issuers of fatwas) are a now common feature in these countries postindependence (Masud et al. 1996: 27). Such state-sponsored figures are frequently perceived to have been suborned by their political masters.[31] In the case of medical regulation, however, a close relation between practitioners, the religious establishment, and the state as in Egypt will no doubt be more effective at establishing and policing such standards than the much more differentiated and informal situation in Lebanon, for instance.[32]

More significant still is the emergence of specialized committees established specifically to overcome what may be perceived as a dangerously confused multiplicity of opinion through the issuing of collectively agreed fatwas (Masud et al. 1996: 27–28; Eich 2008): most influential have been those instituted by the Muslim World League at Mecca and the Organization of the Islamic Conference in Jeddah. Here consensus is actively sought; and, one might suggest, the more conservative opinion would seem almost inevitable to emerge as the compromise.[33]

Further, where Egyptian state mufti Shaykh 'Ali Jad al-Haqq Jad al-Haqq's (1997[1980]) influential fatwa on IVF was still framed, somewhat artificially no doubt, as a response to a series of questions from a medical practitioner in the classic mold, the output of these committees is impersonal and more bureaucratic in form: a numbered series of points and prescriptions (see, e.g., Clarke 2009: 100–101). As Eich (this volume) points out, these committee prescriptions are not, in his term, "retrospective," addressing real, individual dilemmas, but rather look forward to the potential consequences of, in this instance, new medical technologies. This looks much more like an attempt at regulation, albeit in this case from without the state: certainly more like the production of a bioethics committee. These committee publications, if still termed fatwas, nominally emerge from a very different institutional base than those of the Shia *maraji'* considered above: more modern perhaps, in Weberian terms, even if less "contemporary" in the terms of public perception in Lebanon.[34]

A putative academic "Islamic bioethics" would thus subsume a number of subtly different genres of Islamic discourse subject to different regimes of religious authority and thus politics: orthodoxy is above all else a relationship of power (Asad 1986). We should both learn to see patterns of opinion in this domain of Islamic jurisprudence as tied to particular styles and projects ("contemporary" ones, for instance) and not to be blind to the great swathes of opinion that do not become constituted as authoritative. But more important still are the ways in which Islamic precepts are translated into coercive patterns of regulation, state, legal, or otherwise. If one wishes to undertake a donor egg procedure in the Middle East, one must travel to Lebanon or Iran (Inhorn et al., this volume). But that possibility exists for very different reasons. Lebanon has no regulation to prevent the practice because of a legislature whose politics frequently turn on religious identity, a diversity of religious traditions accompanied by a rhetoric of mutual respect, and the lack of agreement between and even within those traditions concerning the ethics of assisted reproduction. Strongly independent practitioners within an almost entirely private medical sector are free to take their own line, and frequently leave ethical decisions to their patients; Shia opinions permitting egg donation are situated within that particular context.

Iran, on the other hand, has not only state-sponsored regulation but also state-supported fertility clinics and research facilities. As Saniei (this volume) documents, these are encouraged in the pursuit of a nationalist agenda: to make Iran a leading site of biomedical research, in this case regarding human embryonic stem cells and with the blessing of the supreme leader, Ayatollah Khamene'i. And as Garmaroudi Naef and Tremayne (this volume) describe, donor embryo and egg treatments have been permitted in Iranian state law following clerical consultation in committee, noteworthy in itself, given my discussion of personalized religious authority above. But the use of donor sperm has not, despite Khamene'i's permission. It is the machinery of the state, even if it is a nominally "Islamic" state, that counts: we should not overread the formal importance of Khamene'i's fatwa, even if it may, in practice, give cover to such procedures, illegal or not (Abbasi-Shavazi et al. 2008). Majority Shia Bahrain, on the other hand, forbids donor procedures altogether (Inhorn, personal comment).

The "Sunni ban" on third-party donation also plays out differently in various national contexts. As Gürtin (this volume) describes, in

Turkey this "restriction" is neither presented as "Islamic"—in keeping with the state's strictly secular positioning—nor indeed as restrictive: Turkey is portrayed, on the contrary, as less restrictive and more progressive than most European contexts, with regard to embryo transfer numbers for example. The prohibition on donor procedures is rather a matter of "culture." We will struggle to read these various contrasts in terms of "religion" alone.

Conclusion

The search for Muslim medical ethics leads readily to the discourse of Islamic religious specialists. But it cannot stop there: such discourse is enmeshed in broader projects and relations of power and authority. Those projects and relations do not necessarily match up with those of globalized biomedical or liberal legal and academic institutions, nor are they homogeneous. To be blind to that would be to fail to see much else clearly—the contrasts between and within Sunni and Shia contexts, for instance. This is not just to make a sociological point, although a focus on such issues is illuminating in that regard, as I hope I have shown. These layers of religious and political authority matter.

States, even if imagined as religious communities, like to set themselves apart, through law as well as borders. Indeed the barriers erected by regulation seem the more solid: people circulate more easily than ethical possibilities in this domain. Infertility patients frequently have to move between different regulatory regimes, styled as "religious" or otherwise, to obtain the services they desire, often with the co-operation of their medical advisors and a wink from society.[35] We cannot understand this in terms of theology alone. Students of Islamic bioethics, whether academics or believers, would do well to embrace the exigencies of international and national as well as religious politics: networks need to be wired up correctly.

Let me end with a pertinent—if tangentially and bizarrely so—example of what happens when they are not. *New Yorker* staff writer George Packer (2006: 109), in his admirable account of America's involvement in Iraq culminating in the invasion of 2003, has a fascinating anecdote regarding the support certain factions of the US administration gave to Iraq's Shia, then still suffering under Saddam Hussein's regime, as recounted by one administration official, a religious Jew in Packer's characterization:

He and his wife had difficulty conceiving a child, and he approached his rabbi to ask if advanced fertility treatments fell within the rules of Orthodox Judaism. The rabbi gave his blessing. But the official wanted to know his reasoning, and the rabbi explained it. When the official went to the Middle East during the Iraq War, he found a Shiite cleric and put the same question to him. Not only did the official get the same answer; the theological reasoning was exactly the same too. Eureka! The experience clinched his belief that the Shia and the Jews, oppressed minorities in the region, could do business, and that traditional Iraqi Shiism (as opposed to the theocratic, totalitarian kind that had taken Iran captive) could lead the way to reorienting the Arab world toward America and Israel.

While the theological parallels may indeed be stimulating,[36] the political analysis was at right angles to reality—with, as Packer goes on to describe in all its terrible detail, the most disastrous of consequences.

Acknowledgments

I owe a great debt of thanks to all those who have helped me in my researches in Lebanon and beyond, far too many to thank individually here. Many thanks are also due to all my colleagues in the workshop at Yale that led to this volume, both for their excellent company and for the rich discussions that have informed the rewriting of this chapter, and to all those who helped in bringing the workshop and this volume to fruition. I must also thank Judith Scheele, who patiently read the chapter in several of its versions, and our anonymous reviewers. None of the above is in any way responsible for anything erroneous or infelicitous here.

Notes

1. At the time of writing, his future, and that of the institution itself, is uncertain following the mass protests against his rule in Iran subsequent to the 2009 presidential elections.
2. The term has academic currency: see the references cited in the note below.
3. Some might argue that even to perceive religious legal positions as more or less restrictive is to adopt a particular and not necessarily helpful perspective, too closely allied to Western liberal preoccupations. But Muslims and Christians in Lebanon do talk in such ways (if not necessarily in those exact words), in the context of fertility treatment at

least—as well they might. "Restrictive" and "unrestrictive" are, I should say, my attempt at reasonably neutral terms of analysis, preferable to "(il)liberal," "conservative," or even "permissive."

4. E.g., the Hastings Center and the Kennedy Institute of Ethics in the U.S. See Jonsen (1998: ix–xi, 20–24, 26–27) and Reich (1994). This is not, incidentally, to deny the importance of religious institutions, and theology, in the development of bioethics in the U.S., for instance (Jonsen 1998: 24–26, 34–64; Jonsen, a pioneer in the field, was himself a Jesuit priest), but to point to the new institutional settings in which they were deployed. Such committees are also, I should say, to be found in the Middle East and Muslim world (Atighetchi 2007: 15–18, 25; Eich 2008; and see below).

5. For a brief discussion of Arabic and Persian renderings of "(Islamic) bioethics," see Sachedina (2009: 17–18). Shanawani and Khalil found 497 references to "Islamic," "Muslim," or "Arab bioethics" in English-language medical literature, primarily with an applied interest in frameworks for ethical compliance (2008: 214–15). Vardit Rispler-Chaim, in her pioneering work in Islamic studies on "Islamic medical ethics" found good cause to concentrate on Islamic legal literature (fatwas in particular) (1993: 3), as have others (Brockopp and Eich 2008: 5), including myself (Clarke 2009). Atighetchi, in his compendium of material on "Islamic bioethics," stresses the need to examine biomedical (and state legal) discourse as well (2007: 13). Brockopp and Eich, in their invaluable collection on "Muslim medical ethics," adopt a more sophisticated approach, wanting to integrate material on the responses of patients, doctors, and religious scholars in order to describe both normative discourse and its diverse applications (2008: ix, 1). Given the varied and contested nature of the relationship between norm and individual practice, they thus prefer the term "Muslim medical ethics" (elsewhere "Muslim bioethics") over "Islamic" (2008: 2, 5). My aim here is less to refine our descriptive terms, or indeed demolish a straw man (as one reviewer suspected), than to consider what an emergent "Islamic bioethics" might entail sociologically. For a serious attempt to rethink what it might entail intellectually, see Sachedina (2009).

6. Lebanese politics can most certainly not be reduced to "sectarianism," and Lebanese people's identities are neither necessarily nor essentially confessional. We are nevertheless especially interested in religious discourse and mobilization here.

7. This is a particular instance. Another recently proposed law on mandatory testing of marrying couples for genetically transmitted diseases was passed and is in effect, for example.

8. Regulation need not be by parliamentary legislation alone, of course. Another important factor is the strongly independent and entrepreneurial nature of the Lebanese medical sector, as elsewhere in the Lebanese economy and by contrast with many other countries within the wider Middle East.

9. Although neither tradition has any official sway among Lebanon's Sunni establishment, and the Sunni family law courts are bound to follow the Hanafi school of their Ottoman predecessors, which is most unfriendly towards *ijtihad.*

10. The hospital was built in 1988 by the Iranian Martyrs' Association around a mosque and serves Hizbullah's interests still more directly: at election time patients and staff are reportedly ferried to and from polling stations (Harik 2006: 275).

11. Such as renowned Lebanese Shia scholar Sayyid Muhsin al-Amin (d. 1952) (Mervin 2000: 229–74). See Deeb (2006: 129–64) for reformist visions of Ashura in contemporary Lebanon. There are many in Lebanon who nevertheless prefer to stick to the "authentic" form (Shaery-Eisenlohr 2008: 119–38).

12. Khamene'i's fatwa collection, *Ajwibat al-istifta'at,* widely available in a number of editions in Lebanon, has a section devoted to "religious occasions" that includes a number of fatwas condemning self-mortification, but without mention of the encouragement of blood donation cited by Shaery-Eisenlohr (Khamene'i 2006: part 2: 120–26).

13. On the ninth night (17 January 2008).

14. Nasrallah's nightly sermons during the commemorations attract a massive television audience, although he almost never appears in public, the risk of assassination being too great. He rather appears on a big screen in a huge auditorium in the southern suburbs; the sermon is simultaneously broadcast on al-Manar, Hezbollah's television station; I work from a DVD copy. The sermon lasted for about an hour in all; I radically summarize it here.

15. Shaykh Muqdad has himself contributed a number of articles on this and related topics for the Hizbullah magazine and positively relishes the challenging nature of some of these positions. In an interview with me in 2008, he noted with satisfaction "His [Khamene'i's] fatwa on cloning [allowing it], that gave rise to an uproar [*thawrah*]." There is, he told me, a book especially devoted to Khamene'i's meetings with doctors to answer their ethical questions, published in Farsi, which Shaykh Muqdad had gone to the effort of translating into Arabic; the manuscript was destroyed along with his old offices in the 2006 war with Israel.

16. Then on its second run through. My rendition throughout is not verbatim, but communicates the substance, and I hope something of the style, of the exchanges.

17. In our (2008) interview regarding Ayatollah Khamene'i's position on IVF, Shaykh Muqdad noted that the issue of the *'awrah* was not a problem in IVF treatment, "because the doctor looks at the inside of the *'awrah* and not the outside—the external form [*al-shakl al-khariji*] is what's forbidden." Cf. Tremayne (this volume).

18. Note then that it is not that the religious authorities' opinions are always followed: far from it. Likewise, not everyone is going to use donor sperm just because Khamene'i allows it (Clarke 2009: 169–71). We

should also note that such an insistence on gendered medical treatment is not necessarily helpful in practice, as Mahmoud (this volume) points out.

19. I am presenting in abbreviated form an argument I have made in more detail elsewhere (Clarke 2010). For the Weberian tradition, it is precisely through the depersonalization, routinization, and rationalization of relations of authority that the modern state emerges. Here, the "contemporary" is presented as not necessarily so. "Governmentality" is Foucault's (1991) expression.

20. To invoke Latour's (1993) characterization of the liberal Western modernity project. Where Western modernities, in Latour's analysis, pursue an untenable isolation of domains deemed proper to "religion," "science," and "politics," this Islamist work of purification acknowledges, indeed vehemently affirms their interpenetration, supposing the equally elusive possibility, indeed necessity, of a social and political domain purged of human moral failing, governed by Islamic precepts, and harnessing science and technology to that right purpose.

21. Not, that is, I think I am right in saying, that one has to take Khamene'i as *marja'* to be a member of Hizbullah, nor that all members or supporters do. Rather, that is the exemplary position and there is considerable pressure to conform to it.

22. And thus his opinions on assisted reproduction seem to be more relevant in Lebanon than they are in Iran (compare e.g. Inhorn 2006 and Clarke 2009 with Garmaroudi Naef and Tremayne, this volume). Khamene'i's frequently repressive attempts to mold Iran's religious classes and institutions to his political will are placing traditional models of religious pedagogy and authority there under almost irresistible pressure (Khalaji 2006). Conversely, the lack of such state-sponsored projects in Lebanon notwithstanding, not every religiously committed Shia there acknowledges the traditional authority of these "sources of imitation" (*maraji' al-taqlid*): as in Iran (Chehabi 2006: 300–301), there are no doubt many who find such "imitation" an outmoded notion in itself.

23. I have written more fully on Fadlallah's "contemporary" approach to jurisprudence elsewhere (Clarke 2010, n.d.).

24. Petition no. 70,324 in the office's archives.

25. This has consequences for marriage prohibitions and thus domestic intimacy: see Clarke (2007b, 2009: 42, 121).

26. As reported in practice in Iran by Soraya Tremayne (2009). See my reference to similar fatwas by Iranian Ayatollah Makarim al-Shirazi, for instance (Clarke 2009: 145n23).

27. As I have documented elsewhere (Clarke 2007b). See also Tremayne 2009 on such practices in Iran.

28. Responses to medical innovation do of course require specialist knowledge, and for such a figure this is generally obtained through personal contacts. For example, Fadlallah issued a fatwa in response to a query

from a widow, ruling that female (self-)masturbation is not prohibited—a characteristic fusion of women's rights, scientism, and sexuality emblematic of "contemporaneity" that attracted controversy and notoriety (Aziz 2001b: 210–11). His reasoning here is that it is not equivalent to male masturbation, no "seed" being ejaculated. This position was adopted after taking medical advice, and I was fortunate enough to talk to one of the doctors who gave that advice. "Fadlallah is a friend," he told me. "He calls and asks questions. Once he rang about the woman's orgasm. A woman, who had lost her husband, and didn't want to commit adultery, had asked if masturbation renders the fast void, like for men. That is, does it produce *janabah* [major ritual pollution]—woman have this in menstruation, but what about vaginal sexual secretion? I told him no, it's like sweating, a transudate, it has no gamete" (Clarke 2009: 147n35).

29. See the note above.
30. As Tappan (this volume) powerfully argues following Sachedina (2009), the reductive format of a fatwa hardly constitutes an ethics of medical practice, even if in many clinical contexts it is taken as sufficient for one. Of course, as Houot (this volume) shows, Islamic religious specialists are not blind to the broader ethical dimensions of jurisprudential opinions either.
31. As was the case regarding Egyptian mufti Tantawi and Ibn Baz of Saudi Arabia's fatwas on American military involvement in the first Gulf War, for instance (Haddad 1996).
32. Lebanon does have a Mufti of the Republic, but he speaks only for Lebanon's Sunnis.
33. Witness the changing position of the Muslim World League's council as regards the transfer of gametes within polygynous marriages (Clarke 2009: 106–7). A similar dynamic might also obtain in the nominally more individualized context of the Shia scholars we have been considering: such major figures need a sizeable staff through which access to them is mediated and who may themselves exercise some form of discretion over which of their master's words are to be foregrounded.
34. Again, the actual institutional framework of a *marja'*'s staff and offices may not in practice be so very different: but it is certainly portrayed as so. There have, I should say, been proposals to reform the institution of the *marja'* along similarly "modern" lines (Aziz 2001a).
35. See, e.g., Inhorn et al. and Gürtin, this volume.
36. See, e.g., Kahn 2000.

References

Abbasi-Shavazi, Mohammad Jalal, Marcia C. Inhorn, Hajiieh Bibi Razeghi-Nasrabad, and Ghasem Toloo. 2008. "The 'Iranian ART Revolution': Infertility, Assisted Reproductive Technology, and Third-Party Donation in the Islamic Republic of Iran." *Journal of Middle East Women's Studies* 4(2): 1–28.

Abisaab, Rula. 2006. "The Cleric as Organic Intellectual: Revolutionary Shi'ism in the Lebanese *Hawza*s." In *Distant Relations: Iran and Lebanon in the Last 500 years*, ed. Houchang Chehabi. London: Centre for Lebanese Studies, in association with I. B. Tauris.

Asad, Talal. 1986. *The Idea of an Anthropology of Islam* (occasional paper). Washington, DC: Center for Contemporary Arab Studies, Georgetown University.

Atighetchi, Dariusch. 2007. *Islamic Bioethics: Problems and Perspectives.* Dordrecht: Springer.

Aziz, Talib. 2001a. "Baqir al-Sadr's Quest for the *Marja'iya.*" In *The Most Learned of the Shi'a: The Institution of the* Marja' Taqlid, ed. Linda Walbridge. Oxford: Oxford University Press.

———. 2001b. "Fadlallah and the Remaking of the *Marja'iya.*" In *The Most Learned of the Shi'a: The Institution of the* Marja' Taqlid, ed. Linda Walbridge. Oxford: Oxford University Press.

Brockopp, Jonathan, and Thomas Eich, eds. 2008. *Muslim Medical Ethics: From Theory to Practice.* Columbia: University of South Carolina Press.

Chehabi, Houchang. 2006. "Iran and Lebanon after Khomeini." In *Distant Relations: Iran and Lebanon in the Last 500 years*, ed. Houchang Chehabi. London: Centre for Lebanese Studies, in association with I. B. Tauris.

Clarke, Morgan. 2007a. "Children of the Revolution: Ayatollah Khamene'i's 'Liberal' Views on *In Vitro* Fertilisation." *British Journal of Middle Eastern Studies* 34(3): 287–303.

———. 2007b. "The Modernity of Milk Kinship." *Social Anthropology* 15(3): 1–18.

———. 2009. *Islam and New Kinship: Reproductive Technology and the Shariah in Lebanon.* New York: Berghahn.

———. 2010. "Neo-calligraphy: Religious Authority and Media Technology in Contemporary Shiite Islam." *Comparative Studies in Society and History* 52(2): 351–83.

———. No date. "*Marja'iyyat* Beirut: Contemporaneity and Tradition in the *Hawza* of Ayatollah Muhammad Husayn Fadlallah." In *Religious Authority in Shi'ite Islam: Knowledge and Authority in the Hawza*, ed. Robert Gleave (forthcoming).

Clarke, Morgan, and Marcia C. Inhorn. 2011. "Mutuality and Immediacy Between *Marja'* and *Muqallid:* Evidence from Male In Vitro Fertilization Patients in Shi'i Lebanon." *International Journal of Middle East Studies* 43(3): 409–27.

Deeb, Lara. 2005. "Living Ashura in Lebanon: Mourning Transformed to Sacrifice." *Comparative Studies of South Asia, Africa and the Middle East* 25(1): 22–37.

———. 2006. *An Enchanted Modern: Gender and Public Piety in Shi'i Lebanon.* Princeton, NJ: Princeton University Press.

Eich, Thomas. 2008. "Decision-making Processes among Contemporary *'Ulama'*: Islamic Embryology and the Discussion of Frozen Embryos." In *Muslim Medical Ethics: From Theory to Practice,* ed. Jonathan Brockopp and Thomas Eich. Columbia: University of South Carolina Press.

Fadlallah, Muhammad Husayn. 1995. "Al-tibb wa-l-din." Unpublished manuscript of lecture given at the Sharq al-Awsat Hospital, 9 September, Beirut.

Fischer, Michael. 1980. *Iran: From Religious Dispute to Revolution.* Cambridge, MA: Harvard University Press.

Foucault, Michel. 1991. "Governmentality." In *The Foucault Effect: Studies in Governmentality,* ed. Graham Burchell, Colin Gordon, and Peter Miller. Chicago: University of Chicago Press.

Gaonkar, Dilip, ed. 2001. *Alternative Modernities.* Durham, NC: Duke University Press.

Haddad, Yvonne. 1996. "Operation Desert Storm and the War of Fatwas." In *Islamic Legal Interpretation: Muftis and Their Fatwas,* ed. Muḥammad K. Masud, Brinkley Messick, and David Powers. Cambridge, MA: Harvard University Press.

Hamdy, Sherine. 2008. "Islamic Legal Ethics in Egypt's Organ Transplant Debate." In *Muslim Medical Ethics: From Theory to Practice,* ed. Jonathan Brockopp and Thomas Eich. Columbia: University of South Carolina Press.

Hamiyah, Siham. 2004. *Al-mar'ah fi-l-fikr al-falsafi al-ijtima'i al-islami: Dirasah fi fikr al-Sayyid Muhammad Husayn Fadl Allah.* Beirut: Dar al-Malak.

Harik, Judith. 2006. "Hizballah's Public and Social Services and Iran." In *Distant Relations: Iran and Lebanon in the Last 500 Years,* ed. Houchang Chehabi. London: Centre for Lebanese Studies, in association with I. B. Tauris.

Inhorn, Marcia C. 2004. "Middle Eastern Masculinities in the Age of New Reproductive Technologies: Male Infertility and Stigma in Egypt and Lebanon." *Medical Anthropology Quarterly* 18(2): 162–82.

———. 2006. "'He Won't Be My Son': Middle Eastern Muslim Men's Discourses of Adoption and Gamete Donation." *Medical Anthropology Quarterly* 20(1): 94–120.

Jad al-Haqq, 'Ali Jad al-Haqq. 1997 [1980]. "*Al-talqih al-sina'i fi-l-islam.*" In *Al-fatawa al-islamiyah,* ed. Ministry of Religious Endowments 9, no. 2. Cairo: Dar al-Ifta' al-Misriyah, 3213–28.

Jonsen, Albert. 1998. *The Birth of Bioethics.* New York: Oxford University Press.

Kahn, Susan Martha. 2000. *Reproducing Jews: A Cultural Account of Assisted Conception in Israel.* Durham, NC: Duke University Press.

Khalaji, Mehdi. 2006. *The Last Marja': Sistani and the End of Traditional Religious Authority in Shiism* (Policy Focus 59). Washington, DC: Washington Institute for Near East Policy.

Khamene'i, 'Ali al-. 2006. *Ajwibat al-istifta'at: Al-'ibadat wa-l-mu'amalat.* Beirut: al-Dar al-Islamiyah.

Latour, Bruno. 1993. *We Have Never Been Modern*, trans. C. Porter. Cambridge, MA: Harvard University Press.

Masud, Muhammad K., Brinkley Messick, and David Powers. 1996. "Muftis, Fatwas and Islamic Legal Interpretation." In *Islamic Legal Interpretation: Muftis and Their Fatwas*, ed. Muhammad K. Masud, Brinkley Messick and David Powers. Cambridge: Harvard University Press.

Mervin, Sabrina. 2000. *Un réformisme chiite: Ulémas et lettrés du Jabal 'Âmil (actuel Liban-Sud) de la fin de l'Empire ottoman à l'indépendance du Liban*. Paris: Karthala.

Packer, George. 2006. *The Assassins' Gate: America in Iraq*. London: Faber and Faber.

Reich, Warren. 1994. "The Word 'Bioethics': Its Birth and the Legacies of Those Who Shaped It." *Kennedy Institute of Ethics Journal* 4(4): 319–35.

Rispler-Chaim, Vardit. 1993. *Islamic Medical Ethics in the Twentieth Century*. Leiden: Brill.

Sachedina, Abdulaziz. 2009. *Islamic Biomedical Ethics: Principles and Applications*. Oxford: Oxford University Press.

Shaery-Eisenlohr, Roschanack. 2008. *Shi'ite Lebanon: Transnational Religion and the Making of Religious Identities*. New York: Columbia University Press.

Shanawani, Hasan, and Mohammad Hassan Khalil. 2008. "Reporting on 'Islamic Bioethics' in the Medical Literature: Where Are the Experts?" In *Muslim Medical Ethics: From Theory to Practice*, ed. Jonathan Brockopp and Thomas Eich. Columbia: University of South Carolina Press.

Sistani, Muhammad Rida al-. 2004. *Wasa'il al-injab al-sina'iyah*. Beirut: Dar al-Mu'arrikh al-'Arabi.

Tremayne, Soraya. 2009. "Law, Ethics and Donor Technologies in Shia Iran." In *Assisting Reproduction, Testing Genes: Global Encounters with New Biotechnologies*, ed. Daphna Birenbaum-Carmeli and Marcia C. Inhorn. New York and Oxford: Berghahn.

Weber, Max. 1978. *Economy and Society: An Outline of Interpretative Sociology*, ed. Guenther Roth and Claus Wittich, trans. Ephraim Fischoff et al. Berkeley: University of California Press.

Chapter 10

Assisted Reproduction in Secular Turkey

Regulation, Rhetoric, and the Role of Religion

Zeynep B. Gürtin

Introduction[1]

In vitro fertilization (IVF) technology—or *tüp bebek* (literally "tube-baby") as it is ubiquitously known—has become one of the most arresting hallmarks of contemporary Turkish society. Ever present in popular media coverage, from celebrity endorsements on daytime television shows to cutting-edge news items on the front pages of daily broadsheets, *tüp bebek* stories regularly pique the national interest and have wide appeal for an emphatically "child-loving" population. With access strictly limited to married couples using their own gametes, assisted reproductive technologies (ARTs) are presented and perceived as modern medicine's (*modern tıp*) efficacious "cure" for the personal, familial, and social tragedy of childlessness.

According to the records of the Ministry of Health, which is responsible for the licensing and registration of ART practice, there are currently 112 IVF centers operating in Turkey.[2] Although many of these are concentrated in the large urban centers of Istanbul, Ankara, and Izmir, clinics offering ARTs have opened throughout the country, extending as far as Diyarbakır in the East, and Trabzon on

the Black Sea coast. The locally welcomed establishment and successful operation of IVF clinics in what are often seen as the most
traditional and conservative (*tutucu* or *muhafazakâr*) areas of the
country is a testament to the widespread desirability of high-tech
fertility treatments, and is interpreted by ART practitioners and the
popular media as an indication of progressing social mores, as well
as national scientific advancement.

Aside from the cultural aptitude of these technologies, the introduction of two funded treatment cycles for all eligible couples
by the state and social security institutions in 2005 and 2006 has
been crucial to the rapid expansion and accelerated growth of this
sector.[3] By 2007, the number of IVF clinics had increased by almost
50 percent,[4] and the number of IVF treatment cycles had doubled.[5]
Indeed, Professor Bülent Tıraş, the president of the Turkish Society
for Obstetrics and Gynecology, estimated that in order to properly
meet demand, IVF numbers would need to rise from the current
40,000 to around 150,000 cycles per year.[6] Some newspaper reports
even spoke of up to "2 million women waiting for *tüp bebek*"[7] across
the nation.

In this chapter, I draw on ethnographic fieldwork conducted in
Turkey since 2006, including formal interviews with Turkey's ART
"experts," and analysis of regulatory materials, legal documents, religious rulings, and assorted popular media coverage, to reflect on
the role that Islam plays (or does not play) in the legislation, discourse, and social practice of ARTs in Turkey. As a staunchly secular
nation with a Muslim population,[8] as well as a country with great
regional variation and enormous socioeconomic divisions, Turkey
often presents paradoxes and hybrids for researchers. Depending on
where the analytic gaze is directed, there are very different stories
that could be told about "Turkish" ARTs, such as the harmony between secular legislation and religious opinion; high efficacy and
successful clinical application; continuing fears and taboos over
"mixing" and donation; or the fast-expanding Cypriot market providing donor gametes for Turkish couples. Shifting the gaze from
one view to another, I examine the assumptions that accompany
different representations, and the political stakes involved in assert-
ing certain frames over others.

I begin the chapter with a detailed ethnographic description of
the atmosphere and events surrounding an international ART conference held in Turkey in 2006. This commentary introduces the
use of the terms "secular," "religious," "restricted," or "progressive"
as rhetorical devices in competing characterizations (which pertain

to Turkey more broadly, as well as to ART practice), and the ways in which they are mobilized by different actors. I then look in detail at the multiple and mixed manifestations of both Islam and secularism, of restrictions and their absence, of progressiveness and conservatism in Turkish ART legislation, its practice and the moral arbitration of Turkish patients. I suggest that hybrid entities such as these cannot be easily understood through explanatory frameworks based on dualities, and instead attempt to elucidate their complexities.

Commentary on a Conference

In April 2006, the second international Science and Moral Philosophy (Ethics) of Assisted Human Reproduction Conference[9] was held in Istanbul, assembling around four hundred international clinicians, embryologists, scientists, ethicists, theologians, and social scientists to discuss the philosophical, legal, and social issues arising from developments in assisted reproduction. The scientific organizing committee for the conference included senior Turkish ART practitioners, as well as Professor Robert Edwards, the pioneer of IVF and chief editor of the scientific journal *Reproductive BioMedicine Online*.

The occurrence of this meeting generated enthusiastic media coverage within Turkey, with various representatives of the ART, academic, and religious communities expressing honor and pride that such a "topical" (*güncel*) and "prestigious" (*prestijli*) conference was to be held in "our country." A popular current affairs discussion program, *Siyaset Meydanı,* aired live in the preceding days, invited members of the conference organizing committee and "the most important" international speakers for a preliminary discussion that was accessible to the wider population. In front of a large and varied studio audience, comprised of successful IVF families professing personal gratitude and involuntarily childless couples eager to benefit from technological advances, the experts—both Turkish and foreign—answered questions and engaged in friendly debates. The program, with its overwhelmingly positive perspectives on IVF, preimplantation genetic diagnosis (PGD), savior siblings, and even "cloning," generated much interest from viewers and lasted for over three hours, much to the surprise of flagging international participants. Robert Edwards in particular was welcomed enthusiastically as "the world-famous scientist and father of *tüp bebek*," and treated as a hero and celebrity. Thanked for "his gifts to science and humanity," Edwards was questioned not only on the history and development of IVF, but also on how he, as an octogenarian, maintained his health and vigor.

The program's host, Ali Kırca, mentioned that the conference had been relocated to Istanbul from Rome on account of "difficulties encountered there, the displeasure of the new Pope regarding these matters and resistance from the Catholic Church," and contrasted this with the honor and warmth with which Turkey "opened its heart and its doors" to this very important and socially significant meeting. He argued, "it would not be an exaggeration to state that the whole of humanity awaits with interest the outcomes of the conference discussions that will lead the way for governments and states to create new legislative structures." Although the meeting attracted very little international media attention, within the national media coverage it was celebrated as a source of pride, and portrayed as proof of both social progress, which made ARTs widely acceptable and debatable within Turkey, and of scientific progress, which included Turkish practitioners at the forefront of a global ART community.

The opening address of the conference was delivered by Professor Mehmet Aydın, a theologian and minister of state with a special interest in cultural and religious issues. His high-profile appearance (albeit delayed and fleeting) was further indication of the national prestige and importance accorded to the meeting, and could be read as the stamp of government approval. During the next two days, there were presentations by renowned "experts" in the field of ARTs from various parts of the world, including, for example, Anand Kumar from India, Mohammed Aboulghar from Egypt, and Yuri Verlinsky from the United States. A large portion of the program, however—a third to be exact—was set aside for Turkish presenters, including scientists, clinicians, and senior academics representing a range of disciplines. As well as two of Turkey's most distinguished ART practitioners, Semra Kahraman and Timur Gürgan, contributions were made by Saim Yeprem, professor of theology and member of the Higher Council of the Presidency of Religious Affairs; eminent philosopher Ionna Kuçuradi; and Yasemin Oğuz, bioethicist and founding member of the Turkish Bioethics Association. The wide variety of topics covered by these Turkish presenters ranged from an analysis of the impact of ARTs on families and society to theological views on the embryo, from questions of professional ethics to regulatory considerations in ARTs.

In an informal conversation over lunch, a Turkish delegate conveyed to me his satisfaction and pleasure at the level of Turkish participation at this meeting, which he evaluated as an ongoing and necessary endeavor to "open Turkey up to the outside." As we ate our lavish buffet lunches on the top floor of the luxury hotel housing the meeting, he added, "There are sometimes misapprehensions about Turkey from abroad, so we need to take responsibility for introducing our country and displaying our *çağdaş*[10] (modern) way of life to outsiders!" For him, this conference provided a great opportunity, not only to represent Turkish ARTs as rapidly advancing and "competing on a global stage," but also to represent Turkey as a modern, secular nation whose progressive characteristics set it apart from its Islamic neighbors. I observed in agreement, as waiters in white uniforms offered wine to delegates engaged in animated English conversations, that save for the minarets punctuating the Bosphorus vista, we might indeed have been in any European metropolis. This indeterminacy of Turkey's identity and affiliation, or what Keyder has referred to as an "ambivalence between inclusion and exclusion" (2006: 72) vis-à-vis its relationship to Europe, had, I suspected, been occupying my lunch companion (and many of the other Turkish delegates), since the somewhat tense discussion that had taken place that morning.

Earlier in the day, Berna Arda, a professor of medical ethics and deontology at the Ankara University School of Medicine, had delivered a paper entitled, "The Importance of Secularism in Medical Ethics: The Turkish Example." During the presentation she argued, "The principle of secularism is essential for scientific practice. Science is an area that requires openness to change itself as well as transforming other things and is independent of belief," (2007: 24) and referenced Turkey as a prototype whose "easily recognized secular legislative basis" for ARTs should be taken as exemplary of good regulation (Arda 2007: 27). Arda provided details of Turkish legislation pertaining to reproduction, as well as details of historical developments that, she argued, rendered Turkey "a unique example in the Islamic world as a democratic, secular, and social state" (Arda 2007: 25). However, following her paper, Belgian bioethicist Guido Pennings questioned Arda's characterization of Turkey's ART legislation as "secular": "I am slightly confused. You are presenting Turkey as a secular society combined with the fact that a lot of restrictions are included in the legislation on assisted reproduction, such as prohibiting the use of donor gametes. It made me wonder how they justify these restrictions if they do not refer to religious reasons? Why do they restrict assisted reproductive treatments to married couples?" Pennings thus asserted an alternative characterization, whereby he drew attention to Turkish "restrictions" on ART practice, and implied that these were based on religious (read Islamic) principles.

This debate—over the competing portrayals of Turkish ART legislation as secular or Islamic—dominated the rest of the discussion period, eliciting input from several Turkish delegates who found Pennings's comments to be a frustrating example of the "misapprehensions about Turkey" referenced by my lunch companion. Such perceptions, particularly those reiterating the role of Islam, were experienced by some Turks as Orientalist attempts to exclude Turkey from Europe by ideologically containing it within the Muslim Middle East. While some respondents appealed to a liberal law on abortion[11] as evidence of Turkey's secular approach to reproductive medicine, or to comparisons with other secular countries such as Germany to defend and illustrate a nation's right to impose moral prohibitions that need not be religiously grounded, Arda introduced a distinction between "religious reasons" and "cultural values" to clarify her position. She stated, "I believe that the Family Planning Law and all legislations on assisted reproductive treatment have secular character in Turkey. Restrictions on treatment to married couples is *not only* based on religious reasons, it is *also* based on cultural, social, and traditional values" (my emphasis). According to this secular discourse, "religion" alone was an unacceptable causal explanation for legislation, whereas "culture" provided a legitimate frame of reference. The point was advanced by Timur Gürgan, who differentiated the dogma of religious ruling from democratic processes, since the latter simply respected "the needs and preference of the majority of the people" (i.e., culture).

The (internal) rhetoric of secularism, modernity, and progress that accompany the proud national coverage of Turkish ARTs had been challenged in this international arena, with a competing view (from the outside) of Turkish ARTs as restrictive, conservative, and guided by religion. Thus, Turkish respondents opposed not only Pennings's definition of their regulations as "restrictive," but also of the charge that the "restrictions" pertained to "religious reasons." Fought over the symbolic territory of the practice of assisted reproduction, the contested characterizations of Turkey's ART legislation as "restrictive" or not, "secular" or "based on religion," were interpreted by all as a broader comment on Turkey's identity and its international position. Responding to the incongruity of internal and external definitions, and aware of the high stakes of such symbolic disagreements, Gürgan added, "I think we should give more information to our European friends to make them understand the Turkish practice of assisted reproduction treatment."

Contested Characterizations

ARTs in Turkey are regulated by the Assisted Reproduction Treatment Centers Directorate, under the Ministry of Health, in accordance with the Statute on Assisted Reproduction Treatment Centers (ÜYTEM).[12] This statute is a comprehensive piece of legislation that provides definitions, makes provisions for the practical regulation of assisted reproduction practice, and details prohibitions (*yasaklar*) as well as all the necessary requirements (including building and physical environment specifications, equipment, materials, and personnel) for clinics to obtain an ART practice license.

The statute provides at its outset a definition of "Assisted Reproduction Treatments" as:

> Procedures, accepted as treatment methods by modern medicine, which involve assisting the fertilization of *the prospective mother's egg* with *her husband's sperm* in various ways, enabling them to fertilize outside of the body when necessary, and transferring the gametes or the embryo back to the *prospective mother's* genital organs. (Item 4f, my emphasis)

This definition is extremely important, not just semantically or symbolically, but for its actual regulatory implication. By referring to the "prospective mother" and her "husband" (rather than to a socially or relationally indeterminate "man" and "woman"), the statute places the marital unit as legally central and clinically indispensable for ART practice. Moreover, by providing this as a definition of ARTs (rather than more explicitly as a definition of their legal application) it collapses the distinction between what is scientifically possible and what is socially acceptable.

The exclusivity of treatment provision to married couples, using their own gametes, is reiterated at the start of Section Five, entitled "Prohibitions":

> The use of the egg and sperm or the embryo of applicants undergoing ART for any other purpose, or in the treatment of other applicants, or the use of those [sperm, eggs, or embryos] obtained from anyone other than the applicants in the treatment of the applicants, or the storage, use, transfer, and sale [of sperm, eggs, or embryos] for any

sort of purpose falling outside the definitions of this legislation, are prohibited. (Item 17)

Thus, while assisted reproduction globally has been associated with the "creation of family *types* that would not otherwise have existed" (Fasouliotis and Schenker 1999: 26, my emphasis), including gay and lesbian families, single mothers by choice, and myriad families formed through third-party reproductive assistance, within Turkey the uses of these technologies have been curtailed to help the reproduction of traditional family types (thought to be) impeded by medical problems. These parameters designate ARTs a simulacrum of "natural" heteronormative procreation and accordingly limit its potential outcomes.

However, although the statute is very specific with regard to who may access ARTs (and whose gametes they may use)—amounting to what Pennings called "a lot of restrictions"—it is rather "unrestrictive" regarding the clinical application of permitted technologies. There is no direct discussion of the status of the embryo, no mention of PGD or PGD with human leukocyte antigen (HLA) typing (i.e., savior siblings), and no reference to the application of selective fetal reduction (often used in cases of high-order multiples). Moreover, where specific prohibitions relating to clinical practice are mentioned, such as regarding the transfer of more than three embryos, these prohibitions are effectively negated by the inclusion of caveats that enable practitioners to exercise expertise and to make transfer decisions dependent upon "age factor, embryo quality, or similar medical imperatives" (Section 5, item 17). Although some contingencies not mentioned in the ÜYTEM statute are covered by other legislation,[13] the situation is nevertheless one of relative freedom, enabling a high degree of professional discretion to ART practitioners.

As a result, reflexive Turkish practitioners are generally happy with the nature of their ART regulation. Moreover, they credit this "lack of restrictions" (as it was described to me in several interviews) as having a beneficial impact on clinical practice and success rates, and as giving them an "edge" in comparison with European providers. Erol Tavmergen, part of the clinical team responsible for Turkey's first IVF baby, explains why he thinks Turkish IVF is so successful and ultimately "more advantageous" (*daha avantajlı*):

> In some countries there are very strict regulations. And these often have a negative impact on pregnancy rates. For example, some countries only allow single embryo transfer, others limit it to two. In some countries there are difficulties choosing the best embryos since regu-

lations require this choice to be made just a day after fertilization. In Turkey, we do not have such restrictions. And this has a positive impact on pregnancy rates. ... Because of these reasons, *tüp bebek* in Turkey is more advantageous than in many other places in the world.[14]

Indeed, although there is considerable variability between the outcomes of different institutions, the better Turkish clinics fare extremely well in global comparisons. Bahçeci Clinic in Istanbul, for example, which provides quality assurance via JCI accreditation and ISO standards,[15] advertises on its website, "While average success rates in America for 2006 were 38 percent, ours are 48 percent,"[16] and others claim figures that are even higher. In another explicit comparison, a senior practitioner contrasts the "meaningless," "restricted," or "nonsensical" legislation in some European countries with the "delicate balance" achieved by Turkish regulation:

> In terms of clinical practice, whatever is practiced abroad in respectable clinics, the exact same thing is "reproduced" here in Turkey. ... But we don't have meaningless legislation. In many locations abroad, it is much more restricted (*sıkıntılı*). In England, for example, there is a specific number of embryos you must transfer; Italy has restrictions, for example, you can only freeze eggs not embryos; Austrian patients are escaping across the border to Prague to avoid their nonsensical (*abuk sabuk*) legislations. There needs to be a balance: patients' chances must be optimized, but it cannot be left uncontrolled either. There should be a "delicate balance." I think it is regulated well in Turkey.[17]

His English-peppered analysis is an apt illustration of how progressiveness and restrictiveness can be variously mapped on different locations, depending on what is identified as a "restriction." This account positions Turkey as "ahead" and Europe as "behind" in the race of social progress via technoscientific or medical application. Indeed, various ART procedures, which may be banned, considered controversial, or subject to ethical or economic restrictions in some jurisdictions (such as PGD, or "savior siblings"; see Jones et al. 2007), are offered in Turkey as an unproblematic part of clinical practice, with competitive success rates and attractive treatment conditions, or at comparatively cheaper prices. In fact, as a result of this, IVF clinics in Turkey (already an established holiday destination) are growing more attractive in the lucrative market for reproductive travel, advertised in one website with the memorable slogan "Excellent Healthcare meets Low Cost & Leisure."[18]

Thus, in the case of Turkish ART legislation, Turkish practitioners see a secular approach and "a lack of restrictions" regarding their clinical practice as enabling them to achieve high success rates and attract foreign patients, where Pennings sees "a lot of restrictions" limiting access to married couples informed by Islamic principles.

Secularism and Islam

While the limitation of ART access solely to married couples using their own gametes is fairly uncommon across the globe, it represents the norm in the (Sunni) Muslim Middle East.[19] In fact, we can contrast the marital focus apparent in the ART legislations of this region (including Turkey) with "Euro-American" legislations, which permit some form of extramarital assisted reproduction, whether by allowing the use of donor sperm or eggs, or surrogacy, or by enabling access to ARTs by unmarried couples, same-sex couples, or single women.[20] It is indeed such comparisons that lead to the characterization of a prohibition on all forms of extramarital reproduction as an "Islamic approach" to ARTs. Although this is an understandable shorthand, it is also overly simplistic, ignoring both the complex intraregional divergences (see this volume passim) and the concurrences that may exist across different religions (as demonstrated in the comparison between Egypt and Italy by Inhorn et al., this volume). Since "Islam is a religion of great diversity" (Inhorn and Sargent 2006: 5), it should not be surprising that ART practice across the Muslim world is subject to differences as well as similarities. Detailed discussions on Islamic approaches to ARTs have taken place both in this volume (see in particular Eich and Houot) and elsewhere in the literature (e.g. Aboulghar et al. 2007; Clarke 2006, 2007, 2008; Inhorn 2003, 2006a, 2006c, 2006d; Serour 1993), documenting both Sunni and Shia reasoning. These accounts show not only how significant differences can exist between Sunni and Shia approaches to donor gametes and surrogacy (see also Garmaroudi Naef, this volume), but also the variety accommodated within each, as well as how apparently convergent outcomes can be the result of distinctly varied processes (Clarke, this volume).

   Turkey, as an ardently secular country whose population is nevertheless Muslim, undeniably presents a high degree of semblance to other Sunni Muslim countries concerning the practice of ARTs. This observation was the basis upon which Pennings made his thorny query. However, the important question is not whether Turkish legislation is similar to (or even the same as) Sunni Muslim rulings, but whether it is *informed and defined by* such religious reasoning. The dispute is over whether "religion" or "culture" is the causal explanation for the legislation's character, the former obviating while the latter accommodating a secular thesis.

Since, as noted by Schenker in a summary of religious perspectives on assisted reproduction, "It is often difficult to dissociate the influence of distinctly religious factors from other cultural conditions" (2005: 310), rather than tease apart religion and culture in an effort to establish which account is "more accurate," it is more productive to try to understand the particular contextual importance of these competing characterizations. This requires some appreciation of the role of secularism—"by and large, the most dominant discourse that forms the basis of public life in Turkey" (Navaro-Yashin 2002: 7)—and its political and ideological significance.

State secularism, or *laiklik*[21] as it is known in Turkey, was crucial to the transformations that accompanied the succession of the obsolete Ottoman Empire by the Republic of Turkey, founded in 1923. A series of thorough reforms, known as Atatürk's Revolution, implemented in the early decades of the republic, replaced Ottoman institutions and traditions with those based on leading European models. These modernizing, or "Westernizing," changes had far-reaching consequences for Turkey's political, economic, and educational systems, as well as for the alphabet, the calendar, and the style of dress. The sultanate and the caliphate were abolished, and the Presidency of Religious Affairs, or Diyanet İşleri Başkanlığı, was founded in 1924. This new organization, one of the first to be created under the new Turkish Parliament (TBMM), was given "the mandate to carry out religious affairs pertaining to faith, worship and moral principles, to inform society on religion and to administer places of worship"[22] in accordance with the principles of secularism.

In addition to this, Parliament constitutionally adopted a stance of active religious neutrality, neither recognizing nor promoting an official state religion. The "will to civilization" (Keyman 1995, 2007) was founded on a central ideology, heavily influenced by the ideas of prominent nationalist Ziya Gökalp (Zürcher 2007), which distinguished between civilization—a rational, international system of knowledge, science, and technology—and culture—the set of values and habits current within a community. Thus the new nation-state could aspire to the ideals of "Western" civilization, while simultaneously maintaining its uniquely Turkish culture. Within this framework, Islam was effectively demarcated from the state and the public sphere, although it could and did continue to maintain its influence and position within the private sphere, as an integral part of "local culture."

Recently, particularly following the 2002 and 2007 elections after which the Justice and Development Party, or AKP,[23] formed unitary governments, discussions on the appropriate role of religion in the public life of Turkey have resurfaced with new immediacy and fervor. The AKP define themselves as "conservative democratic" and deny an Islamic agenda, although Yavuz and other commentators have accused them of a "politics of camouflage," arguing that "Islamic ideas and an Islamic worldview are still included in the identity of its leadership and might also be included in the AKP's deep-seated philosophy" (2009: 3). The party has widespread public support, but also faces a great deal of opposition, particularly from the Kemalist military, security forces, and their sympathizers who suspect that the AKP is smuggling Islam in through the back door and seek to defend the republic's secular character.

Thus, what is termed an everyday Islamization or growing public religiosity (Yavuz 2009) on the one hand is met on the other with a growing privatization and commodification of secular state ideology (Özyürek 2004). As people ascribe themselves into the binary camps of Islamism and Secularism (although not necessarily employing those labels[24]), views over religion and state become fundamental elements of self-identification and group identity (see Navaro-Yashin 2002; White 2002). Claims to modernity are made by both camps: the former reappropriating it and applying an unassimilative critique from within (Göle 1996), while the latter identify themselves as possessing universal mores and modes of behavior that transcend locality (Navaro-Yashin 2002).

In this context, which ties modernity to democracy, to suggest that religion defines Turkish legislation is unacceptable, not only to secularists, but to both parties. Secular democratic regulation is meant to reflect the wishes and morals of the majority, rather than an obedience to religious authority. However, the former may itself be guided by religion, or secular ethics, or a range of factors that could be subsumed under the broad concept of "culture." Accepting the role of culture in informing and influencing the views of the majority is a means to explain how "religious reasoning" may be reflected in "secular" legislation through democratic processes.

Religious Authorities on ARTs

Diyanet, as Turkey's highest religious authority, is the official body charged with providing information about religious rulings, prohibitions, and morality to the country's religious leaders, as well as to the general public. According to Diyanet, ARTs should receive encouragement, as long as the procedures do not damage the sanctity of the family or threaten the four central concerns of protecting inheritance, preventing incest, the prohibition of adulterous relations, and the preservation of lineage. They reason that since children, as blessings, are Allah's endowment, the treatment seeking of involuntarily childless couples does not contradict a sense of fate or destiny. Moreover, as articulated by Saim Yeprem, theologian and member of Diyanet's Higher Council:

> Islam neither considers scientific research an intervention in God's job, nor does it encumber freedom of research. It rather regards scientific research as discovering laws of nature to figure out the works of God (which is called *al-sunnatullah* in Islamic literature) in the universe (2007: 47).

Although he adds that this does not mean that "scientific research has full freedom without warnings from religious and moral values to put its findings into practice" (2007: 47), these views are nevertheless furthered to obviate an antithesis between science and religion, sometimes colloquialized by Christian theologians as "playing God," and enables Islam to be represented as scientifically "progressive."

Indeed, Diyanet has explicitly supported ARTs as practiced in Turkey in its public releases[25] and has even opened its own hospital in Istanbul, providing a range of treatments including ARTs. Speaking at the opening ceremony, Professor Ali Bardakoğlu, Diyanet's president, stated that education and health were Diyanet's biggest priorities, and added: "We want to keep up with scientific and technological advancements, presenting the latest in technological developments to the public, and we want to help those that are in need."[26] Asked to comment specifically on the IVF unit within the hospital, he added: "We will support all treatments within the framework of our religion. ... The aims of religion and medicine are the same: to make people happier on this earth." Bardakoğlu's statements, and of course the practical act of funding the hospital, thus created a medicine-religion nexus, presenting Islamic and biomedical responses to infertility as commensurate, and as naturally cooperating to meet humanitarian needs (cf. Clarke, this volume).

Some time later, when twins conceived after treatment at the clinic were born to a forty-two-year-old imam and his wife from Samsun, newspapers reported the birth as "Diyanet's first *tüp bebekleri* (tube babies)" and quoted the imam as saying, "We were comforted by Diyanet's statements, and we came to this hospital with a clear conscience."[27] Indeed, more generally, practitioners credit Diyanet's support for not only alleviating concerns around IVF but also for promoting treatment seeking among couples "who in the past did not come for *tüp bebek* for fear of religion."[28] Some IVF clinics, such as the Maya clinic in Ankara for example, even provide summaries and direct links to Diyanet's *fetva* (Arabic: fatwa) on their websites' information pages.

This close relationship, or parity, between what is seen as Islamic morality and progressive science is also implicitly or directly contrasted with the stance of other religions, particularly Catholicism (see also Clarke, and Inhorn et al., this volume). For example, the Turkish media coverage of the Vatican's December 2008 document on biotechnology provides a series of oppositions between "restrictive" Catholic and "permissive" Islamic rulings on IVF and stem cells, with headlines such as "Vatican Finds It Abominable, but Diyanet Gives Approval"[29] or "Papa and Diyanet of Very Different Opinions."[30] In these accounts, in contradistinction to Catholicism, Islam is presented as permissive and progressive, or in Clarke's terms (this volume) as a contemporary religion capable of "keeping up with the times."

Moreover, when Islamic prohibitions are discussed, these are represented not as dogmatic injunctions, but as informed or intuitive safeguards against dreadful consequences. Newspaper reports and Diyanet statements that explain the rulings of Islam, regarding, for example, "bank babies" (babies born of sperm donation), stress potential social and psychological maladies as reasons for the restrictions. Adherence to these rulings then, is not necessarily sought through a priori submission but via an appreciation of the rationale underlying the decisions. For example, Diyanet's latest and most detailed announcement on ARTs, dated 1 March 2006, summarizes the stance on sperm donation in the following way:

> In short, in addition to being *haram,* the giving or taking of sperm from a sperm bank is a social tragedy. Because one of the five common principles of all divine religions is the preservation of lineage. This is one of the most important reasons why *zina* is considered *haram.* This practice can result in the degeneration of lineage, the birth of children whose lineage is unclear, the strategic spread of diseases by way of sperm, and many other similar social tragedies. Therefore it is not permissible (*caiz*).

Saim Yeprem explains in a press statement that although a child born of donation should *not* be considered a *veled-i zina* (child of adultery, bastard) since the situation is not exactly adulterous, donor procedures nevertheless beckon widespread social catastrophe and are therefore both religiously and socially unacceptable:

> [T]here are *even bigger* problems here than there are with children who are born of *zina*. Because with *zina,* the child's mother and father are evident. With these [third-party assisted reproduction technologies] the child's grandfather may be its father, its aunt its mother, a person can even give birth to their own sibling, their grandfather's child. So technically this is not *zina*, but it is entirely against the Islamic principle of the preservation of genealogy.[31]

Diyanet's rulings, then, are presented as a dynamic engagement with advancing scientific possibilities, with theologians providing reasoning to inform people's own decision making. The regular presence of Diyanet's opinions in popular media coverage of ARTs, Internet patient forums, and even on the websites of IVF clinics, suggests a high level of importance and authority that patients attribute to these. Indeed, popular discourses regarding ARTs in Turkey portray an ideal synchrony between legal regulation, religious rulings, and public opinion.

Moral Arbitration by ART Patients

The "perfect match" between legislation and religious rulings on ARTs in Turkey are often taken to accurately represent not just the opinions of ordinary Turkish citizens, but also of infertile couples who may be unable to conceive using the available technologies. Regulators and commentators regularly defend the restrictions on ART access and on third-party reproductive assistance with vociferous claims that Turkish persons would not wish to use donor gametes and would not desire reproduction outside marriage. Using donor sperm, donor eggs, or surrogates, or trying to establish new family forms through single parenthood or homosexual unions, is defined broadly as "unsuitable to our culture" (*bizim kültürümüze yakışmaz*) and dismissed as something that happens only in "other" Western nations.

However, actual studies of public attitudes reveal a rather different picture. According to the only survey of Turkish public opinion regarding egg donation, conducted with four hundred participants, only 15 percent showed complete objection to egg donation as part of ART practice (Isikoglu et al. 2006). Moreover, the survey also suggested that people did not have very accurate knowledge of religious rulings on the matter, with 55.6 percent of women and 65.5 percent of men believing (wrongly) that "Islam does not prevent the use of donor eggs." This latter finding is rather surprising, particularly in light of the information that 67 percent of the survey participants considered themselves to be religious, and should act as a warning against inferring individual attitudes from religious affiliation. However, the permissive public attitudes towards egg donation in Turkey should not be read simply as arising from ignorance of religious rulings either, and may require more nuanced explanations. Similarly, the great asymmetry between infertile women's hypothetical acceptance of donor eggs (23.3 percent) and donor sperm (3.4 percent) in another Turkish study (Baykal et al. 2008) also begs further explanation and cannot be understood purely with reference to the symmetrically prohibitive Islamic rulings on gamete donation.[32] Moreover, the complicated picture in which some Turkish couples are willing to consider and accept third-party reproductive assistance can be observed not just in hypothetical surveys but in their actual behavior.

Despite cultural fears of "mixing" in clinics and taboos that undoubtedly persist with regard to sperm donation, there is nevertheless demand for ART treatments involving third-party reproductive assistance from Turkish couples who have failed to conceive with standard IVF cycles. Many practitioners confided to me during private conversations that they had encountered patients who had requested "secret solutions." Although all of the practitioners I interviewed reiterated that they would never consider partaking in illegal practices, in one case, widely dubbed the "Çukurova Sperm Scandal," Professor Dr. İsmet Köker was found guilty of "impregnating women who came to his clinic with sperm from strangers"[33] and in 2006, was sentenced to the maximum three years imprisonment for the offence of "abusing professional power" (*görevi kötüye kullanmak*). The couples had been complicit in their covert treatments, although the medical students and junior doctors from whom semen samples were procured claimed to be entirely ignorant of the true purpose of their donations. It is important to point out that if murmured reports of the high volume of demand for Dr. Köker's unorthodox "solution" are accurate, then Turkish male infertility patients are highly unusual in their acceptance of sperm donation (albeit as a last resort under covert circumstances), since among Muslim Middle Eastern men more generally, this remains an unacceptable option (cf. Inhorn 2006b).

Practitioners who reflected on their own experiences with demands for covert treatments spoke of their "surprisingly common" occurrence. In their accounts, such demands were somewhat understandable from "Westernized" patients, seen to possess an "open mind" and to transcend religious prohibitions, but were particularly remarkable when voiced by (what they considered to be) "conservative" (read religious) persons. Such patients, who did not display the "religious," or "cultural" aversions to donation expected of them by others, presented a contradiction. One practitioner explained this apparent paradox with reference to the stronger imperative and social pressure among the "conservative" population to have children:

> It is interesting that so many patients do consider it. People you wouldn't imagine. … Of course, they imagine that at the end of the day no one will know about it—his wife will be pregnant. There is a lot of social pressure, pressure from the family, from the wider kin group, imagine you've been married for ten years or twenty years and there is still no child! … What is more interesting is that [demand for donor gametes] is more common among the covered (*kapalı*) population, how should we call them, the conservative (*tutucu*) population, because they are also subjected to more social pressure [to have children].[34]

According to this interpretation, such patients were willing to trade the (discrediting) stigma (Goffman 1963) of childlessness for the (discreditable) stigma of using donation, in the hopes of effectively hiding the latter. This desire to keep donation hidden was also used to explain a lack of any public demand for the legalization of donor gamete practices:

> I think the target population is very passive with regards to this, they do not express themselves. They feel a great pressure against openly expressing themselves. For example, we never hear anyone campaigning for the legalization of donor gametes . … Nobody openly voices these claims, because they are reluctant. Even within their own families they are reluctant to own up to such desires. They prefer to pursue it in secret.[35]

These desires to "pursue donation in secret" are increasingly leading Turkish couples to demonstrate "moral pluralism in motion" (Pennings 2002) through reproductive travel, mostly to Northern

Cyprus. Although newspapers sporadically run "moral panic" or "in-dividual success" stories of around "2,000–3,000 couples a year"[36] that resort to donor conception abroad, such travel is coordinated to be largely invisible and conducted with extreme discretion. Turkish clinics, spurred on by demand, have formed partnerships with Cy-priot clinics, or have even opened Cypriot "branches," which allows them to retain a large proportion of the profits and to facilitate the smooth cross-border treatment of their patients. Although Marcia Inhorn has written about Sunni Muslim patients "quietly slipping across transnational borders" (2007: 193) to obtain donor gametes in neighboring Shia countries, I am not aware of any other country in which such a developed institutional infrastructure exists to aid these legal trespasses. One practitioner and member of the ÜYTEM Directorate (which regulates ARTs) summarized the current stance of the Turkish authorities, who are turning a blind eye to this prac-tice, as entirely hypocritical:

> Illegal matters are not discussed in Turkey. They are forbidden, be-cause they are illegal. … It is illegal to shoot a man, so it is also an offense to carry a gun. But our approach to this area is this: you can carry a gun in Turkey, but if you are going to shoot the man, go and do it in Cyprus![37]

The supralegal choreography—incorporating the movement of finances, expertise, gametes, patients, treatment cycles, and even clinic brands in and out of national borders—serves both to meet the needs of patients who require these treatments and provide a resolution without upsetting the impression of a perfect legal-reli-gious-public harmony in Turkey regarding ART practice. Unlike in Lebanon or Iran, where a plurality of opinions afford practitioners the ability to manage allegiances in order to meet patient demands (see Inhorn et al., and Tappan, this volume), practitioners and pa-tients in Turkey achieve maneuverability from within an apparent consensus. A nurse who coordinates a large donor treatment pro-gram between Turkey and Cyprus told me that, under these covert conditions, a much wider section of the population than one would have imagined "look warmly" upon the idea of donation.

Another practitioner described to me in detail her own observa-tions of a group of women that had just undergone egg donation in Cyprus:

> Three days ago I went to Cyprus … and on my way back I ran into one of my patients at the airport; a covered patient. She said to me,

"You told me it was not possible for me to have children, so I came to Cyprus for donor eggs. You see the large crowd of women over there, we all came for donor eggs at the same time, we all had our transfers on the same day, and now we are returning home." I turned and looked at the group, and I am telling you with all sincerity that out of thirty women, twenty-three to twenty-four of them were covered, some in full black sheets (*çarşaf*). I mean when you look at it, the external appearance and the religious beliefs signified by that appearance and the practice that has just taken place are in exact opposition to each other. But they partake in secret. Hence, here we see that the desire for a child overcomes religious beliefs, or cultural traditions, pressures, or anything else.[38]

As noted by Tappan (this volume) it is not possible, or analytically perceptive, to characterize such actions as religious or nonreligious; instead, we should seek to understand how patients *approach* both ARTs and religion. These women were prepared to engage in "reproductive resistance" (Inhorn et al., this volume) against the legal prohibitions of their country and the rulings of their religion in the cross-border pursuit of much-longed-for children. However, we do not yet know enough about the "hidden lives" of these Turkish "moral pioneers" (Rapp 1999) to judge whether successful donor treatments will bring the fulfillment they anticipate and the happiness they imagine (see Tremayne, this volume).

Conclusion

Looking to comment on the role played by Islam in the legislation, discourse, and social practice of ARTs in secular Turkey necessarily involves a certain degree of disentangling, not only between the views of different actors, rhetoric and reality, public and private, but also between the categories of analysis and the categories of informants. The contextual importance on particular formulations of the relationships between religion, politics, and science—as well as the significance of their delineation—results in a series of hybrid phenomena and competing characterizations.

Depending on the vantage point (and political inclination), Turkish ART legislation may be viewed variously as "liberal" or "restrictive," "secular" or "Islamic," based on "cultural values" or "religious reasons." In these rhetorical conflicts, it is rather inconsequential to assign accuracy or legitimacy to one side over the other, and rather more valuable to ask how such opposing views are conjured, and what is at stake in their assertion and propagation. Although it may not be practically possible to disaggregate "culture" from "religion" within the secular politics of Turkey, the latter is unacceptable as a causal explanation of state regulation, whereas the former can be used to mobilize democratic aspirations. These discourses, which may be used and understood rather differently by internal and external commentators, pertain to sensitive questions about Turkey's identity and its international affiliation.

Moreover, seemingly incongruent manifestations, such as "a lot of restrictions" on access to ARTs coupled with a "lack of restrictions" regarding their clinical application (e.g., including PGD and fetal reduction), can be explained with reference to the same underlying elements. In this case, core "family values" (Kağıçıbaşı and Ataca 2005), highly espoused in Turkey, valorize (if not mandate) the reproduction in stable families of *healthy* children who are biologically related to both their parents. The ability of ARTs to address these fundamental desires within Turkish society has been crucial in both their widespread acceptance, and the particular forms given to the constraints of their practice.

"Restrictive" and "progressive," as tropes, are so heavily laden with broader connotations that, in general, whenever they are advanced as part of reflexive comparisons, the speaker invariably positions themselves as the latter. This is no less true for Pennings than it is for the Turkish practitioners, or for the newspaper articles that compare Diyanet's rulings with those of the Vatican. Frameworks constructed on such dualities—or indeed on the lesser burdened binaries of conservative/liberal, traditional/innovative, or religious/nonreligious—do not provide much help in exploring hybrid phenomena, such as Diyanet's IVF clinic or "covered" patients pursuing donor gametes across national borders.

The myriad negotiations of Islam and secularism, and of competing social pressures, may engender differences between appearance and actions, or stated and hidden intentions. A cultural context that highly values procreation, yet also highly stigmatizes third-party reproductive assistance (in particular sperm donation), can generate a heterogeneity of compromises. Thus, the seeming consensus on "marital" parameters for ARTs between legislation, religious rulings, and public opinion also harbors silent dissent and clandestine transgressions, at both a personal level, as patients request "secret solutions," and at the level of national infrastructure, as supralegal choreographies coordinate the movements of ARTs, gametes, and patients.

Faced with these hybrids and competing characterizations, my aim has not been to label Turkish ARTs as one thing or another, but to ask which aspects of this cultural context—including religion, international relations, and personal moral arbitration—determine the ways in which a global technology is assembled (Ong and Collier 2005) in particular formations, or how "local moral worlds" (Kleinman 1992) are shaping and curtailing its local application (Inhorn 2002). Attending to the role of religion in this secular context—to competing discourses on the character, position, and significance of Islam, as well to its manifestations in social practices—reveals a rich mine of information, and warns against the pitfalls of cursory glances.

Acknowledgments

This chapter draws on material from my ESRC-funded doctoral research, which would not have been possible without the help of many facilitators and countless willing informants, to whom I remain deeply thankful. I am grateful to Marcia Inhorn and Soraya Tremayne for inviting me to Yale in September 2009; I have benefited enormously from the wonderful discussions at that workshop and from continuing exchanges with my new colleagues. I would also like to thank Charlotte Faircloth, Yael Navaro-Yashin, and especially Mustafa Gürtin for their thorough reading and insightful comments on earlier versions. Needless to say, any remaining errors are my own.

Notes

1. Subsequent to the completion of this chapter in January 2010, Turkey's statute regulating assisted reproduction was updated. The March 2010 amendments introduced several important changes, most significantly restricting embryo transfer numbers and prohibiting reproductive travel and its facilitation for the purposes of gamete donation. Although it is yet unclear how these changes, which are currently under debate, will affect practitioners and patients, they are likely to have significant consequences. This chapter must therefore be read as describing a particular period of assisted reproduction practice in Turkey, which will already be history by the time it is published.

2. These figures refer to the "Ministry of Health Licensed Assisted Reproduction Treatment Centers List, June 2009" available from the Ministry of Health website, http://www.saglik.gov.tr.

3. Criteria for eligibility include that the couple must be married for a minimum of three years and have no living children. It also specifies the age of the woman as 23–39. Social security institutions contribute 80 percent of the drug costs, and 70 percent of the costs for the first, and 75 percent for the second cycle of medically indicated IVF treatment.

4. There were 66 licensed clinics at the end of 2005; this had grown to 91 clinics at the end of 2007.

5. Exact data for the number of IVF treatment cycles undertaken per year are not available for Turkey, so I rely on the informed estimates of the Turkish Society of Reproductive Medicine (TSRM).

6. *Hürriyet*, 31 January 2008.

7. *Radikal*, 13 August 2007.

8. The Turkish census does not collect detailed data on religious affiliation, although estimates suggest that between 95–99 percent of Turkey's population self-define (at least nominally) as Muslim. Of these around 75 percent belong to the Sunni-Hanafi branch of Islam, with the Alevi and Twelver Shia forming significant minorities. Religiosity varies greatly within the population.

9. The full conference proceedings have been published as a special supplement of *Reproductive BioMedicine Online*, edited by Robert Edwards (2007). When providing direct quotes from the meeting, I have relied on discussion transcriptions and published versions of the papers as they appear in this publication.

10. The word *çağdaş* carries strong ideological undertones. It literally translates as "contemporary," but is also employed to mean "modern" and "civilized". Navaro-Yashin (2002) explains that the word has Eurocentric connotations, with certain Kemalist sectors of society employing it to reference themselves and their aspirations in contradistinction to Islamists.

11. The 1983 Law on Population Planning (Official Gazette no. 18059, 27 May 1983) states in Item 5, "As long as there are no medical drawbacks for the health of the mother, until the tenth week of pregnancy, the womb may be evacuated upon request." The termination of more advanced pregnancies is also possible, but these require medical or health-related justifications (Aydın 1999).

12. A structure for the regulation of assisted reproduction in Turkey was first introduced in 1987, under the title "Statute on Centres for In Vitro Fertilization and Embryo Transfer" (Official Gazette 19551, 21 August 1987). This was superseded by "The Statute on Assisted Reproduction Treatment Centers" (ÜYTEM, Official Gazette 22822, 19 November 1996), which has subsequently been amended four times with the latest changes made in 2005 (Official Gazette 25869, 8 July 2005). All of the references to the statute provided in this chapter refer to its current version. All issues of the Official Gazette may be accessed through the online Official Gazette archives at: http://rega.basbakanlik.gov.tr/.

13. For example, the law emerging from Turkey's approval of the Convention of Human Rights and Biomedicine of December 2003 (Law no. 5013, Official Gazette 25311, 9 December 2003) allows embryo research, but forbids the creation of embryos solely for research purposes (item 18.2), and states that the use of assisted reproduction for sex selection should be avoided, except as a means to avoid serious sex-linked disorders. The Statute on Centers for Genetic Disease Diagnosis (Official Gazette 23368, 10 June 1998) also forbids sex determination except in the case of sex-linked diseases, which would cover the use of PGD for social sex selection (item 17). See also Uysal (2003) and Arısoy et al. (2008).

14. *Yeni Asya*, 23 April 2008.

15. The International Organization for Standardization (ISO) and Joint Commission International (JCI) are both standard-setting bodies. The former is an international organization setting quality standards in a wide variety of industrial and commercial areas, and the latter is a predominantly United States–based body that operates voluntary accreditation programs in healthcare settings. A clinic's ability to meet these standards can guarantee a certain level of quality and enable international comparisons.

16. http://www.bahceci.com.

17. Quote from senior ART practitioner, Expert Interview number 39 conducted by author.

18. http://www.ivfturkey.com.

19. Of the fifty-seven countries included in the International Federation of Fertility Societies (IFFS) survey by Jones et al. (2007), only Turkey and four other nations (Egypt, Morocco, the Republic of the Philippines, and Tunisia) completely prohibit the use of third-party assistance and access to ARTs by unmarried individuals. However, many Middle Eastern nations that also practice ARTs within such parameters were not included as part of this survey (e.g. Bahrain, Jordan, Saudi Arabia, Sudan, Syria, UAE).

20. There is a great range of ART legislations, accommodating both large differences and fine distinctions between jurisdictions. Various countries may allow all or some of these "extramarital" forms of assisted reproduction in myriad configurations; for example, some countries may allow certain forms of third-party assistance (e.g., sperm donation and surrogacy) but not others (e.g., egg donation), or allow the use of donor gametes only under particular conditions of anonymity and disclosure. For details, see Jones et al. (2007).

21. The Turkish concept of *laiklik* is distinct from both the French *laïcité* and American religious freedom (usually accepted as referring to freedom *from* and freedom *of* religion respectively), and is more specifically concerned with a *control of* religion by the state. However, the growing diversification and difference within Turkish politics in recent years has

led to competing meanings of secularism that encompass all of these. For a detailed discussion, see Yavuz 2009.

22. See "The Structure, Mission and Social Function of the Presidency of Religious Affairs" published in English on Diyanet's website, http://www.diyanet.gov.tr/english/weboku.asp?id=787&yid=31&sayfa=2 .

23. The Adalet ve Kalkınma Partisi is usually abbreviated as AKP by scholars, since the official party abbreviation AK Party is seen as too politically loaded. In Turkish *ak* means "white" and has connotations of purity and honesty.

24. "Islamist" and "secularist" are commonly used labels in academic writing, although people assigned to these groups are more likely to refer to themselves respectively as "conservative" (*muhafazakâr*) and "pious" (*mütedeyyin*) or as laic (*laik*), Ataturkist (*Atatürçkü*), and Kemalist. Each side imagines themselves to be completely different from "the other," though White observes, "While these [identities] appear as competing dyads in Turkish public life, in the factualness of everyday life they form a continuum" (2002: 8).

25. For example, "*Tüp Bebek*" dated 1 May 2002 and "Islamic Assessment of Today's Medical Developments in *Tüp Bebek* and Stem-cell Research" dated 1 March 2006, both available from their website: http://www.diyanet.gov.tr.

26. *Akşam*, 29 December 2005.

27. *Sabah*, 11 February 2007.

28. *Star Gazete*, 24 November 2007.

29. *Sabah*, 14 December 2008.

30. *Star Gazete*, 14 December 2008.

31. *Şok Gazetesi*, 02 July 2007.

32. Delaney's (1991) "seed and soil" thesis may give us a way to understand such an asymmetry in attitudes towards donor eggs and donor sperm. Based on her ethnography of an Anatolian village, anthropologist Carol Delaney argues for the existence of monogenetic procreation metaphors within the cosmology of Turkish village society, whereby the man's "seed" is recognised as the generative component in procreation, and the woman's embodied involvement as nongenerative nurture, akin to the role of the "soil" in agriculture. While I did not encounter these terminologies or explanations in my interviews with infertility patients, I would agree that the man's contribution to the identity of the child was often emphasized. See also Inhorn for a detailed discussion of gamete donation in Sunni and Shia Islam (2006d), and a brief summary of Muslim patients' views on donation (this volume).

33. *NTV-MSNBC*, 24 November 2006 and *Hürriyet*, 23 October 2009.

34. Quote from senior ART practitioner, Expert Interview number 29 conducted by author.

35. Quote from senior ART practitioner, Expert Interview number 18 conducted by author.

36. *Aktüel*, 13–19 April 2006; *Sabah*, 19 December 2005.

37. Quote from senior ART practitioner, Expert Interview number 38 conducted by author.
38. Quote from senior ART practitioner, Expert Interview number 18 conducted by author.

References

Aboulghar, Mohamed, Gamal Serour, and Ragaa T. Mansour. 2007. "Ethical Aspects and Regulation of Assisted Reproduction in the Arabic-speaking World." *Reproductive BioMedicine Online* 14(1): 143–46.

Arda, Berna. 2007. "The Importance of Secularism in Medical Ethics: The Turkish Example." *Reproductive BioMedicine Online* 14(1): 24–28.

Arısoy, Y., Ç. Eresen, and V. Ö. Özbek. 2008. "Yeni Yasal Düzenlemeler ve Moleküler Genetik İncelemeler" [New Laws and Molecular Genetic Tests: Review]. *Türkiye Klinikleri J Med Sci* 28: 178–81.

Aydın, Erdem. 1999. "Bioethics Regulations in Turkey." *Journal of Medical Ethics* 25: 404–7.

Baykal, Baris, Cern Korkmaz, Seyit T. Ceyhan, Umit Goktolga, and Iskender Baser. 2008. "Opinions of Infertile Turkish Women on Gamete Donations and Gestational Surrogacy." *Fertility and Sterility* 89: 817–22.

Clarke, Morgan. 2006. "Islam, Kinship and New Reproductive Technology." *Anthropology Today* 22: 17–22.

———. 2007. "Kinship, Propriety and Assisted Reproduction in the Middle East." *Anthropology of the Middle East* 2(1): 71–91.

———. 2008. "New Kinship, Islam, and the Liberal Tradition: Sexual Morality and New Reproductive Technology in Lebanon." *Journal of the Royal Anthropological Institute* 14: 143–69.

Delaney, Carol. 1991. *The Seed and the Soil: Gender and Cosmology in Turkish Village Society.* Berkeley: University of California Press.

Edwards, Robert G, ed. 2007. "Ethics, Law and Moral Philosophy of Reproductive Medicine." *Reproductive BioMedicine Online* 14(1): 29–31.

Fasouliotis, Sozos J., and Joseph G. Schenker. 1999. "Social Aspects in Assisted Reproduction." *Human Reproduction Update* 5: 26–39.

Goffman, Erving. 1963. *Stigma: Notes on the Management of Spoiled Identity.* New York: Touchstone.

Göle, Nilufer. 1996. *The Forbidden Modern: Civilization and Veiling.* Ann Arbor: University of Michigan Press.

Inhorn, Marcia C. 2002. "The 'Local' Confronts the 'Global': Infertile Bodies and New Reproductive Technologies in Egypt." In *Infertility around the Globe: New Thinking on Childlessness, Gender, and Reproductive Technologies,* ed. Marcia C. Inhorn and Frank van Balen. Berkeley: University of California Press.

———. 2003. *Local Babies, Global Science: Gender, Religion, and In Vitro Fertilization in Egypt.* New York: Routledge.

―――. 2006a. "*Fatwas* and ARTs: IVF and Gamete Donation in Sunni vs. Shi'a Islam." *Journal of Gender, Race and Justice* 9: 291–317.

―――. 2006b. "'He Won't Be My Son': Middle Eastern Muslim Men's Discourses of Adoption and Gamete Donation." *Medical Anthropology Quarterly* 20: 94–120.

―――. 2006c. "Islam, IVF and Everyday Life in the Middle East: The Making of Sunni versus Shi'ite Test-Tube Babies." *Anthropology of the Middle East* 1(1): 42–50.

―――. 2006d. "Making Muslim Babies: IVF and Gamete Donation in Sunni versus Shi'a Islam." *Culture, Medicine and Psychiatry* 30: 427–50.

―――. 2007. "Reproductive Disruptions and Assisted Reproductive Technologies in the Muslim World." In *Reproductive Disruptions: Gender, Technology and Biopolitics in the New Millennium,* ed. Marcia C. Inhorn. New York: Berghahn.

Inhorn, Marcia C. and Carolyn F. Sargent. 2006. "Introduction to Medical Anthropology in the Muslim World." *Medical Anthropology Quarterly* 20(1): 1–12.

Isikoglu, M., Y. Senol, M. Berkkanoglu, K. Ozgur, L. Donmez, and A. Stones-Abbasi. 2006. "Public Opinion Regarding Oocyte Donation in Turkey: First Data from a Secular Population among the Islamic World." *Human Reproduction* 21(1): 318–23.

Jones, Howard W., Jean Cohen, Ian Cooke, and Roger Kempers. 2007. "IFFS Surveillance 07." *Fertility and Sterility* 87(4): S1–S67 (Supplement 1).

Kâğıtçıbaşı, Çigdem and Bilge Ataca. 2005. "Value of Children and Family Change: A Three-Decade Portrait From Turkey." *Applied Psychology* 54: 317–37.

Keyder, Çaglar. 2006. "Moving in from the Margins? Turkey in Europe." *Diogenes* 53(2): 72–81.

Keyman, Fuat. E. 1995. "On the Relation between Global Modernity and Nationalism: The Crisis of Hegemony and the Rise of Islamic Identity." *New Perspectives on Turkey* 13: 93–120.

―――. 2007. "Modernity, Secularism and Islam: The Case of Turkey." *Theory, Culture & Society* 24: 215–23.

Kleinman, Arthur. 1992. "Local Worlds of Suffering: An Interpersonal Focus for Ethnographies of Illness Experience." *Qualitative Health Research* 2: 127–34.

Navaro-Yashin, Yael. 2002. *Faces of the State: Secularism and Public Life in Turkey.* Princeton, NJ: Princeton University Press.

Ong, Aihwa, and Stephen J. Collier, eds. 2005. *Global Assemblages: Technology, Politics, and Ethics as Anthropological Problems.* Oxford: Blackwell Publishing.

Özyürek, Esra. 2004. "Miniaturizing Atatürk: Privatisation of State Imagery and Ideology of the State in Turkey." *American Ethnologist* 3(3): 374–91.

Pennings, Guido. 2002. "Reproductive Tourism as Moral Pluralism in Motion." *Journal of Medical Ethics* 28: 337–41.

Rapp, Rayna. 1999. *Testing Women, Testing the Fetus.* New York: Routledge.

Schenker, Joseph G. 2005. "Assisted Reproductive Practice: Religious Perspectives." *Reproductive BioMedicine Online* 3: 310–19.

Serour, Gamal I. 1993. "Bioethics in Artificial Reproduction in the Muslim World." *Bioethics* 7: 207–17.

Uysal, P. 2003. "In Vitro Fertilizasyon-Embriyo Transfer (IVF-ET) ve Etik" [In-Vitro Fertilization-Embryo Transfer (IVF-ET) and Ethics]. *Türkiye Klinikleri Tıp Etiği-Hukuku-Tarihi* 11: 41–44.

White, Jenny. 2002. *Islamist Mobilization in Turkey: A Study in Vernacular Politics.* Seattle: University of Washington Press.

Yavuz, Hakan M. 2004. "Is There a Turkish Islam? The Emergence of Convergence and Consensus." *Journal of Muslim Minority Affairs* 24: 213–32.

———. 2009. *Secularism and Muslim Democracy in Turkey.* Cambridge: Cambridge University Press.

Yeprem, Saim. 2007. "Current Assisted Reproduction Treatment Practices from an Islamic Perspective." *Reproductive BioMedicine Online* 14: 44–47.

Zürcher, Eric. J. 2007. *Turkey: A Modern History.* London: I. B. Tauris.

CONTRIBUTORS

P. Sean Brotherton is Associate Professor of Anthropology at the University of Chicago. His main interests are concerned with the critical study of health, medicine, the state, subjectivity, psychoanalysis, and the body. Over the past decade, he has been conducting ethnographic research on bodily practices, economic reform, and state power in Cuba's primary health sector. He has published several articles and chapters on his research, including his first book, *Revolutionary Medicine: Health and the Body in Post-Soviet Cuba* (Duke University Press, 2012). More recently he completed a project on Cuba's medical humanitarian missions throughout the Americas as a lens to explore the emergent logics and counter-practices that are taking shape in relation to larger enterprise of global health. His latest research explores psychoanalysis as an interpretative and therapeutic framework in the multiple spheres of quotidian life in Buenos Aires, Argentina.

Morgan Clarke is Lecturer in Social Anthropology at the University of Oxford and Fellow of Keble College. He was previously Simon Research Fellow in the Department of Middle Eastern Studies at the University of Manchester and British Academy Postdoctoral Fellow in the Department of Social Anthropology at the University of Cambridge. He is the author of *Islam and New Kinship: Reproductive Technology and the Shariah in Lebanon* (Berghahn Books, 2009) and a number of other articles on Islamic bioethics and anthropological theory. He has a special interest in contemporary Islamic legal discourse and authority, and is currently working on an ethnography of Lebanon's shariah courts.

Thomas Eich is Professor at the Asia Africa Institute at Hamburg University, Germany. He received his academic training in Bamberg, Damascus, and Freiburg, with his PhD from Bochum University focused on the social history of the late Ottoman Empire. Since 2003, he has been conducting research about contemporary Sunni legal debates on bioethics, especially cloning, pre-marital counseling, abortion, pre-natal diagnosis, genetic research, and reproductive medicine. He is author of *Islamische Bioethik* (Wiesbaden 2005) and co-editor with Jon E. Brockopp of *Muslim Medical Ethics: From Theory to Practice* (University of South Carolina Press 2008).

Narges Erami is Assistant Professor of Anthropology at Yale University. Her work is centered in the Holy city of Qum in Iran. She primarily works on the relationship between economy and religion and how it is played out in rituals of everyday life. Her first book length manuscript entitled *The Soul of the Bazaar: Knowledge and Authority Amongst the Carpet Merchants of Qum* introduces readers to the social world of carpet merchants and the process of self-fashioning through the acquisition of specialized knowledge. Her current research continues to be focused in Qum, examining the cultural production of authority and knowledge through publications of Islamic texts and their global circulation. She received her PhD from Columbia University in 2009.

Frank Griffel is Professor of Islamic Studies and Chair of the Council on Middle East Studies at Yale University, where he teaches courses on Islamic intellectual history, Islamic theology and philosophy, and developments in contemporary Muslim thought. He is author of *Al-Ghazali's Philosophical Theology* (Oxford University Press 2009), *Apostasy and Tolerance in Islam* (in German, Brill 2000), as well as numerous articles in academic journals. Together with Abbas Amanat, he edited *Shari'a: Islamic Law in the Contemporary Period* (Stanford University Press 2007). In 2003-2004, he was Mellon Fellow at the Institute for Advanced Study in Princeton, and in 2007 a Carnegie Scholar.

Zeynep B. Gürtin is a Research Fellow at the Centre for Family Research, University of Cambridge. Her PhD thesis examines the cultural constructions of IVF in Turkey, analyzing current regulation, commercial structures and media discourses, alongside an exploration of patients' attitudes and experiences. Her post-doctoral project concerns egg-sharing, a particular form of egg donation, and explores the experiences of donors and recipients in a London IVF clinic. She is co-convener of the Cambridge Interdisciplinary Reproduction Forum, and lectures at the University of Cambridge on the social and psychological aspects of assisted reproductive technologies, gender and reproduction, and bioethics.

Sandra Houot is an Associate Researcher at the Centre of Cultures and Religious Studies (CECR) at the Catholic University of Lyon, France. She is also a temporary lecturer at the Ecole Pratique des Hautes Etudes (EPHE) of Paris, where her teaching focuses on the bioethical issues in contemporary Islam. Her research program concerns contemporary religion, with a focus on Islamic discourse. Her work shows the pluralization of contemporary Islamic discourse via the particularities of scholars causing these discursive productions, and she has published articles concerning the shift from religious to secular ethics. Houot received her PhD in Arabic and History from La Sorbonne.

Marcia C. Inhorn is the William K. Lanman, Jr. Professor of Anthropology and International Affairs in the Department of Anthropology and The Whitney and Betty MacMillan Center for International and Area Studies at Yale University, where she has also served as Chair of the Council on Middle East Studies. A medical anthropologist and specialist on Middle Eastern gender, religion, and health, Inhorn has conducted ethnographic research on the social impact of infertility and assisted reproductive technologies in Egypt, Lebanon, the United Arab Emirates, and Arab America over the past 25 years. She is the author of four books on the subject, including *The New Arab Man: Emergent Masculinities, Technologies, and Islam in the Middle East* (Princeton U Press, 2012), *Local Babies, Global Science: Gender, Religion, and In Vitro Fertilization in Egypt* (Routledge, 2003), *Infertility and Patriarchy: The Cultural Politics of Gender and Family Life in Egypt* (U Pennsylvania Press, 1996) and *Quest for Conception: Gender, Infertility, and Egyptian Medical Traditions* (Un Pennsylvania Press, 1994), which have won the AAA's Eileen Basker Prize and the Diana Forsythe Prize for outstanding feminist anthropological research in the areas of gender, health, science, technology, and biomedicine. She is also the editor or co-editor of eight books. Inhorn has been a visiting faculty member at the American University of Beirut, Lebanon, and the American University of Sharjah, United Arab Emirates, where she has conducted studies on "Middle Eastern Masculinities in the Age of New Reproductive Technologies" and "Globalization and Reproductive Tourism in the Arab World." In the fall of 2010, she was the first Diane Middlebrook and Carl Djerassi Visiting Professor at the Centre for Gender Studies at the University of Cambridge. Inhorn is also is the current and founding editor of *JMEWS (Journal of Middle East Women's Studies)* of the Association of Middle East Women's Studies, Associate Editor of *Global Public Health,* and co-editor of the Berghahn Book series on "Fertility, Reproduction, and Sexuality." She is the past-president of the Society for Medical Anthropology (SMA) of the American Anthropological Association and current member of the executive board of the Middle East Studies Association (MESA).

Farouk Mahmoud is currently a Consultant Obstetrician, Gynaecologist and Infertility Specialist in London. In 2009, he also completed a PhD on Islamic perspectives on assisted reproductive technologies, focusing on the implications of divergences in shariah interpretation. His special interests are infertility medicine and its bioethical and religious perspectives. He graduated in medicine in Sri Lanka and received his post-graduate training at Charing Cross Hospital, London. During this period, he completed the qualifying examinations both in obstetrics and gynaecology (MRCOG) and in surgery (FRCS). Following a brief spell in Kuala Lumpur as Lecturer at the University of Malaysia, he worked as a Consultant Gynaecologist in Gisborne, New Zealand for 8 years, Sydney, Australia for 15 years and the UK for 6 years. During this time he was conferred fellowship degrees from the Royal Colleges of Australia-New Zealand (FRANZCOG) and the UK (FRCOG).

Shirin Garmaroudi Naef is currently a doctoral fellow in the Research Training Group "Bioethics" at the International Centre for Ethics in the Sciences and Humanities (IZEW), University of Tübingen, funded by the German Research Foundation (DFG). Her doctoral project focuses on the use of assisted reproductive technologies in Iranian society from an anthropological perspective, including legal, ethical and jurisprudential aspects and social dynamics. Since 2005, she has been conducting ethnographic research on assisted reproductive technologies and infertility treatments in Iran. She studied Theatre in Tehran, earned her BA in English Language Translation from the Azad University, Tehran in 2000, and her MA in Social Anthropology and Islamic Studies at the University of Berne, Switzerland in 2008. Her thesis was titled "Sibling Intimacy in the

Age of Assisted Reproduction: An Ethnography of New Reproductive Technologies in Iran." Her areas of interest and research include assisted reproductive technologies, anthropological theories, reproduction and kinship studies, bioethics, Shia jurisprudence (*fiqh*) and theology, Persian drama and theatre.

Pasquale Patrizio is Professor of Obstetrics and Gynecology at Yale University and is the Director of both the Yale Fertility Center and the Reproductive Endocrinology clinical practice. His clinical interests include infertility (female and male), IVF, egg donation, gestational surrogacy, and preservation of fertility in cancer patients. Among his many research interests are whole ovary cryopreservation, egg freezing, genetics of oocytes, isolation and freezing of male germ cells, and ethical issues in assisted reproduction. He is a co-author with Marcia Inhorn of research on the ethics of reproductive tourism. Dr. Patrizio is Board Certified in OB/GYN and Reproductive Endocrinology and Infertility and is an active participant in bioethical discussions, following receipt of a Masters in Bioethics at the University of Pennsylvania under the mentorship of Arthur Caplan.

Mansooreh Saniei is currently doing her PhD in Biomedicine and Society Studies at King's College London. In her PhD project, she is working on ethics and the regulatory policy of human embryonic stem cell research in Iran (funded by a Wellcome Trust Biomedical Ethics Developing Countries Studentship). She has a background in bioethics from the Erasmus Mundus Masters Program. She also has a Masters degree in Nursing Education from Shaheed Beheshti University, Iran. Saniei has spent five years working as a researcher and counsellor in social policy and ethics in health and medicine at Shaheed Beheshti University, combining this with nursing teaching at different universities in Iran. Her main research interests are cross-cultural research, sociology and ethics of bioscience, as well as the regulatory policy of biotechnology in Muslim and Middle Eastern countries.

Gamal I. Serour is Professor, former Chairman of Obstetrics and Gynecology, and former Dean, Faculty of Medicine, Al Azhar University, Egypt. He is also the past President of the International Federation of Gynecology and Obstetrics (FIGO). Since 1990, he has served as Director of the International Islamic Centre for Population Studies and Research at Al Azhar University. In this capacity, he leads the Centre's work on reproductive health, population policy, population education, women's rights, empowerment of women, sexual health, children's rights, and medical ethics in developing countries, particularly in the Muslim world, through projects and programs funded by UNFPA, WHO, UNESCO, UNICEF, Ford Foundation, among other organizations. He has organized and chaired workshops for doctors, researchers, midwives, community leaders, and policy makers from Egypt, Syria, Yemen, Gambia, Maldives, Guinea Bissau, Somalia, Bangladesh, Thailand, India, Pakistan, the Philippines and Palestine. His current and previous affiliations include Member of the WHO Scientific Group on Recent Advances in ART, the IPPF International Medical Advisory Panel (2000–2002), the Intergovernmental Bioethics Committee UNESCO (1999-2005) and International Bioethics Committee UNESCO (IBC) (2006–2009), as well as treasurer and member of the Board of Directors of the International Association of Bioethics (IAB) (1992–1999). Serour established the Al Azhar endoscopy and microsurgery training unit in 1974, which later became the Al Azhar-JPIEGO (Johns Hopkins University) regional training center for physicians from Asia and Africa. With two of his colleagues, he established the first IVF Center in Egypt and delivered the first IVF baby in Egypt in July 1987. He continues to advise IVF centers internationally. In 2004, he established an ART unit at Al Azhar University to serve low-income Egyptians; it is also a research and a training unit. He has authored and co-authored numerous papers published in international, regional and national journals and has edited various books. He is a reviewer for several international journals, and often addresses scientific meetings. Serour obtained his M.D. at Cairo University in 1963. He has received numerous national awards and honorary memberships in obstetrics and gynecology societies worldwide.

Robert Tappan is an Assistant Professor in the Department of Philosophy and Religious Studies at Towson University. He earned his PhD in Islamic Studies at the University of Virginia. As part of his dissertation research, he spent nine months in Qom, Iran, where he investigated Islamic views of assisted reproductive technology. His areas of interest include Islamic ethics, theology, and law, particularly in the areas of biomedical ethics, animal and environmental ethics, and the ethics of warfare.

Soraya Tremayne is a social anthropologist and the Founding Director of the Fertility and Reproduction Studies Group at the University of Oxford, where she has also served as Research Associate in the Institute of Social and Cultural Anthropology, and the Director of The Centre for Cross-Cultural Research, Queen Elizabeth House. For the past fifteen years, she has carried out research on reproduction and sexuality in Iran. Her current research focuses on assisted reproductive technologies and Islam in Iran. She is Founding Editor of the Fertility, Reproduction, and Sexuality series at Berghahn Books, and editor of several books in the series, including *Managing Reproductive Life: Cross-Cultural Themes in Fertility and Sexuality* and with Maya Unnithan-Kumar *Fatness and the Maternal Body: Women's Experiences of Corporeality and the Shaping of Social Policy.*

INDEX

CPSIA information can be obtained
at www.ICGtesting.com
Printed in the USA
LVOW03s0854120417
530545LV00007B/26/P